ROMAN TOILETS

B A B E S C H

Annual Papers on Mediterranean Archaeology

Supplement 19 — 2011

BABESCH FOUNDATION
Stichting Bulletin Antieke Beschaving

ROMAN TOILETS

Their Archaeology and Cultural History

Edited by

Gemma C.M. Jansen, Ann Olga Koloski-Ostrow and Eric M. Moormann

With contributions by

Jesús Acero, Horst Aspöck, Domenico Camardo, Ingrid Feuereis, Miko Flohr, Adam Goldwater, Melle Aude Gräzer, Elly N.A. Heirbaut, J. Barry Hobson, Stefanie Hoss, Andrew K.G. Jones, Anne-Marie Jouquand, Zena Kamash, Jens Koehler, Günther Karl Kunst, Antonella Merletto, Carlo Molle, Richard Neudecker, Eddie Owens, Beatrix Petznek, Silvia Radbauer, Roman Sauer, Jacques Seigne, Günther E. Thüry, Monika Trümper, Jeroen Van Vaerenbergh, Kathleen Wheeler, Andrew Wilson, Nancy Zibman, and Gabriel Zuchtriegel

PEETERS

Leuven - Paris - Walpole, MA

2011

BABESCH Supplement Series
edited by
G.J. van Wijngaarden

Photo on the cover:
Defecating pygmee in the frigidarium *of the Sarno Baths (VIII 2, 17-21) in Pompeii (photo S.T.A.M. Mols).*

ISBN 978-90-429-2541-0
ISSN 0165-9367
D/2011/0602/95

Contents

Preface and Acknowledgments

The editors are extremely grateful to the scholars who came to the Ancient Roman Toilet Workshop, organized by us and held both at the Royal Dutch Institute in Rome and at the American Academy in Rome, from June 23-25, 2007. Not everyone who came to the 2007 workshop in Rome was able to write something for this book, but there were some who contributed greatly in other ways, especially to the lively debates and discussions we had, and we wish to acknowledge them here with our gratitude: Mark Bradley, Valerie Curtis, Anne Hervé-Moretti, Manfred Horstmanshoff, Hubertus Manderscheid, Loes L. Raimond-Waarts, and Gilbert Wiplinger. On the other hand, some people were not able to come to the workshop, but they later learned about the project and submitted chapters or sections of chapters. In the end we had a large group of contributors from several different countries and continents and without their strong intellectual commitment at the workshop itself and to the subsequent research and preparation of their submissions on the wide variety of topics represented here, we could never have achieved the high level of collaboration and cohesiveness evident in these pages.

In addition, we wish to thank most warmly the Royal Dutch Institute in Rome for the use of their facilities and for much generous hospitality during the first two days of our workshop. We enjoyed comfortable accommodation, the fine library, the lovely landscape, and excellent discussion rooms. We are particularly grateful to interim director, dr. Gert Jan Burgers, and to Janet Mente, head librarian. Likewise, the staff at the American Academy in Rome, most especially Professor Thomas A.J. McGinn, then the Andrew W. Mellon Professor-in-Charge of the School of Classical Studies, warmly welcomed us, offered us a hearty lunch, gave us free reign of the gardens, and provided a fine conference room for our deliberations. We are also grateful to various members of the Department of Classics at Radboud University in Nijmegen, The Netherlands, and to the editorial staff at BABESCH who assisted us in improving the manuscript.

Gemma C.M. Jansen, Ann Olga Koloski-Ostrow & Eric M. Moormann

1

Introduction

Gemma C.M. Jansen, Ann Olga Koloski-Ostrow & Eric M. Moormann

We felt that this is an opportune moment to produce a handbook on Roman toilets. Such a book offers not only a timely recognition of the growth of interest in all matters concerning Greek and Roman daily life, but it offers an overdue acknowledgement that Roman toilets, perhaps more than any other facet of Mediterranean archaeology, have always fascinated legions of non-specialists, while specialists have tended to avoid the topic.

Many subfields related to Roman daily life, especially those considered ancient technologies, have recently been very well treated: for example, daily practices of mining and metallurgy, stone-working, woodworking, agriculture, food production, engineering and construction, hydraulics and water supply, trade, textile production, ceramic and glass production, land and sea transport, warfare and fortification, and many more minor technologies such as time-keeping, writing, and book production. Quite surprisingly, however, until now a text of sufficient authority and accessibility that includes a comprehensive treatment of ancient sanitation, another major hallmark of Roman daily life, has been lacking. The amateur enthusiast, in fact, would be hard-pressed to find any suitably detailed guide to ancient waste management systems for any period in any language, even if he or she were to look in Dutch, French, German, Italian, or Spanish, let alone English, publications. Toilets are strangely underrepresented in the standard archaeological guides (cf. Filippo Coarelli's *Laterza* guides to Rome, Rome's environs, and Lazio, for example), and are usually treated perfunctorily in both single-volume travel guides and scholarly studies of Rome and other Mediterranean cities.

This handbook, therefore, in the first instance, has been designed to fill this gap with the aim (daunting, perhaps, but achievable, we think) of providing both non-specialists and specialists alike with a reasonably comprehensive introduction to Roman toilets and toilet matters in the ancient Mediterranean. Chapters and case studies include Punic, Egyptian, ancient Near Eastern, Greek, and Roman toilets and sanitary systems from a wide variety of settings (public, domestic, urban, suburban, rural, military, and private), both for study in their own right and for comparative purposes.

While the bulk of evidence presented here is clearly on the Greco-Roman period, we know that the Greeks and Romans appreciated and learned from pre-classical periods and cultures, so we felt it was important to explore these older roots to sanitary systems as well. We started our work with several very basic questions: Where is the evidence for sanitary matters? What is the evidence - archaeological and literary? What do we think we know about toilets and waste management from the ancient Mediterranean? What has new research (in archaeology or literature) recently revealed to help us with what we do or do not know?

One of the barriers to working on ancient sanitation derives from the very nature of classical archaeology and its role. The field has long concerned itself with the high culture of the Greek and Roman world. Its principal aim has traditionally been to show how highly civilized the Greeks and Romans were and how studying their world can enlighten us moderns. Such a focused aim for classical archaeology helps to explain why interest in toilets (and other really probing questions about daily life whose answers may not always reveal a 'pretty picture' of ancient culture) is still only gradually taking hold.

The research topic of lavatories and human excretory habits has another barrier to overcome as well: that of the taboo of the subject. As Roman toilet customs have constantly been considered an embarrassing subject, a subject to be passed over as quickly as possible, or preferably not be mentioned at all, we can easily understand why this field of research is still in its infancy and why the study of this important aspect of Roman daily life has remained, as it were, in the back seat.

When taboos are put aside, it becomes apparent that Roman sanitary practice can reveal many barely known Roman habits and traditions. We can learn not only what toilets looked like and how they functioned, but much about attitudes towards hygiene, the level of privacy various facilities had, and about the Romans' own taboos that encircled acts of urination and defecation. Some caution is necessary, however. Modern authors on such topics must constantly be aware of our own biased views. No one is free from his or her own cultural values regarding sanitation. This fact is clearly demonstrated in the following short section on the history of Roman toilet research.

1.1 History of Research on Sanitation

The first archaeologists who came across Roman toilets seemed to have an immediate ambivalence towards them. On the one hand, these toilets looked similar to their own, therefore, they did not seem worth mentioning. They were not seen as an expression of the high cultural achievements of Roman society. Early excavators of Pompeii, like Giuseppe Fiorelli, only very briefly mentioned the toilets they found and with no overall analysis.

On the other hand, as early as the 18th century, some scholars did recognize the existence of Roman toilets, and they found a small place in the famous encyclopedia of the time by Daremberg and Saglio.[1] But several excavators were blinded by the longstanding taboos about topics like toilets. They did not even recognize what they were digging up in some cases. Richard Neudecker[2] lists some amusing interpretations. The toilet in the *macellum* of Pozzuoli was regarded a medical steam bath, and it was thought that, because the steam was so strong, one had to sit down as it was emitted into the room. The excavator of the toilet underneath the Domus Transitoria in Rome thought it was a machine chamber of a hydraulic lift. Neudecker found that other toilets were regarded as chairs for medical treatment, bath showers, or prison installations.

In the 20th century the attitude gradually changed, and we can find some milestones in Roman toilet research. The researchers, however, were not all archaeologists or historians, and it is not surprising that a physician was among the first to point out the importance of this research. In the 1920s the Danish physician Hølger Mygind wrote several articles about Roman Pompeii of which two were devoted completely to the water supply and sanitation of the town. In one of these articles Mygind was the first to make an analysis of the total ensemble of toilets, drains, and sewers in one Roman town.[3] He believed that the hygienic standards of a people tell something about the level of their civilization, and from this point of view he wondered why a study of this subject had not been conducted for Pompeii before.

He investigated both toilets *in situ* and those mentioned in the literature. His work is very thorough, and he had a keen eye for solid observation and analysis. His final conclusion is: 'Von einem ästhetischen und hygienischen Gesichtspunkt aus betrachtet, war die Einrichtung des Abtritts des privaten pompejanischen Hauses allerdings nicht lobenswert [...].'[4] It seems that he was disturbed by his own conclusion and in his last paragraph he tried to weaken it by comparing the toilets of Pompeii with those found in Rome (of which there were hardly any at that time) and with toilets in contemporary Italy (that are also located in or near kitchens, as are the house toilets of Pompeii). In comparison with those later toilets, according to Mygind, the toilets of Pompeii were a great step forward.

During the Fascist era, when large-scale excavations were carried out in Italy, dozens of toilets came to light. Amedeo Maiuri excavated many of them in Herculaneum and in Pompeii. Guido Calza discovered dozens more in Ostia, when he was excavating large areas of the city in the preparation for the great exhibition 'Esposizione Universale di Roma', which was scheduled to open in 1942, but, in fact, never took place.

Ostia became the model example for archaeology in the Fascist regime, and was used as a demonstration of how a Roman town functioned and to prove that Italians had descended from an impressively civilized ancient people. In the Fascist programmatic plan to 'resurrect' the glories of antiquity, careful restoration of buildings was a key ingredient. As a part of this plan, the toilet near the Forum baths was fully restored (we could even say 'overly' restored), and given a prominent role in 'making a positive impression' in behalf of the Romans (*fig. 1.1*). The toilet was heavily reconstructed for the specific reason of emphasizing how technically advanced and hygienic the Romans really were. Neudecker calls

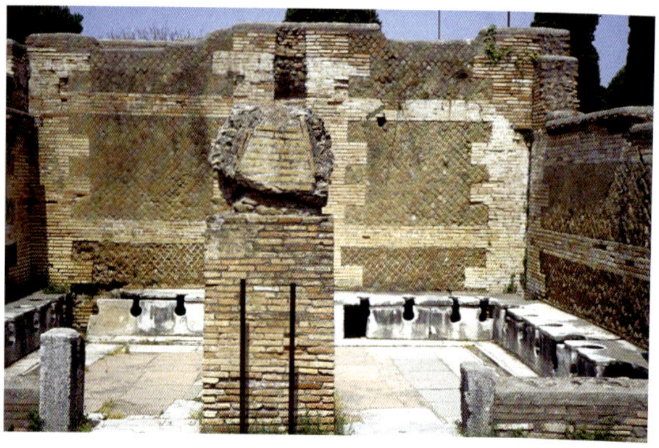

Fig. 1.1. Ostia, famous toilet near Forum Baths (I xii, 1) (photo A.O. Koloski-Ostrow).

it 'neo-imperialistic pride for Roman toilet civilization'.[5] Perhaps because of the role that the Fascist regime gave it, the Ostia Forum toilet is still one of the most well known Roman toilets that we have.

Many more decades passed before Alex Scobie, an ancient historian and classicist from New Zealand, wrote his pioneering article 'Slums, Sanitation and Mortality in the Roman World' (1986). The aim of his study was 'to try to estimate, as accurately as available evidence permits, how sanitary and unsanitary Roman towns were'.[6] Fully aware that literary evidence on the subject is extremely meager, he complained that archaeologists rarely concerned themselves with sewers and latrines. He had to base his archaeological discussion on the available evidence, which itself was very modest, little more than was available for Mygind's earlier study. This meant that he had to work with few classical texts and not very many excavated latrines. He concluded, not surprisingly, that the inhabitants of ancient Rome lived in an extremely unsanitary environment.[7]

So far, the first and only book (before this handbook) that is completely devoted to Roman latrines is by the archaeologist Richard Neudecker (1994). Because Neudecker wrote his book eight years after Scobie's seminal article, he had more archaeological information available to him and more awareness of the problems related to the topic. In addition to his careful treatment of what he called *Prachtlatrinen*, very beautifully decorated and appointed latrines of the late first and second centuries, Neudecker expanded the scope of the sanitary discussion. Based on the archaeological remains of toilets, he tried to establish the vision and attitude of the Romans toward toilets and their personal hygiene. His work now has to be the starting point for all current latrine research. Ann Olga Koloski-Ostrow's *The Archaeology of Sanitation in Roman Italy: Water, Sewers, and Toilets* (forthcoming, University of North Carolina Press) covers toilets before the luxury latrines were constructed. Barry Hobson's *Latrinae et Foricae: Toilets in the Roman World* (2009) gives an overview of Roman toilets across the Mediterranean with particular focus on Pompeii.

More or less along the lines of these developments are the new contributions of very recent decades. Koloski-Ostrow and Gemma Jansen have published articles respectively on public and private toilets. Their work fits into a research exchange in which there is more scholarly interest in dirt generally. *Sordes Urbis* by Xavier Dupré Raventós (2000), presenting the papers of a conference in Rome in 1996, is a major breakthrough as dirt and filth are in the center of the debate. Also the German scholar Günther E. Thüry (2001) published a book on dirt in antiquity: *Müll und Marmorsäulen: Siedlungshygiene in der römischen Antike*.

In addition to these pioneering articles and books, others have offered important contributions as well. In recent years researchers have been gathering facts about latrines (what did the toilets look like? how did they operate?). Because of this work, toilets have finally started to receive more mention in books on Roman daily life and on water systems. See, for example, the chapter of Andrew I. Wilson (2000) on drainage in the *Handbook of Ancient Water Technology*, or chapters by Nathalie de Haan, Jansen, Koloski-Ostrow, and Wilson that consider water in the context of urban sanitation in, *Water Use and Hydraulics in the Roman City* (2001), edited by Koloski-Ostrow.

Researchers are now turning to even more probing questions, beyond the sheer facts we know about the ruins, such as 'what can these toilets tell us about Roman feelings towards hygiene and privacy?'[8] and 'what can the toilets tell us about daily life in general?'[9] Jansen and Koloski-Ostrow discuss for the first time what is really going on in a Roman toilet. This is quite a break from former studies, which tended to describe toilets as if no one ever used them. Jeroen Van Vaerenbergh takes the issue even further and dares to ask whether the toilets even functioned according to their design. He brings the filthier side of Roman society into even more precise focus.[10]

1.2 The Need for a Book on Roman Toilets and the Roman Toilet Workshop (Rome, June 23-25, 2007)

Due to all these changes in research and to the fact that more toilets have come to light in urban contexts, there is a current need both for an assessment of results of recent research and for a set of guidelines on how to study these toilets. As the researchers of Roman toilets live and work in different parts of the world, there is not a common idea on how to approach this subject. This relatively new field of research needs a clear vision more than ever. That is why a three-day expert meeting was organized in Rome in the summer of 2007 in order to discuss the latest results of work on toilets, to put forward the more pressing research questions, and to compose a book on the subject.

All participants submitted thoughts and ideas about what they wanted to discuss and these were put together into a summary booklet in preparation for the meeting in Rome. These ideas covered a surprisingly broad and diverse range of topics and themes. They ranged from urine collection, to the discovery of chamber pots in *Carnuntum*, to Fortuna paintings in toilets that aimed to scare off the demons lingering there. The booklet provided rich material for starting the meeting and for beginning the work on this book. Most of the experts who participated are archaeologists, but historians, an architect, and a biologist were also present. Many are citizens of countries all over Europe and two were from United States. Not all are specialists in Roman sanitation, but several devote their research to Greek toilets and some even to Egyptian, Punic or Medieval toilets. The meeting had the character of a brainstorming session more than a conference for the presentation of polished papers. In the famous Dutch tradition, a lot of talking took place. We used a method that consists of several rounds of discussion based on the equal participation of all (*figs 1.2-3*). After all groups had the opportunity to complete their debates, we made a visit to the toilets of Ostia and a tour of a small section of the Cloaca Maxima in Rome (*figs 1.4-5*). When the fieldtrips were over, participants presented the outline of the book and different parts were assigned to different authors for writing over the next year. The finished product is the book before you.

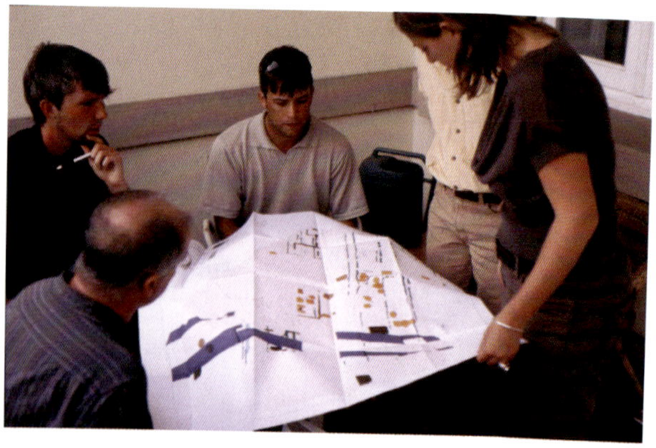

Fig. 1.2. Rome 2007, discussion group on cesspits and sewers (photo G.C.M. Jansen).

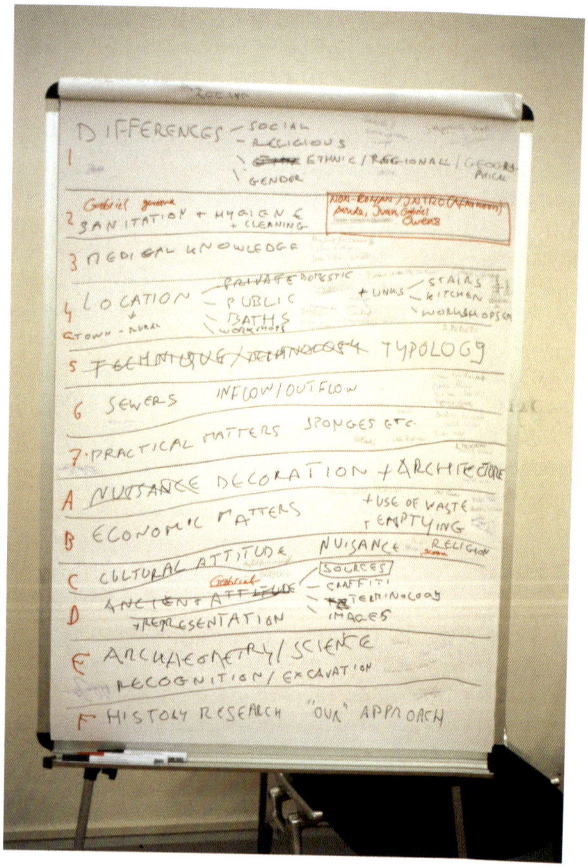

Fig. 1.3. Rome 2007, defining main theme's for the book (photo G.C.M. Jansen).

1.3 Observations about Stylistic Choices and How to Use this Book

Since the authors of the following chapters are international (they come to the topic at hand from the perspective of different training and different scholarly traditions), we editors realized that we would have to make a number of choices about the style, formatting, spelling, and terminology used throughout the book. We decided to standardize these points as much as possible to eliminate confusions and inconsistencies. We have used American (as opposed to British) spelling. In Latin spelling, we have used 'v' for 'w' sounds, for example *privatus* as opposed to *priuatus*. All dates appear with BC or AD. We understand multi-seat toilets accessible in public areas as 'public' toilets. These can also be called 'latrines'. Smaller toilets (with one, two, or a few seats in them) accessible from within private properties are called 'private'. These matters can be complicated, however, and we have asked our authors to be ever vigilant and sensitive to possible confusions or inconsistencies.

While we asked our authors to give us detailed evidence for their claims, we requested analytical

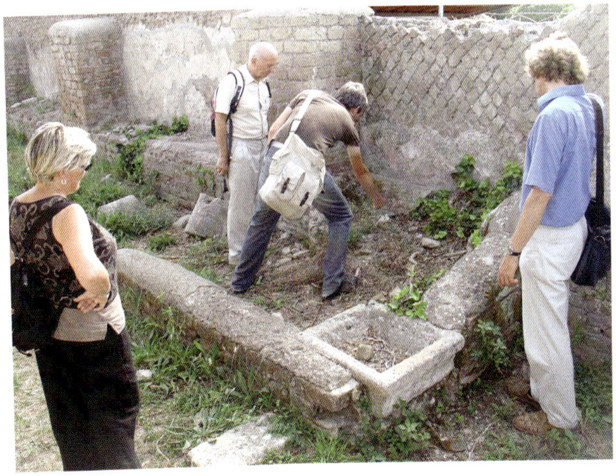

Fig. 1.4. Ostia 2007, discussion group during field trip (photo G. Wiplinger).

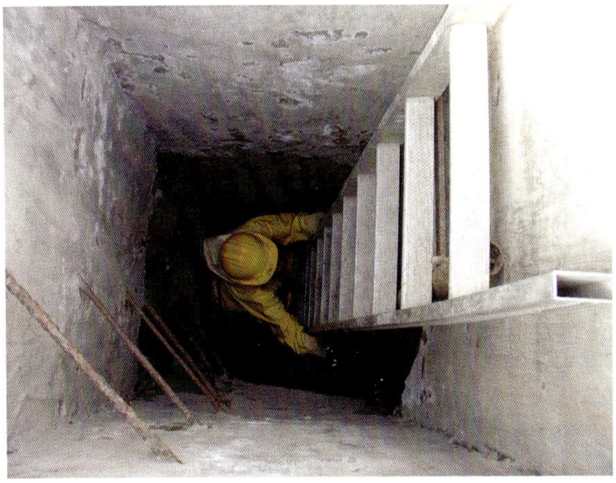

Fig. 1.5. Rome 2007, entering the Cloaca Maxima (photo G. Wiplinger).

analyses of whatever problems they were treating, as opposed to purely descriptive points of view. With this in mind, in several of the following chapters and sections of chapters, we approved case studies to accompany the more general analytical narratives to strengthen arguments with detailed excavation reports or research results. We think these case studies offer exciting avenues for future research efforts to be intensified.

Editors and authors of many books before ours have argued with fierce conviction about the importance of their works. We too, however, want to convince all of our readers that the cultural and archaeological history of toilets (especially in ancient Rome) is indispensable for a true appreciation of antiquity. And while all such claims are rarely true, in this case we believe they are. The modern world cannot plausibly hope to understand urban infrastructure (including aqueducts, sewers, roads, baths, plumbing, and toilets) without some grasp of urban sanitation and the facilities necessary to provide it.

We know that we have not covered all possible topics related to toilets in this book. Astute readers will notice, no doubt, many omissions: the famous Knossos toilet system; Bronze Age precursors to toilets of the Hellenistic and Roman periods; discussion of ancient medical and philosophical texts that deal with faeces and urine; treatment of late antique and Byzantine toilets. Still, we ask our readers to hold on to your seats (excuse the pun) for a reading adventure that will overturn many well-established ideas. For example, the notion that visiting a toilet was a social event or that the sponge tied to a stick and used for cleaning was the only cleaning device available in a Roman toilet come under attack. In addition, we think this book offers a great variety of ideas (large and small) that are new, and many facts about ancient Roman toilets and sanitation that were unknown before their presentation here.

Notes

1 Daremberg/Saglio 1912, 9.
2 Neudecker 1994, 8-9.
3 Mygind 1921, 251-385.
4 Mygind 1921, 319.
5 Neudecker 1994, 9.
6 Scobie 1986, 399.
7 Scobie 1986, 417.
8 Jansen 2000a and 2003.
9 Koloski-Ostrow 1996 and 2000.
10 Van Vaerenbergh 2006.

2

Archaeometry: Methods and Analysis

2.1 Introductory Comments (*Andrew K.G. Jones*)

Although some archaeologists view sewers, drains and latrines as dull utilitarian structures, when excavated carefully and sampled adequately, they usually prove to be very rich sources of both cultural and bioarchaeological data. Recent developments in scientific archaeology[1] mean that there is now a plethora of investigative techniques that can be applied to the contents of drains, sewers and latrines. Before considering the range of data available and the practical methods that could be used to investigate these features, it is important to consider the academic research aims underpinning each project, and what kinds of evidence are likely to be preserved.

It is common for excavation projects to seek information on a wide range of topics which might include:

- What agricultural products were being utilized on the site?
- What was the environmental setting of the site and how has it changed over time?
- Is there evidence for food production, consumption and waste disposal?
- Is there evidence for the general state of health and sanitation of the population who lived at the site?
- Is it possible to identify social status from the finds?

To answer such questions requires the integration of several sources of evidence, some gained from conventional archaeological analysis of buildings and associated assemblages of artefacts. Today bioarchaeological data are increasingly significant. The close scrutiny of groups of animal bones, assemblages of charred seeds, wood and preserved plant tissues, typically from anoxic waterlogged contexts, parasite ova, ancient DNA and stable isotope analysis can provide new insights and interpretations of archaeological discoveries.

Scientific research is most useful when it fits into a research framework that is clearly identified and agreed by the project team. Large archaeological projects now include specialist staff experienced in the analysis of animal and plant remains from excavation and these individuals are fundamental in helping to design the research questions and sampling strategies used.[2] To answer the research questions listed above, and others, it is necessary to analyse material from closely dated features likely to contain a wide variety of animal, plant and mineral materials. Sewers, drains and latrines often are important features on excavations because they can usually be very closely dated. Drains become clogged with effluent, are damaged and repaired, and become redundant when buildings are altered, so their use-phase fills are often deposited over a well-defined period of time.

Many Roman and post Roman sewers, drains and latrines are built from limestone, a calcareous stone that gradually dissolves in rainwater. This has two important implications for the analysis of animal and plant remains. First, the imported limestone may alter the acidity of local soils and sediments, enabling new species to colonise the area and favouring the preservation of biological materials that may not survive elsewhere on site. Second, limestone, and water from limestone regions, can be the source of relatively fast-forming calcium rich deposits such as flowstone and tufas. These often incorporate biological and other materials in hard amorphous deposits, preserving organic materials which might otherwise not persist. Recent work in Pompeii has demonstrated that more than 90% of samples collected from intra-mural ceramic down-pipes contained eggs of the common human intestine parasite whipworm *Trichuris trichiura* (Love 2007). Thus it is a *sine qua non* of 21st-century archaeology that sewers, drains and latrines should be carefully excavated and analysed.

2.2 Multi-Disciplinary Research Questions and Methods, Taphonomy (*Elly Heirbaut & Kathleen Wheeler*)

Research Questions

Toilets are an undeniably important feature of daily life. A strategy for the disposal of human waste and effluvia is a necessary fact of life for people living in densely-populated settings. In our modern world, the First World flushing toilet is often ignored as a critical component of personal and social health and hygiene - we take for granted our hardy porcelain bowls that whisk away our waste as if by magic. Of course, it was not always so, and New World 19th-century municipal records are replete with admonishments and regulations for controlling household privies and city sewers. Archaeologists have a unique perspective on the development and enhancement of human sanitation systems over time and space.

For antiquity, archaeologists often have far less archival evidence to work with, as literary sources about toilets and (regulations on) the use of toilets are limited. The main sources of information for the archaeologist are the physical traces of the feature itself and the deposits within it, which can contain a wealth of information on architectural, economical and social levels. In addition, they provide data on nourishment, diet and diseases, and represent ideas on cultural attitudes towards health, disease and hygiene. The question is how to get all this information out of the structures?

Schiffer's[3] behavioral scheme reminds archaeologists to consider the human behaviors in the construction, use/maintenance, and abandonment of features we recover in the archaeological record. These distinct use-phases are further applied to a social theory of architectural design articulated by McGuire and Schiffer,[4] where they outlined the process of decision-making archaeologists should consider in examining the archaeological landscape. In terms of toilets, research questions can be organized by these three main human behaviors of construction, use and abandonment.

For the purposes of discussion of research and methods, human sanitation systems are organized into two gross classes - (1) the containment system and (2) the flushing system. The first can be considered a most elegant-in-its-simplicity adaptation to the problem of human waste disposal and can range from a single-use, simple hole in the ground, to a wood-lined cesspit. The obvious flaw to the containment system is that when it reaches capacity, the feature needs either to be emptied or abandoned and replaced. The flushing system involves an input of water that permits an outflow of effluvia and solid waste; flushing systems can also be simple (as in the case of household septic tanks), but they are inherently more complex in that they require a water source and involve pipe connections for both inlet and outlet. Flushing eliminates the drawback of containment systems, in that they are constantly moving wastes out of the immediate living space. Design flaws in a flushing system can result in breaks in pipes or blockages and smelly back-ups.

The research questions which follow are at least partly explored in subsequent chapters of the book, particularly as they pertain to Roman-period toilets. Some authors bring case studies from other times and places, including the New World, Egypt, and the Far East. Research questions can be raised at any point in the analysis of ancient sanitation systems, but it is of greatest benefit to define them in advance of the fieldwork.

Research Questions Pertaining to the Construction *of Toilet Facilities*

Toilets are a specific type of structure, demanding specific construction methods and infrastructure, and often assigned to specific places in the urban landscape. Even within civil and military settlements, a wide variety among toilet facilities and their construction can be determined. The most basic questions to resolve are: What kind of system (self-contained or flushing) will be built? Where will the facilities be located? What kinds of decisions are involved in the physical location of sanitation systems?

The type and complexity of the social structure will affect the research questions related to human decisions pertaining to the construction of toilets. At the simplest level, a single household may dig a latrine, toilet pit, or privy in a portion of their landholding, while at the most complex level of social organization, municipalities will engage in elaborate civil engineering to install below-ground facilities. The same goes for military camps, where the layout was carefully planned by military engineers, and depending on whether these camps were temporary or permanent, different construction methods and materials may have been applied.

In the first example - that of a single household - archaeologists may ask where are the toilet pits dug. Were they located inside the house, and if yes, where are they located within the general floor plan of the dwelling? Plotting the location of toilets on ground plans of private houses can generate information on the spatial use inside houses and rooms. Were specific rooms or locations reserved for toilets? And what about toilets on the second floor? How do archaeologists reconstruct the floor plan of upper stories when only a ground floor foundation remains?

Or was the toilet pit dug *outside* the house and on the premises? If so, what was its relation to the dwelling? To the garden? To any outbuilding? The specific setting of the toilet can give information on the spatial use of, and infrastructure on the premises. Over time, or between households, can archaeologists detect a recurring pattern of location? Are features placed close to the dwelling, or away from it? Are they placed in proximity to a fence or property line? Are they located in such a manner to be downwind from the prevailing wind?

For flushing systems, locations of the single toilet must always be in relation to the sewer, in how it connects, and how it is flushed. Was the toilet flushed with a bucket of water, or was there another system?

In urban contexts, defecation and urination becomes a matter of social concern when space is constrained and jointly shared. At this level of social organization, archaeologists are likely to discern both public and private (exploited by private persons) toilets. Where are public facilities found, in relation to temples and churches? To theaters or other entertainment venues? To city halls or municipal headquarters? To other public buildings such as baths, or to buildings with a more industrial connotation such as tanneries? Can we deduce principles of aesthetics from a pattern of toilet placement - were toilets hidden, as if they were ugly? Or were they quite public, as if a mark of civic or personal pride? Might we interpret remoteness of a sign of olfactory response to repugnant smells? What can we discern about local concepts of sanitation by noting where human sanitation systems are placed on the urban landscape? Are they conveniently located (numerous and easily accessible from main streets)? Or are they tucked away down alleys or in remote areas? If this was the case, were they signposted so that people could easily find them or was their location common knowledge?

The second facet of construction is how are toilets constructed in terms of production costs, energy expended, or materials used? Who is responsible for construction? Do facilities require a separate class of engineers to design and specialized workers to build them? If there are specialized designers and laborers, we should find consistency in layout, configuration, and choice of materials. If households are responsible for individual containment systems, we might find considerable variability across time and space.

But what if (almost) nothing has remained? What if toilets and their infrastructure were completely built in perishable materials, and no portion of the physical structure has remained? What if only discolorations of the soil are visible? Is it still possible to draw some conclusions, or is all lost? Needless to say it will be more difficult, but nevertheless it is not a lost cause. Detailed documentation of whatever is left can still offer significant information, not only on the construction of these facilities but also on their functioning.

Research Questions Pertaining to the Use and Maintenance *of Toilet Facilities*

The two processes of use and maintenance are considered together, because they are interrelated and correspond to the time that systems are in use, including those operations necessary for the continued use (i.e. maintenance) of the system. Maintenance may also consist of cleaning, repairing, upgrading, or replacement of components. The most basic research questions begin with how are the toilets used? Who uses toilets? Is there differentiation between one kind of toilet and another? Related to these questions, archaeologists also have to consider more social and cultural aspects of toilet use. Are toilets unisex? Or are some facilities reserved for one sex or the other? How is sexual segregation articulated in the archaeological record?

In considering the use of toilets, archaeologists from historic periods *may* have access to texts informing on the necessities/advantages of regular bowel movements; proper cleansing techniques; and the requirement of hand washing after each visit to the toilet. These archives (including poetry, paintings, etchings, municipal records) are augmented by the physical traces of toilet behavior, beginning with the remains of human excrement.

In containment systems, use processes are represented by the accumulation of organic nightsoil deposits, which are the result of primary deposition (on-the-spot defecation) or secondary deposition through emptying of chamber pots. Residues within containment systems can be subject to parasitological study to reveal aspects of diet and disease; these can be applied to a household level of analysis, then compared against other households in the same neighborhood or time period.[5]

But these are not the only deposits archaeologists may find. Evidence from the 1st-century Roman settlement *Oppidum Batavorum* at Nijmegen shows small channels conducting water discharge into the cesspits. This 'gray' water was probably carrying refuse material (e. g. kitchen waste). The containment systems were thus not only used as a toilet, but functioned also as a 'garbage bin'. The same goes for some New World privies, where human excrement is not the only material found in privy vaults - they can become receptacles for any number of unwanted or shameful items - including broken tableware, alcohol bottles, drug paraphernalia, dead pets (cats), and neonates or aborted fetuses (Pena/Demnon 2000). Because American law equated the concealment of an illegitimate birth with murder - whether born alive or not - the need to secretly dispose of still- or newborns is illustrated at an 1840s privy on Block 160 in the gritty Five Points neighborhood of New York. The bones of twin neonates were discovered in the privy shaft behind a brothel, and the author finds 'the evidence that the remains represent a case of infanticide is convincing'.[6]

Analysis of faunal and botanical samples from these deposits can provide a better understanding of the eating habits and agricultural occupations of a community. Bone fragments, seeds, and sometimes flour can be used to reconstruct diets, data that again can be used in the study of food supply and provenance (local production versus import). When enough data are collected, archaeologists may possibly see diachronic developments and trends, at the neighborhood, regional, or global levels.

Other questions could be raised about how non-excrement is introduced into the containment system. Did privy users periodically sweep small loads of trash into the shaft? How do we explain large deposits of still serviceable ceramics and glasses? Were they part of the toilet equipment or are they to be considered as trash? Are there inorganic deposits, such as sand or lime that may be defined as deodorizing agents? If household items are dumped into a containment system, could artifacts from a later episode of deposition sink through a fluid matrix and become commingled with earlier materials?

Of course, archaeologists will be challenged at times to distinguish between use-phase deposits and those created after site abandonment. To determine which finds belong to the use phase of the toilet, and which finds to the abandonment phase, archaeologists in the field must pay attention to distinguishing layers belonging to different phases. Artifacts within primary deposits can not only be used for dating purposes, but they hold a strong potential for understanding many aspects of practice during the use phase of a feature. Moreover, 'they encode information upon the societies that produced and consumed them'.[7] Study of these artifacts by amongst others categorizing and comparing them may reveal differences between deposits, in which phenomena as chronological variation, social identity, supply connections, consumption patterns, etc. can be recognized.[8] Artifacts within secondary deposits (material used to fill abandoned cesspits or material that has sagged into the cesspit after abandonment), although containing as much information on societies as those in primary deposits, cannot be used for analyses mentioned above. Nevertheless, they have their value for resolving other questions, for instance for analyses of the premises, and will be discussed further below.

In flushing systems, organic materials are often not allowed to accumulate, but tiny samples may be collected from crevices between mortared stones. Research questions applied to these contexts will be not household-specific, but may be generalized across a population at large. Can we see anything pertaining to common diseases or intestinal micro-organisms in these samples? How was the maintenance of sewer systems taken care of? Were materials with a longer durability used? Were specific coatings applied to the walls of these systems?

In the maintenance of containment systems, the obvious question is: what happens when the container is full? Who defines when capacity is reached? Information on this topic during antiquity is hard to find, however, in late-18th-century Boston, Massachusetts, health ordinances required privy owners '...to empty all privies whose contents are within 18 inches of the surface'.[9] In Portsmouth, New Hampshire during the same time period, it was time to clean when the contents were within a foot of the ground surface, while in Lowell, Massachusetts, '...contents shall never be within two feet of the surface of the ground'.[10]

Privy cleaning is a subtractive process resulting in the depletion of accumulated deposits; it is a behavior that removes in a single episode materials collecting over time. In the careful excavation of privy vaults, one can detect truncated deposits along the sides of privy walls[11] - these are the results of vault cleaning, which create a new surface or interface in Harris' terms.[12] Evidence from Nijmegen shows that cesspits were emptied several times before they were abandoned (see case study p. 87).

Following the cleaning process, the archaeologist must ask whether the contents are scraped out and carted elsewhere. For antiquity, it is difficult to grasp how and when this was done. Other questions archaeologists must consider are how was the emptying of cesspits organized (by private persons or by the municipality) and what was ordure used for? In 19th-century United States, most cities had a cooperative arrangement with their rural outlying communities - nightsoil from urban privies made its way to agricultural fields of farms and fields.[13] Will some settlements place the excrement directly on local agricultural fields? And could this behavior serve as an analog for processes during Antiquity? What are the mechanisms of transport? Who does the cleaning? In several New England cities, health ordinances required regular cleaning by persons licensed by a Board of Health.[14] In ancient times, would a slave be required to clean public toilets?

In flushing systems, toilets located on the ground floor could be linked to sewer systems, but how was the removal of waste material from toilets from upper stories arranged?

For the continued use of containment systems, maintenance behaviors could include the replacement of planking of privy walls and the replacement of corner posts. Maintenance can consist of additive processes, such as the deposition of non-organic layers (e. g. sand or lime) for the purpose of deodorizing.

Research Questions Pertaining to the Abandonment *of Toilet Facilities*

Abandonment pertains to the artifacts and features left behind after a site has been deserted. Taphonomy is the study of all formation processes affecting archaeological deposits between discard and excavation. Originally, the term was only used in palaeontology to describe the transition of bones into fossils, but nowadays archaeologists use this term for all archaeological finds. In order to understand our archaeological record, one must be aware that a whole series of post-depositional processes, both cultural and natural, have affected and sometimes even altered this record. In the case of toilets, cesspits and their contents one has to consider processes as construction, use and maintenance, and processes that took place after abandonment of the feature, for example destruction or decay.

What survives in the archaeological record depends not only on taphonomic processes, but also on the materials itself. Usually, inorganic materials survive better than organic materials, and stone is one of the best examples of an inorganic material that - while not undestructible - fares well against climatic, chemical or biological processes. Fired clay (pottery) also preserves well in the archaeological record. Although stone and pottery can be much affected by cultural formation processes, these inorganic materials can better maintain their integrity against natural formation processes (apart from natural disasters).

Preservation of metal objects and organic materials is more complicated and depends on multiple factors, one of which is the matrix, usually sediment or soil, in which the organic materials are buried. Clay deposits are favourable for preservation. In these deposits an oxygen-free environment (anaerobic environment) is created, vital for survival of metal objects and organic materials such as wood, bone, leather and textiles. Sandy soils, on the other hand, almost always have a deleterious effect on preservation of organics and metal. Unless the organic remains are situated permanently under groundwater level (which again creates an anaerobic environment), these soils are often well oxygenated, and the percolation of rainwater as well as the fluctuation of groundwater levels allow a quick decay of organic materials, resulting in discolorations of the soil on places where these materials once used to be. Moreover, sandy soils are often acidic, leading to a fast deterioration of organic materials, specifically bones and wood.[15]

The archaeological excavation itself is also a post-depositional process that has a very destructive influence on the archaeological record. Therefore, it is of utmost importance that everything is very carefully documented during the excavation process.

In urban settings, it is important to understand how continuous occupation at sites is comprised of both outgoing and incoming groups. One will leave behind the abandoned, or de facto, refuse, and the incoming inhabitant must find the means to deal with it. In rural environments, space is obviously much less of a factor, in that a newcomer to a rural site might simply fill the old toilet shaft and build a new one for himself. With so much open space, however, archaeologists may be hard-pressed to predict where to find containment systems from one household or generation to the next. In some instances, much of the archaeological record may have disappeared. Only when archaeologists try to understand the genesis of a context, and all the processes that have altered this context and the archaeological record within it, they can reconstruct and interpret past behavior as fully as possible.

As this book makes clear, we already know a great deal about toilets. Still, many aspects slip through our fingers. Resolving one question does not only provide new and exciting information, but also results automatically in generating many new and important questions.

2.3 Logistics for the Recognition and Excavation of Toilets

Archaeologists are often aware that privies can be veritable treasure troves, but sometimes our methodology defeats our ability to interpret fully these features. The following set of methods is offered with the aim of retrieving archaeological data on each of the formation processes - construction, use/maintenance, and abandonment - described above. These formation processes can only be elaborated with an excavation strategy designed to delineate discrete deposits.

In the case of containment systems, excavation methods typically consist of excavation from within the privy vault or cesspit (*fig. 2.1*). Where these features are small and deep, safety issues are raised; in the United States, archaeologists are subject to compliance to Occupational Safety and Health Administration (OSHA) that prescribe against excavations in excess of 1.3 m without shoring. From a purely methodological point of view, however, excavation in such a manner requires standing within/on top of the same deposits one is trying to excavate. The flaws to this approach are further exacerbated through the excavation by arbitrary levels, where deposits that might otherwise be separated are mixed. Wheeler[16] has previously noted that each deposit is the result of a distinct behavior that can be defined with thoughtful excavation. If the separation is not detected in the field, it is unlikely that deposits or artifacts can be distinguished in the lab.

For containment systems, archaeologists are urged to excavate features in stratigraphic units - not by arbitrary levels - and the stratigraphic units organized in a Harris matrix.[17] Where excavation by arbitrary levels cannot be avoided, the excavation of sanitation facilities can be greatly aided by keeping in mind the concepts of the Harris system of stratification, especially the recognition and recording of the horizontal plan. The goal for the archaeologist utilizing Harris' principles is that the three dimensions of a deposit are recorded in the field. The horizontal plan is attached to the vertical profile both in the field and the lab. An example of relating horizontal with vertical boundaries of deposits is shown in *figs 2.2-3*.

The key components of the Harris methodology of recording and analysis consist of the matrix itself (the series of boxes and lines that indicate the stratigraphic relation between deposits), the use of the vertical profile, and the use of the horizontal plan. Even if the Harris matrix is not fully operationalized, these three essential concepts can help in the decoding of the privy depositional sequence by forcing us to remember the three-dimensional aspect of archaeology by visualizing it, excavating it, and recording it.

Toilets constructed in perishable building materials such as wood are often not always recognizable in the archaeological record. As stated above, not all environmental conditions are favorable to guarantee the preservation of these materials in the soil. Wooden structures built in a wetland environment have a good chance of being preserved, while in sandy contexts, wooden structures, if not preserved under groundwater level, are completely decayed. What remains is often little more than a discoloration in the soil where posts or wooden casings once stood. Recognition of these toilets/cesspits is therefore not obvious. Even more difficult to recognize are toilets where no wooden casing had been placed in the soil. In these cases only one of several seats were put on top of a pit. This has been the case for several toilets found in Cologne.[18]

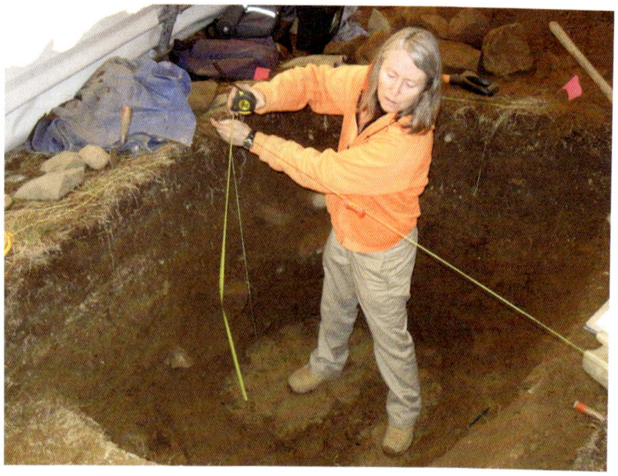

Fig. 2.1. Kathleen Wheeler measuring interior dimensions of a small wood-lined privy from the Neal Garrison site (ME 143-006) in Eliot, Maine (photo M. Carter, Independent Archaeological Consulting, LLC, Portsmouth, NH, USA).

However difficult, there are some indicators which could be useful in recognizing and interpreting features as toilets/cesspits. In some cases the original filling, nightsoil, has (partly) remained. This can be distinguished by cess inclusions, a humous texture, layers rich in phosphates and the fact that it is rather loose. Sometimes thin layers of ash or sand cover the nightsoil, probably to avoid stench. This has been established at several sites, for instance Zurzach,[19] Augst[20] and Usk.[21] Moreover, cesspits have not only been used as toilets, but also as rubbish pits. Besides nightsoil, one can also find many other materials such as pottery, bone fragments, charcoal and other waste material.

In other cases no original deposits are found, as these cesspits were completely emptied. Recogni-

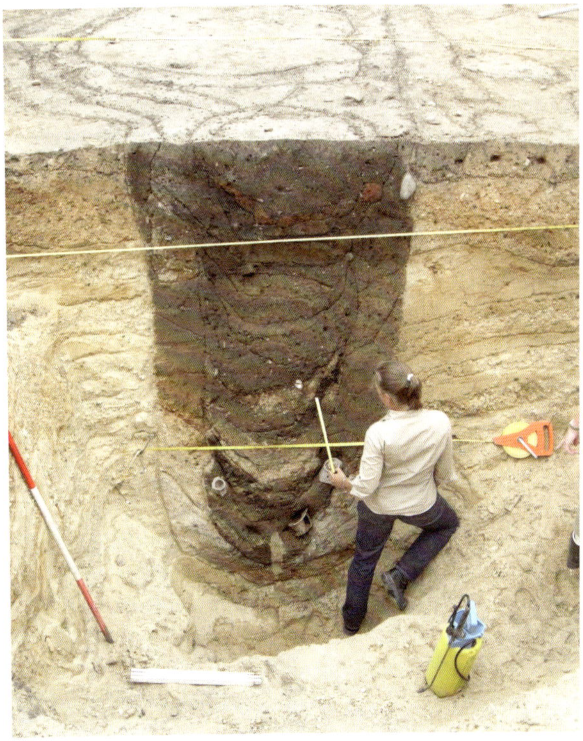

Fig. 2.2. Nijmegen-St. Josephhof, recording cesspit deposits. Note at the top of photo how the horizontal limits of deposits have been scored and correlated to vertical limits (photo N. van Hoorn, Bureau Archeologie en Monumenten van de gemeente Nijmegen).

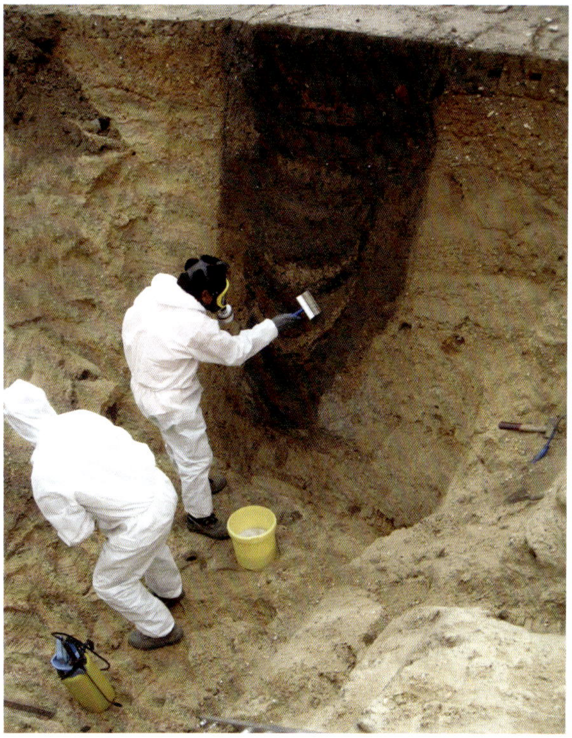

Fig. 2.3. Nijmegen-St. Josephhof, application of a lacquer peel in progress (photo N. van Hoorn, Bureau Archeologie en Monumenten van de gemeente Nijmegen).

tion and interpretation of these cesspits is very difficult, and can usually only be done after the excavation itself, or when one is experienced in this field or has excavated several others of this type of cesspits. Parameters for recognition are not easily offered, but the depth of the feature may be one key piece of evidence. Most cesspits have been dug much deeper than any other feature, with the exception of wells. The distinction between one and the other cannot be easily made as both consist of a wooden casing in a pit. It seems, however, that casings for wells are most often excavated as a funnel-shaped pit, whereas pits dug for a cesspit casing seem to have more vertical sides. Another indication may be found in the presence of infrastructural elements, such as cesspools which are connected with the cesspits via small overflow ducts, and small ditches which flow into the cesspits and might have transported effluent water. Finally, toilets sited outside houses would have been fitted within a small roofed toilet building to hide people from view. At Usk (South-Wales) cesspits were found, surrounded by many postholes. Based on these, small buildings were reconstructed.[22] Similar toilet buildings were found at Ellingen.[23] At Nijmegen, small rectangular foundation trenches were found surrounding the cesspits, indicating that here also small toilet houses were built.[24]

Excavating these decomposed wooden constructions needs a lot of thought. It is not possible to excavate them from the inside, as could be done with stone-built toilets or preserved wooden toilets. Because so little is left, it is of outmost importance to document as many details as possible. The best way to achieve this, is to excavate them in quadrants, documenting both the plans and the cross-sections in detail. While going down, one has to try to excavate stratigraphical units instead of arbitrary levels. In this way, a better reconstruction of the deposition of the contents and the finds within, but also of the chronological framework of the deposits can be made. Much attention has to go to matching the plans and the sections, in order to make a three-dimensional reconstruction.

It is crucial to investigate surrounding infrastructural elements connected with the cesspits simultaneously, for example by determining how overflow ducts are constructed (at the same time as the cesspit or later, just one or many at different levels, etc.) or by measuring the absolute depth of ditches or overflow ducts in order to know the course. If this is not done, one risks losing much important information. After all, this may the only way in which archaeologists can gain insight into the construction and functioning of these systems.

Furthermore, one must purposefully and scrupulously search for elements that contribute to the knowledge of the construction of cesspits. In sandy areas, iron nails used in the construction are often corroded, but nevertheless quite well preserved. Mapping them three-dimensionally provides information on how the wooden casing was put together. Absence of nails can mean that they have perished, but it could also indicate that sections of the casing were secured together in a different way, perhaps by using wooden pins and staples or by using the outer pressure of the soil to keep the planks in place. Therefore, it is very important to look for possible remains of building elements either in soil discolorations or in the remains of wooden fragments.

Artifacts, as argued above, should be meticulously pinpointed within these units. If they can be used for dating, it allows archaeologists not only to put the layers in a chronological sequence, but also to date the period of use of the toilet/cesspit. Even if there is no original filling, it is important to know exactly where finds were located. Were they imbedded in layers dating immediately after the toilet/cesspit was abandoned, or were they located in the sagging? One must take into account that finds coming from the latter are rather to be interpreted as refuse material. Analysis of these finds will not yield much information about the use or dating of the toilet/cesspit, but can be involved in the analysis of the premises.

The context of artifacts largely determines what has been preserved of botanical, faunal and other residues, and what has not. Keeping this in mind, questions of sampling strategy on site during the excavation should be formulated in advance, but should also be adjusted to every new context that is encountered.

2.4 Analysis (*Andrew K.G. Jones*)

To understand the relationship between deposits, one of the simplest ways is to identify sherds of ceramics and glass in different contexts that join together (crossmend). If the bulk of the vessel comes from one particular layer, and there is some downward movement of small sherds, we can determine these to be the result of natural formation processes of gravity, sinking, and possibly bioturbation from rodent burrowing. We do not have to assume that two layers are related just because sherds crossmend between them.

Range of Evidence Available

Sewers, drains and latrines are particularly rich contexts for recovering evidence of the dietary sources of the occupants of ancient sites. Several kinds of waste are deposited, most obviously and perhaps of most interest to archaeologists are human urine and faeces. While faeces are composed largely of water and bacteria, partly digested foodstuffs and other ingested materials can also survive. While seeds and pollen grains are the most easily identified plant remains, experienced palaeobotanists are capable of recognising a wide range of residues - bran fragments, fruit skins[25] and most recently starch granules.[26] Animal remains present in human faeces can include fragments of fish and other small bones, insect remains, and eggs of intestinal parasites.[27] It is also important to remember that human faeces are a source of nourishment for many animals and plants that may be attracted to drains, rats and other rodents, and a wide variety of decomposer organisms, notably fungi, insects, especially subterranean coleopterans, earthworms, molluscs, mites, etc. and evidence for the remains of these organisms should be anticipated.

In addition to human excreta, kitchen wastes, notably mammal and bird bones, eggshell, fish scales, mollusc shell, and vegetable wastes, are often discarded into latrines and other waste systems.

Finally, latrines, sewers and drains are also convenient places for depositing a wide range of other domestic rubbish and builders' waste.

Careful stratigraphic excavation (see chapter 2.3) with the meticulous collection of samples of sediments and other deposits is essential if excavators are to distinguish between deposits that were formed by people dumping rubbish, and deposits that accumulated during the use of the features.

Practicalities of Sampling and Processing in the Field

The overarching aim of all sampling strategies is to collect representative samples for field or laboratory analysis. Archaeological deposits contain a bewildering range of macroscopic finds, from huge pieces of building materials, large bones of domestic animals, small bones of rodents, birds, reptiles and fishes and seeds. In addition, there are smaller remains such as pollen grains, parasite ova and fungal spores that are only visible with aid of microscopes.

This section outlines the terminology and techniques used to recover samples of these objects. While the terminology applied to sampling is confusing and varies according to the traditions of archaeological teams, there is a widespread consensus that a range of samples should be collected from archaeological deposits in order that representative assemblages of cultural and bioarchaeological materials are recovered. While hand-collection of large finds such as mammal bones and pottery will continue, there is a growing band of archaeological researchers who recognise that excavators are rather unreliable in what they recover. Several classic studies demonstrate variability between individual excavators e.g. Levitan and, long ago, Payne demonstrated very significant differences in the assemblages of ceramics and large mammal bones collected by hand from the trench and with the aid of coarse sieving.[28]

The prerequisites for all sampling procedures are: a simple, but clear recording pro forma; a sample numbering system so that each sample and all its separate finds can be identified; clean tools and containers; water proof labels; indelible markers and meticulous excavators.

Coarse sieving, with a maximum mesh size of 8 mm, and minimum mesh size of 2 mm, is a practical method for recovering small bones, bone fragments, marine molluscs, charcoal and artefacts such as pottery, metal work etc. Here the aim is to sieve large volumes of sediment to recover unbiased assemblages of finds.

The coarser the mesh size used, the faster it is to process material. Likewise dry sandy deposits can be sieved much more quickly than clay rich sediments. The choice of mesh size will determine the size of objects recovered and the rate of processing. Excavators need to use a flexible approach to sampling. It is rarely desirable or practical to sieve all material on a 2 mm mesh. At the Anglo-American Project in Pompeii where sediments are usually dry and friable, the excavators have sieved all excavated sediments to 5 mm on large swinging sieves to recover pottery, animal bones, molluscs etc. Where it is impractical to sieve the entire deposit, it is recommended that large samples, at least 100 litres, preferably more, should be processed using this method. It is always possible to discard material once it is known that it does not add anything new to the corpus of evidence the site is producing. It is essential that this material is processed *during the excavation*, rather than stockpiled for future processing.

While coarse sieving is essential for retrieving representative samples of large finds such as mammal bones, a very large number of researchers have recognized that small objects, such as seeds and small fish vertebrae, are not recovered on coarse sieves. As a result a variety of sieving apparatus, often incorporating the use of 1-millimetre aperture (or finer) nylon or polyester bolting cloth (mesh), have been devised. This kind of sample processing has several names - flotation, bulk sieving, and wet sieving are all applied.

While methods vary in detail, typically the mesh is suspended in clean water, and samples added to the water and the soil gently disaggregated by hand or with the aid of gentle mechanical devices (*fig. 2.4*). This allows light particles, such as charred grains, small mollusc shells and other floating particles to be skimmed off the surface of the now dirty water. The gentle agitation helps all soil and other dense particles less than 1 mm in size to be removed from the sample, leaving a relatively small amount of cleaned earth residues. These can then be air-dried, sieving into fractions typically >4 mm, <4>2 mm, <2>1 mm, <1 mm fractions. These can then be sorted for small bones, fish scales, charred seeds etc. by site staff using forceps. It is rarely necessary to sort all fractions, but clear records need to be kept showing exactly what has been collected for each

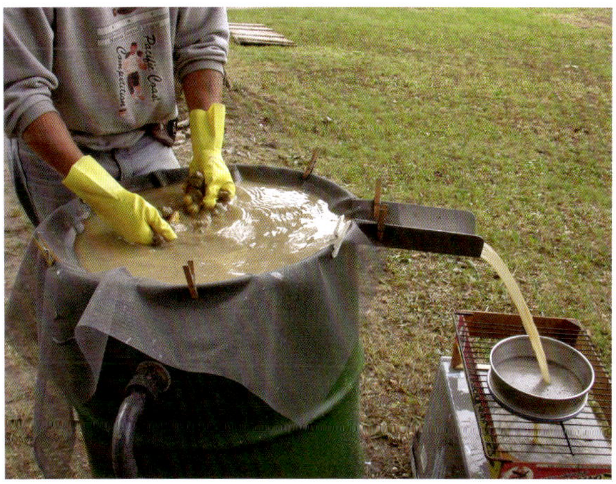

Fig. 2.4. Carnuntum, *flotation device (photo S. Radbauer).*

sample. There is a great deal of variation in how this technique is used on site depending on the range of materials present in the sediments being examined.

Some palaeobotanists insist on the use of 250-micron aperture mesh to collect floating particles and 500 aperture mesh for the heavy fraction. This is to ensure that small charred seeds and chaff particles are recovered.

As with coarse sieving, this technique is best carried out in the field in order to avoid the accumulation of daunting backlogs.

Practicalities of Sampling and Processing in the Laboratory

While field-based coarse and bulk sieving techniques are practical and efficient ways of processing much material from sewers, drains and latrines, these features are likely to contain minute traces of biological materials and chemical traces that can only be investigated thoroughly in the laboratory. Several reasons preclude the analysis of these samples in the field. First, and perhaps most important, is that few field projects can provide a processing environment that will minimize the problem of contamination. Parasite ova, pollen and DNA traces are invisible to the naked eye and small specks of contaminating dust may introduce alien species into the sample. Other factors include security and logistical needs for high-powered transmission microscopes, spectrometers and other equipment.

A widespread practice is to collect a single sample, typically weighing approximately 10 kg that can be subjected to a wide range of laboratory-based analyses. It is important to establish that the sediments being sampled do contain at least some identifiable traces, and this is best done on site. Careful observation, with a hand lens, of the processing of bulk sieved samples is perhaps the simplest way to check. Modern practice is to collect this sample, often termed 'General Biological Analysis' (GBA) sample in 10-litre plastic food containers with a tightly sealing lid.

The GBA is usually sufficient to allow a palaeobotanist and an entomologist, palynologist and parasitologist all to examine a separate sub-sample or series of sub-samples in the laboratory. The details of laboratory processing methods, all of which involve the use of laboratory-grade sieves, vary across the disciplines, and most analysts have developed their own preferred processing procedure.

The processing of GBA samples for insect and

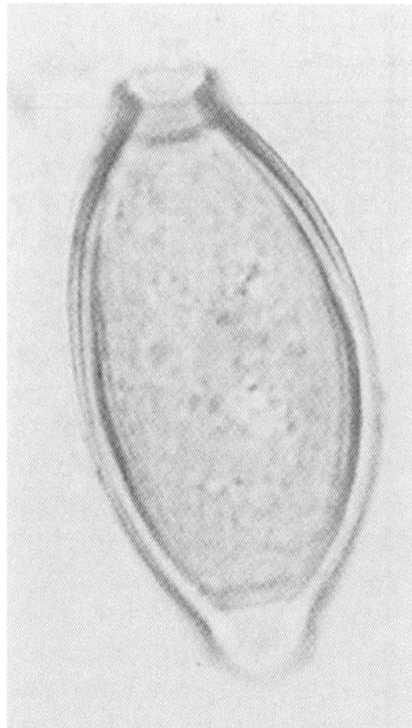

Fig. 2.5. Well preserved Trichuris *ovum recovered from an archaeological context. Note the presence of polar plugs. Size approximately 57 microns by 26 microns (photo A.K.G. Jones).*

plant remains has been clearly discussed.[29] A 1-kg sample is gently washed in a clean domestic bucket and disaggregated on a 300 micron aperture laboratory sieve in tap water. Boiling the sediment and the addition of chemicals such as sodium carbonate can facilitate this process. Once free from particles smaller than 300 microns, the wet residues are mixed with domestic paraffin and cold water is added. The paraffin will adhere to insect cuticles and some seeds and will float on the surface. After a period of settlement, the floating insect remains can be decanted into the sieve, washed in detergent and stored in laboratory ethanol for identification. The residues can then be washed through a tower of sieves, typically 4 mm, 2 mm, 1 mm and 300 microns and scanned for plant remains.

Microscopic analysis of samples requires much smaller amounts of earth and have been developed from procedures used by medical and veterinary parasitologists.[30] Three grams of earth can be disaggregated in 42 millilitres of deionised water and passed through a 250- micron aperture sieve. The filtrate can then be examined on standard microscope slides on a transmission microscope. Parasite ova are generally fairly large - 30-100 microns - and are usually present in faecal samples in large numbers and can be identified by a combination of morphological features and measurement (*figs 2.5-9*). Dainton (1992) developed simplified techniques for examining smaller samples of earth, and this is particularly useful when highly organic waterlogged faecal deposits are encountered. When sediments contain noticeable amounts of mineral particles, however, it is wise to exam-

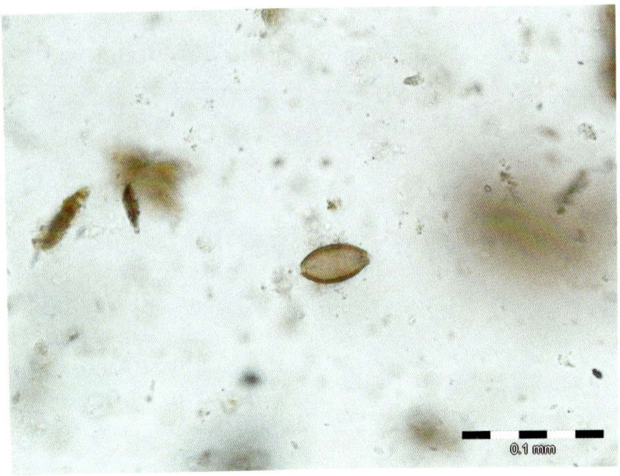

Fig. 2.6. Moderately well preserved Trichuris *ovum lacking polar plugs recovered from an archaeological context (photo A.K.G. Jones).*

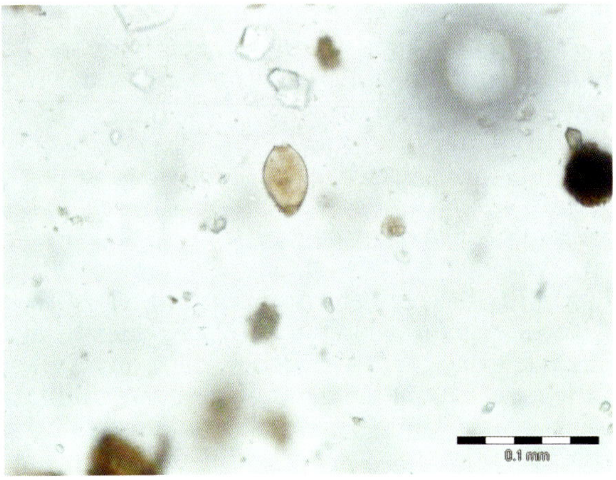

Fig. 2.7. Poorly preserved Trichuris *ovum recovered from an archaeological context. Note thin wall and absence of polar plugs (photo A.K.G. Jones).*

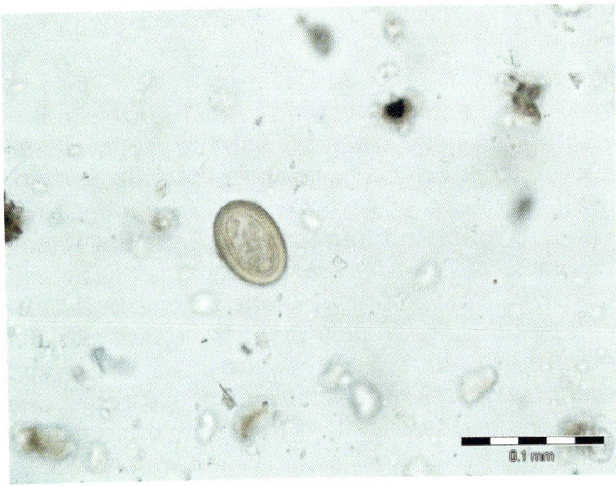

Fig. 2.8. Is it a parasite ovum? An object that is consistent with a decorticated fertilized Ascaris *ovum recovered from an archaeological context (photo A.K.G. Jones).*

ine at least 3 grams. Parasitologists have also developed techniques for finding parasite ova in 1 kg and larger samples of earth,[31] and these may be applicable to archaeological materials.

When tufa and other calcareous deposits are encountered, acid, normally 1 molar hydrochloric acid is essential in order to break down the samples and release microfossils.

Pollen grains, fungal spores and a host of other microfossils may survive in faecal deposits. While some of these are likely to derive from ingested foods, some are also likely to be chance finds causually ingested or objects that become associated with faecal matter, and the interpretation of

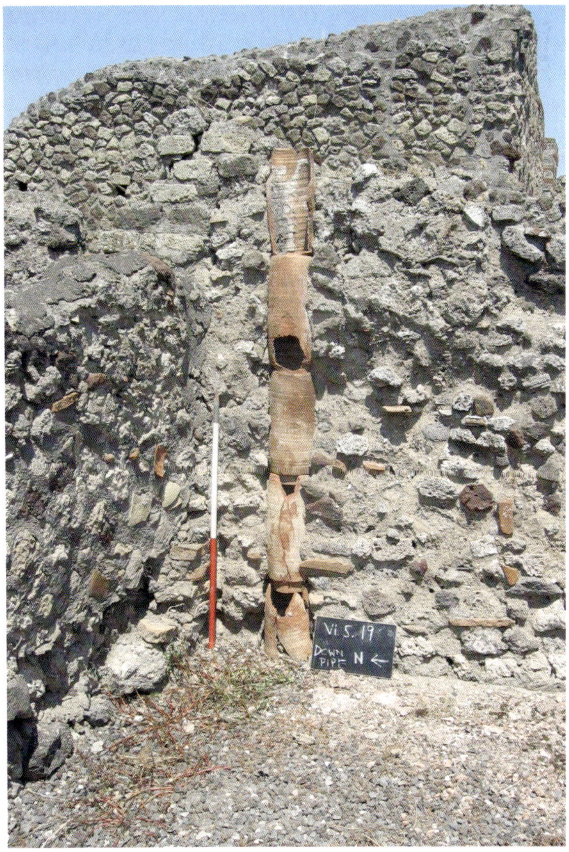

Fig. 2.9. Pompeii VI 5, 19: a ceramic down pipe. The uppermost broken tubulus *shows traces of a white calcareous deposit. Samples from other down pipes have been shown to yield parasite ova on microscopic analysis (photo B. Hobson).*

these remains is often challenging. To summarise, the advice of specialist analysts can be very helpful in determining the precise details of sampling and sieving procedures.

Case Study: Earlier Studies Done Well and What We Can Learn - *Carnuntum (Silvia Radbauer & Günther Karl Kunst)*

In the Roman civil town of *Carnuntum* (Lower Austria), the former capital of Pannonia, archaeological investigations have been going on for over fifty years. At *Carnuntum*, founded as a military camp in the Claudian period, urban development started in the civil town towards the end of the 1st/beginning of the 2nd century AD, saw important restructuring in the Hadrian and Severian periods and possibly came to an end in the Late Roman era.[32] Recent excavations, carried out by the Archaeological Park Carnuntum, are taking place in the so-called *Insula* VI, situated on a terrace gently sloping northward in the direction of the Danube riverbed. *Insula* VI, comprising both public and private buildings, is delimited on all four sides by stone-paved streets.

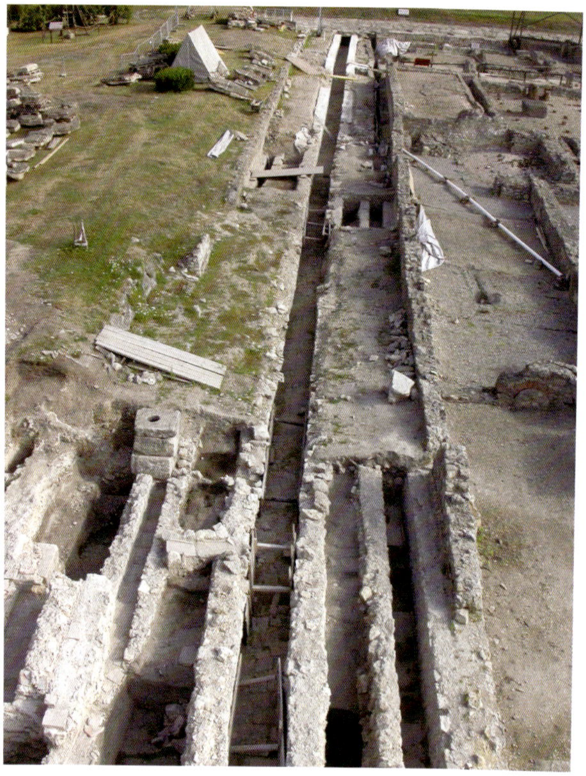

Fig. 2.10. Carnuntum, *overview of the* Weststraße *with sewer K14 in the center; structures in the left foreground belong to the freshwater supply system and a street latrine; to the right, a part of a former second century sewer; wall and stone structures to the right, along the street, belong to the bath and the latrine (photo S. Radbauer).*

In 2002-2003, research excavations in the substructure of the so-called western street (*Weststraße*), passing by the urban bathhouse, yielded important features concerning street development and the former water supply and sewer systems.[33] While the fresh water system saw only minor changes, the sewers belong to two different stages. K14, which was taken for an example here, belongs to this second stage and is related to a reconstruction phase taking place in this part of the town around AD 200 (*fig. 2.10*). It is a solid structure with a rectangular cross-section (breadth 0.90 m, depth up to 1 m) with stonewalls and a ground with two lines of brick plates. The construction was covered with the stone pavement of the street. After it was filled gradually with thin sandy layers very rich in artefacts and biological materials, it clogged up by a massive mudflow some time in the last decades of the 3rd century AD (*fig. 2.11)* and was abandoned. K14 can be traced along the whole length of 75 m of the excavated part of the *Weststraße.*

The stratigraphical method was applied in the excavation of the backfill of the sewer. Some pragmatism, however, in the documentation of these special structures appeared useful. Due to the considerable recorded length of K14, a vertical control profile was inserted every 3 m. This procedure facilitated the recognition and documentation of the internal structure of each unit. Great care was taken in avoiding standing upon undocumented surfaces of layers. Documentation of individual strata and channel walls was carried out according to Harris, with detailed drawings and photographs of the tops of the strata and the recording of certain artefact groups (e.g. coins, needles, concentrations of potsherds). All objects were retrieved according to the strata, with an additional horizontal separation every 3 m and in the case of evident deposits.

Artefacts and faunal macro remains were collected by hand, but in a rather meticulous fashion. The dry-sieving of the whole backfill was unfeasible because of its sedimentary texture and also for economic reasons. However, soil samples were taken systematically.[34] To avoid a disruption of the primary context, the basic data (including state of preservation and specimen counts) of all objects from each unit were recorded before they were handed over to the specialists. Likewise, some effort was

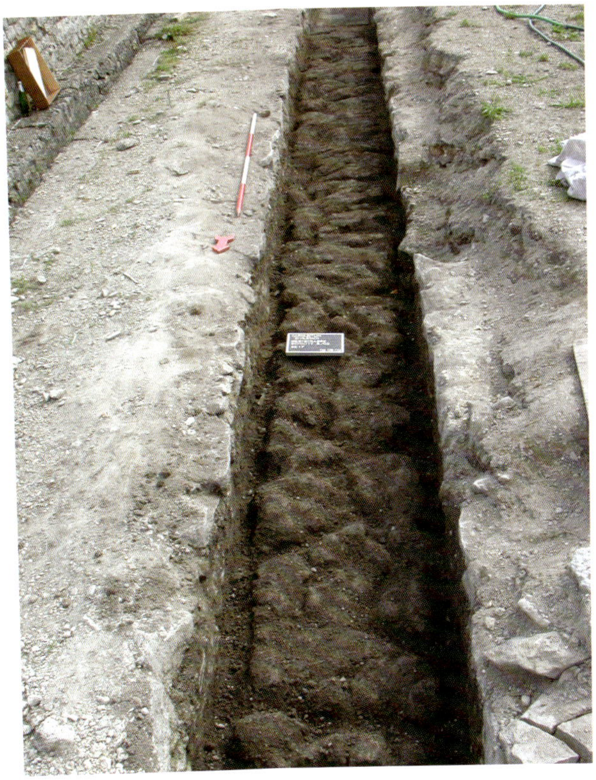

Fig. 2.11. Carnuntum, Weststraße, *sewer K14: surface of the muddy top layer from the 3rd century AD (photo S. Radbauer).*

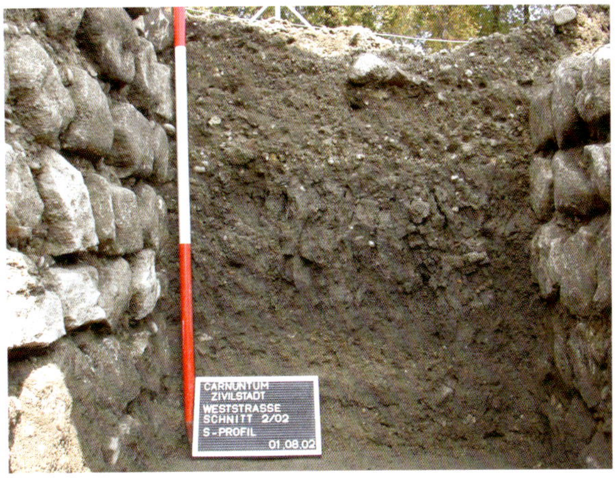

Fig. 2.12. Carnuntum, Weststraße, *section of backfill of sewer K14; from top: recent sandy earth with gravels (to bottom of topmost stone row on the right); homogenous muddy layer with coagulated clusters (to bottom of third stone row on the right); thin sandy layers down to the brick plates, which contained most of the settlement waste (photo S. Radbauer).*

expended in identifying cross-mending ceramic fragments from different sections of the same unit, thus recording eventual dispersal patterns.

Within the sandy layer, the material appears to be rather equally distributed, with no local concentrations or blockings if not in the area of the crossings with the respective outlets from the buildings (*fig. 2.12*). Potsherds and glass fragments cross-mend across a distance of over 20 m and very few complete vessels could be restored. A longitudinal dispersal pattern, probably caused by the water current, is also indicated by the spatial distribution of the bones of several neonate and very young human individuals. The animal bone assemblage from this context, comprising several thousand determinable specimens, consists of butchery waste (e.g. head and hoof parts from cattle) and consumption refuse proper with a high amount of ribs. Due to the high species diversity and the constant presence of the remains of rodents, wild birds, fishes and land snails, specialists had to be contacted.

For archaeobotanical, microfaunal and parasitological studies, soil samples were taken from all sediments of the sewer. In accordance with the specialists, samples of 40 litres were drawn systematically every 10 m, and additionally at crossings and connection points with side channels and from complete vessels. Botanical flotation samples were treated according to standard procedure using a flotation tank, a steady water current and a set of sieves with a minimal mesh width of 2-1-0.5-0.25 mm.[35] Charred and mineralised plant remains and shells of small land snails were obtained from the sieves. Weakly mineralised fruit seeds from grapes and figs and charred cereal grains figured most prominently among the finds. Great effort was also put into the collection and analysis of the heavy fraction from the coarse mesh within the tanks.

A considerable amount of microvertebrates (fish, rodents, birds), small molluscs and certain artefact groups (e.g. gems) could be retrieved from this residue of the soil samples. Naturally, from certain species and groups like the black rat, passerine birds and small freshwater fishes, the majority of the material results from these samples. Furthermore, control samples were stored for eventual future studies, including palynological analysis. A lack of local academic tradition is responsible for the fact that, at the moment, no special investigations were carried out on certain groups like insects and on the microanalysis of the soil thin-sections.[36] For the parasitological studies carried out, see case study chapter 11 (p. 163).

Regarding building materials, samples from the mortar coatings of the channel walls were taken every 20 m. Thin-sections from these mortar fragments reveal their composition and texture and allow for the discrimination of different construction teams involved in the completion of the sewer and during renovation works. The wooden coating of the outlet of an adjacent public latrine leading into K14 was determined as coniferous wood and restored for exhibition purposes. Thin layers from the wooden surface were identified as incrustation of urine stone scalings (see case study pp. 97-98). The origin of the pottery could be evaluated by archaeometrical studies (thin sections and heavy mineral analysis). Further investigations involve the determination of vessel contents (colour remains; metal remains from crucibles) and of the slag remains.

Doubtlessly, the biological remains result from adjacent households, inns and butcher's shops. A private/public dichotomy can also be defined for the artefacts. Again, table- and kitchenware, chamber pots and glass vessels point to the domestic sphere, and some small finds may have been lost in the bath. There is, however, a considerable amount of rubbish resulting from craft activities like metal and bone working, and, most of all, of building debris. The social status of the local population, according to the finds, appears rather high if compared to the adjacent military area.

As mentioned, the majority of the items, several thousand artifacts and animal bones, can be ascribed to the bottom sandy-layer, while the muddy top-layer was comparatively poor in finds. Because of this sedimentary sequence, some questions remain concerning the nature of the backfill: Was it a common practice to get rid of solid waste by dumping it into the sanitation system (including the dead bodies of small children), and how far was this practice a tolerated or even a defined function of K14? A repeated cleaning of the sewer system can be deduced from the archaeological remains, suggesting an assemblage rather closed chronologically, belonging to the last decades of the 3rd century only. It is, however, impossible to tell if the assemblage accumulated in the course of a few months or of several years.

Notes

1 See Brothwell/Pollard 2005.
2 See Richardon et al. 1997.
3 Schiffer 1987, 25-140.
4 McGuire/Schiffer 1983, 227-303.
5 See Fisher et al. 2007.
6 Crist 2000, 408-419.
7 Willis/Hingley 2007, 2.
8 Willis/Hingley 2007.
9 Barlow 1992,137. In fact, the notice was signed by none other than Paul Revere, who was serving as Boston President of the Board of Health in 1799.
10 Bell 1987, 60.
11 Wheeler 2000, 14-15.
12 Harris 1989, 11.
13 Roberts/Barrett 1984.
14 Barlow 1992; Bell 1987; Bilicki 1996; Heck/Bilicki 1996.
15 Meeussen et al. 1997.
16 Wheeler 2000, 3
17 Harris 1979; 1989, 34
18 Bridger 1989.
19 Hänggi et al. 1994.
20 Hufschmid/Sütterlin 1992.
21 Manning 1981.
22 Greene 1979.
23 Zanier 1992.
24 At the moment of writing, the analysis of the results of the excavation at Nijmegen-Josephhof is in progress (Bureau Archeologie en Monumenten van de gemeente Nijmegen, Elly Heirbaut & Harry van Enckevort).
25 Hall/Kenward 1990.
26 Torrence/Barton 2006.
27 Follett 1967.
28 Levithan 1983; Payne 1972.
29 Hall/Kenward/Jones 1984.
30 Jones 1983.
31 Burden et al. 1976.
32 Kandler et al. 2004.
33 The excavations took place during the project 'Carnuntum - Zivilstadt', directed by F. Humer in the Open-Air-Museum Petronell. The project was financed by the Government of the State of Lower Austria - Department for Culture Affairs and the Archaeological Park Carnuntum.
34 Evans/O'Connor 1999; Brothwell/Pollard 2001; O'Connor 2003, for a detailed discussion of sampling and recovery.
35 Jacomet/Kreuz 1999.
36 Evans/O'Connor 1999.

3

Non-Roman Forerunners

3.1 Latrines domestiques d'époque pharaonique: tentative de reconstitution des dispositifs et des pratiques *(Aude Gräzer)*

Que reste-t-il des latrines égyptiennes?

Malgré un climat d'ordinaire favorable à la préservation des vestiges, rares sont pourtant ceux relatifs à ce type d'installation.[1] Les seuls vestiges de dispositifs de latrines à avoir survécu en contexte domestique se concentrent sur l'actuel site de Tell el-Amarna, où le roi Akhenaton fit édifier sa ville (18e dynastie). Découvertes dans la partie privée des maisons individuelles dites «de plan amarnien»,[2] ces latrines consistaient en un siège maçonné à usage individuel (*fig. 3.1*),[3] composé de deux murets bas de briques crues, parallèles l'un à l'autre et légèrement inclinés vers un espace central, laissé libre pour recevoir un récipient dont seule l'empreinte a parfois pu être relevée.[4] Dépourvu d'évacuation et enduit de plâtre (tout comme les murs contre lesquels il venait s'appuyer), ce siège impliquait, après usage, un nettoyage à l'eau et la vidange manuelle du «pot de chambre», dont le contenu avait peut-être été préalablement asséché par du sable; solution encore mise en pratique de nos jours dans les latrines les plus rudimentaires. Ce siège était généralement dissimulé derrière un mur-paravent, de façon à rester parfaitement invisible depuis la porte.

La découverte, aux abords de la maison T35.20, d'une plaque de calcaire (*fig.* 3.2), concave pour s'asseoir et pourvue en son centre d'une fente en forme de trou de serrure, suggère que les latrines se composaient parfois de parties amovibles.[5]

La position de ce siège dans l'habitation amarnienne, en connexion avec la salle d'eau où se trouvait déjà un équipement sanitaire permettant de se doucher, vient confirmer son identification. Latrines et douche se partageaient alors le même espace[6] ou bien se trouvaient réparties dans deux pièces successives (l'accès aux latrines étant conditionné par la salle d'eau),[7] voire dans deux pièces contiguës.[8] Cette proximité spatiale induit probablement un lien fonctionnel entre les deux dispositifs.

En dehors d'Amarna, aucun vestige de tels sièges n'a cependant pu être mis au jour, si ce n'est en contexte funéraire, dans des mastabas de la nécropole nord de Saqqara, datés des 2e et 3e dynasties. En annexe de la chambre mortuaire des tombes n° 2302, 2307 et 2337, on identifia à chaque fois un siège de latrines derrière son muret bas, par comparaison avec les dispositifs alors fraîchement mis au jour sur le site d'Amarna.[9] Leur présence dans ces tombes doit-elle être considérée comme l'indice que des sièges de briques étaient déjà en usage dans l'habitat des premières dynasties?

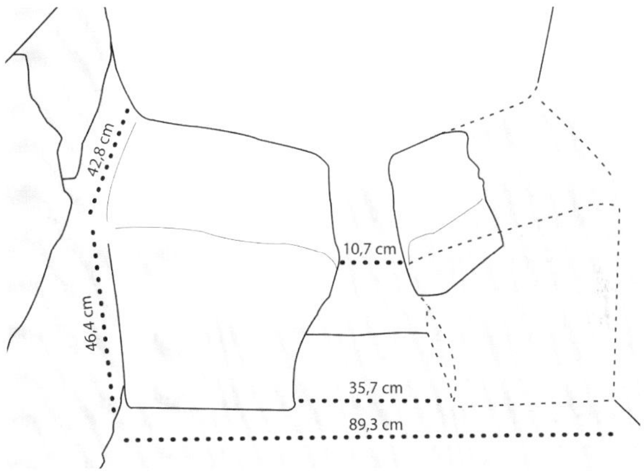

Fig. 3.1. Tell el-Amarna, Maison O48.1, siège de latrines (briques encore partiellement enduites de plâtre) (d'après une photographie et un relevé proposant une restitution des parties endommagées, respectivement publiés dans Borchardt 1912, 20, fig. 13 et Borchardt/Ricke 1980, 194, fig. 28; dessin de A. Gräzer).

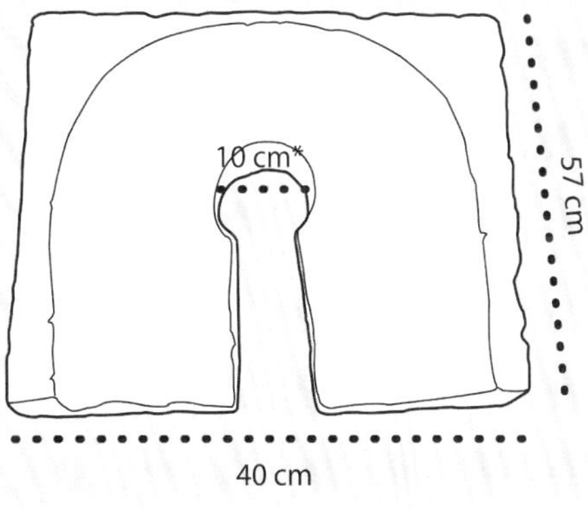

Fig. 3.2. Tell el-Amarna, Abords de la Maison T35.20, lunette de latrines (calcaire, Le Caire, Musée égyptien, JE 55.520) (d'après une photographie publiée dans Freed et al. 1999, 253, fig. 165: dessin de A. Gräzer).

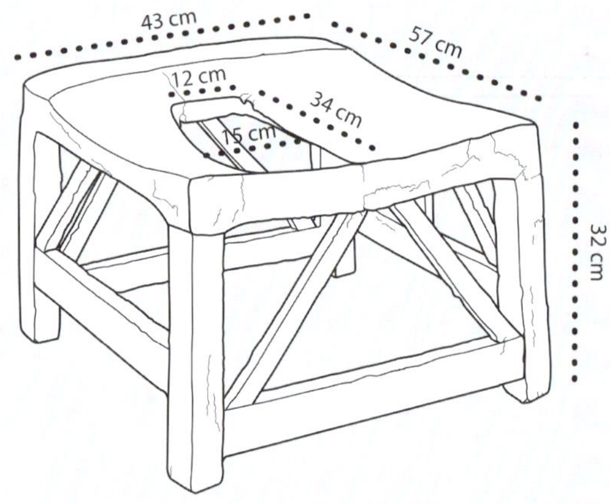

Fig. 3.3. *Deir el-Médina, Tombe de Kha, tabouret percé (bois peint en blanc, Turin, Musée égyptien, salle III, inv. Suppl. 8513) (d'après une photographie publiée dans Donadoni Roveri 1987, 146, fig. 193; dessin de A. Gräzer).*

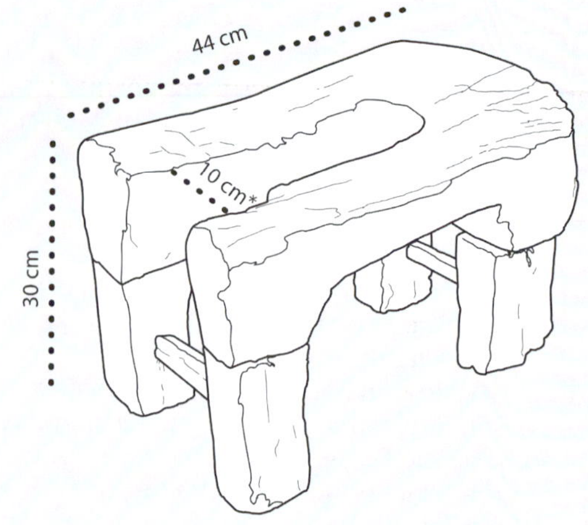

Fig. 3.4. Gourna, Tombe de Khnoummose (n° 253), tabouret percé (bois peint en blanc, Le Caire, Musée égyptien, JE 56.353) (d'après une photographie publiée dans Pillet 1952, 91, fig. 8; dessin de A. Gräzer).

Or, comment expliquer l'absence totale de vestiges de latrines dans d'autres habitations aisées voire royales, où pourtant d'autres installations sophistiquées telles que les plaques de douche ont été conservées? L'ancienneté des fouilles de la plupart des sites d'habitat n'est sans doute pas seule responsable de cette lacune. L'absence de latrines est probablement à imputer aux matériaux choisis pour les construire: à Amarna par exemple, nombreuses sont les maisons à posséder, en annexe de la douche,[10] un emplacement indubitablement vierge de tout équipement. Un simple pot de chambre voire un siège amovible en matériaux légers ont dû y prendre place. Or, le hasard veut que des tabourets percés (*figs 3.3-4*) aient justement été conservés parmi le mobilier funéraire de deux tombes de particuliers de la 18e dynastie,[11] approxivement contemporains des habitants d'Amarna. Il s'agit de deux tabourets de bois, recouverts d'un enduit blanc (dont la nature reste à déterminer), aux pieds consolidés par des traverses et à l'assise pourvue en son centre d'une fente dont la largeur avoisine les 10 à 15 cm. Leurs dimensions somme toute assez réduites - en particulier celles de la fente - concordent tout à fait avec celles relevées sur les sièges de briques et la lunette de calcaire (*figs 3.1-2*) mais récusent la fonction qui leur a parfois été attribuée de siège d'accouchement, en référence aux grandes chaises percées utilisées encore récemment dans l'Égypte islamique.[12]

Tout Egyptien possédait-il des sièges de latrines?

La concentration de vestiges à Amarna rend ce site d'autant plus intéressant pour le sujet qui nous occupe qu'elle permet de se faire une idée de la proportion de maisons - à l'échelle d'un site urbain - à avoir été pourvues d'un espace faisant office de «lieu d'aisance», et d'un équipement fixe ou mobile (*fig. 3.5*). Sur un échantillon de 586 habitations,[13] seules 90 maisons (15%) ont livré, au moins à l'état de traces, des installations hydrauliques à vocation sanitaire (plaque de douche,

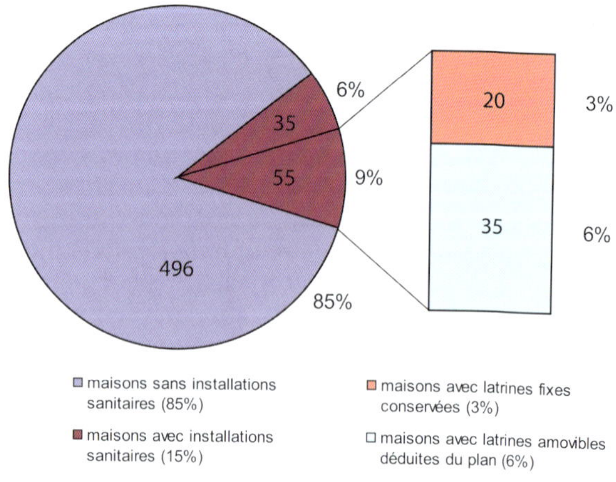

Fig. 3.5. Tell el-Amarna, proportion de latrines (fixes et mobiles) pour un échantillon de 586 habitations non royales retrouvées sur le site (A. Gräzer).

«lustration slab», etc.).[14] Parmi celles-ci, au moins 55 maisons (9%) ont dû être pourvues de latrines privatives: 20 d'entre elles (3%) arboraient les sièges maçonnés précédemment décrits tandis que les 35 autres (6%) devaient comporter des sièges de bois (dont l'emplacement a pu être identifié sur le plan). Si l'on en croit l'étude menée par C. Tietze sur ces maisons, l'existence d'une pièce voire d'un équipement, dédiés aux latrines, n'aurait en tous cas concerné que les maisons de moyen et haut niveaux.[15]

La question se pose donc quant aux moyens mis en œuvre dans les demeures de niveau inférieur, qui devaient représenter le cas le plus répandu. Très probablement, on devait faire usage - comme pour la toilette corporelle[16] - d'ustensiles que l'on sortait au moment de leur utilisation et que l'on rangeait ensuite, mais la documentation est insuffisante pour déterminer par exemple la forme ou la matière de ces «pots de chambre».

L'archéologie montre également que les anciens Egyptiens se rendaient parfois à l'extérieur pour se soulager : dans un terrain vague, comme le prouve la fouille du niveau d'abandon d'une maison d'Éléphantine où furent identifiés des excréments humains.[17] Or, justement, il est important de souligner que, même dans les fouilles récentes de sites d'habitat, la découverte de fèces humaines demeure exceptionnelle. La rareté de ces matières doit donc être considérée comme une donnée significative.

Le «devenir» des excréments

Les latrines égyptiennes étant vidées manuellement, on s'interroge en effet sur les moyens mis en oeuvre pour prendre en charge les excréments collectés ainsi que sur leurs zones de rejets. Existait-il par exemple une organisation à échelle urbaine pour en gérer l'évacuation hors des zones habitées?[18] L'hypothèse est séduisante mais ne trouve malheureusement aucun écho dans l'archéologie ou la documentation textuelle. En l'absence de documents, il semble donc plus pertinent de considérer que ces matières étaient simplement rejetées à proximité des habitations[19] et de chercher à déterminer la cause de leur disparition. Peut-on ainsi envisager que les excréments humains aient pu être recyclés, au même titre que les excréments animaux, dont on sait qu'ils étaient utilisés comme combustible, le bois étant une denrée rare et précieuse?[20] Le caractère «impur» aux yeux des Égyptiens des excréments humains, de même que leur composition - pauvre en matières combustibles -, s'accorde cependant mal avec une telle hypothèse.

Autre possibilité qui semble aussi la plus convaincante: les Égyptiens ont peut-être tiré parti de la tendance coprophage de certains animaux en leur faisant assurer un rôle d'«éboueurs». L'archéologie a effectivement révélé une cohabitation entre les habitants des villes égyptiennes et leurs animaux domestiques: notamment un grand nombre de chèvres et de porcs,[21] qui circulaient en toute liberté dans les zones d'habitat. Cette situation est notamment attestée au cours du Moyen Empire et de la Deuxième Période Intermédiaire dans la ville d'Éléphantine.[22] Les fouilles récentes menées sur le site de Tell el-Amarna (Nouvel Empire) ont permis d'identifier, aux abords du «Walled Village», des enclos où étaient élevées des truies le temps de leur gestation.[23] Une analyse de la couche de résidus alimentaires qui recouvrait encore le sol de ces porcheries temporaires montre que ces animaux étaient nourris grâce à une préparation composée de céréales auxquelles avaient été incorporés les déchets provenant des poubelles du village tout proche, notamment des matières fécales identifiées comme humaines.[24]

Silence sur les latrines : pourquoi une telle omission?

Dans l'iconographie égyptienne, les latrines sont quasi-inexistantes. Dans les représentations de maisons d'époque amarnienne, où les Égyptiens décrivent pour la première fois avec précision l'intérieur des habitations (nous permettant de reconnaître par exemple la salle d'eau avec sa plaque de douche derrière un mur-paravent), les latrines se réduisent à une pièce contiguë à la salle d'eau, munie d'un mur-paravent mais absolument vide de tout équipement.[25] Cette omission apparemment volontaire du siège de latrines, même si l'on a manifestement tenu à représenter la pièce où il se trouvait, traduit probablement l'embarras des anciens Égyptiens à évoquer explicitement l'action qui y était étroitement associée.[26]

Le rapport aux excréments

Même si elle a dû être effective, cette pudeur n'est cependant pas le seul facteur dont il faille tenir compte pour caractériser le comportement des anciens Égyptiens vis-à-vis de la défécation. La manière dont sont mentionnés les excréments, dans des textes principalement funéraires ou médicaux, tend à démontrer que ces derniers posaient également un problème d'ordre symbolique aux Égyptiens, problème qui a dû avoir un certain impact sur les pratiques d'hygiène quotidiennes. Plusieurs termes sont attestés pour décrire les déjections humaines: «l'urine» est désignée par le terme descriptif *wsšt* (littéralement «ce qui est uriné»)[27] tandis que les matières fécales pouvaient être évoquées par le terme *ḥwꜣꜣt* («matières en putréfaction») ou par les euphémismes *ḥs* («ce qui est loué (?)») et *ḥtp-kꜣ* («ce qui apaise/soulage le *ka*»).[28] En tant qu'excrétions corporelles, les matières fécales et l'urine étaient considérées comme des matières potentiellement dangereuses mais dont l'action néfaste pouvait être enrayée grâce à une purification, qui a dû se traduire au quotidien par une toilette corporelle systématique.[29] Dans les maisons amarniennes, l'emplacement des latrines, en connexion étroite avec la salle d'eau (parfois même à l'arrière de celle-ci), suggère un passage obligé par la douche et donc des ablutions pour se débarrasser de ces *excreta*.[30]

Le contact avec la saleté au sens large a d'ailleurs été utilisé comme critère pour déprécier certains métiers, ce qu'illustre notamment le texte dit de la «Satire des métiers».[31] Ce choix descriptif nous laisse en tous cas imaginer le statut peu enviable du serviteur chargé de vider le pot de chambre, dans les maisonnées suffisamment aisées pour disposer d'un personnel domestique; serviteur qui a dû exister mais dont nous ne savons malheureusement rien puisque son rôle n'est jamais évoqué.[32]

Signalons pour finir qu'en contexte funéraire, l'excrément constituait un danger pour la sécurité du défunt. En effet, toutes les substances putrescibles, telles les humeurs et liquides corporels que la momification et le rite funéraire avaient pour but de neutraliser, étaient susceptibles de mettre en péril l'état de pureté du défunt et du même coup sa survie dans l'au-delà. Dans les textes funéraires, les passages où le défunt certifie ne pas avoir été corrompu par les excréments, ni en les touchant ni en les consommant, sont donc nombreux.[33] Le risque d'en être réduit à manger et à boire ses propres déjections fait d'ailleurs figure de *Leitmotiv* dans certains textes qui décrivent l'au-delà comme un monde «à l'envers», où les fonctions du corps (celles de l'anus et de la bouche) sont inversées.[34]

Cette inquiétude, qui tient parfois presque de la hantise dans la littérature funéraire, pourrait donc expliquer pourquoi certains Égyptiens auraient tenu à placer des dispositifs de latrines dans leur tombe.[35]

3.2 Five Early Stone Toilet Seats in Jerusalem
(Stefanie Hoss)

Five stone toilet seats have been found in Jerusalem.[36] According to the excavators, they are made of large single blocks of the local limestone, scooped out in such a way as to create a hollow for a seat and leave ridges on three sides. With one exception they have two openings at the top. The larger opening (ca 15 cm in diameter) is in the middle of the hollow and leads straight down. The second opening is smaller (ca 3 cm in diameter), set slightly to the front and empties to one side. The excavators suggest that the latter hole was used for male urination. One stone seat has a keyhole-shaped hole instead, with only the round part going the whole way through the stone.

Two of these seats were found in their original position during the 1978-1985 excavations of the Ophel hill.[37] The seat with the keyhole-shaped hole was found in area E3, positioned over a cesspit and located in a small cubicle attached to a house, dated to the 7th to 6th century BC (*fig. 3.6*). The other seat was found in a small cubicle attached to the so-called 'House of Ahiel' in area G and had been in use at the time of the Babylonian destruction of the city in 586 BC. It also was found placed over a cesspit, which in this case was lined with plaster. Next to the seat, a small ceramic bowl was found, interpreted by the excavators as having contained either water for washing the hands or having been used for the pouring of liming agents into the cesspit. Three other seats of similar form come from earlier excavations of the Ophel hill, but were found in destruction debris.[38]

The deposits in the cesspit of the area G toilet were micromorphologically analyzed and found to contain faecal matter mixed with calcareous ash.[39] Other soil samples were analyzed for pollen

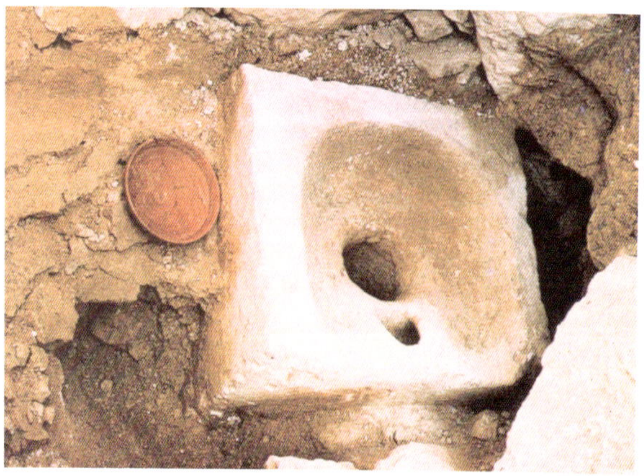

Fig. 3.6. Jerusalem, Stone Toilet Seat in original context: a small cubicle attached to the so-called House of Ahiel in area G in the 1978-1985 excavations of the Ophel hill (after Cahill et al. 1991, p. 66).

and parasites. The pollen analysis showed that most of the pollen came from just four plant families: the mustard, carrot, mint and composite (or daisy) families, which each have several edible members from which the pollen could have come.[40]

The analysis of the parasites revealed unusually large numbers of eggs from both the tapeworm (*taenia*) and whipworm (*trichuris trichura*). While the tapeworm eggs according to the authors attest to the consumption of poorly cooked beef or pork, the whipworm eggs seem to suggest poor hygiene, such as eating unwashed vegetables that had been fertilized with human waste. The authors connect both circumstances with shortages brought about by the siege of Jerusalem by the Babylonians in 586 BC. They conclude with the statement that both pollen and parasite analysis can be successfully applied to soil samples from the Near East.

While the large block seats seem unique to Jerusalem, thin slabs of stone with large, keyhole-shaped openings set above shallow pits identified as toilets have been found elsewhere in the Near East, for instance at Buseirah (Southern Jordan), in a stratum dating from the 8th to the 7th century BC.[41]

Toilets are also known from the Hellenistic period in Palestine, for example from a 3rd-2nd century BC house at Beth Yerah on the shores of the Sea of Galilee and from the community at Qumran near the Dead Sea (1st century BC).[42]

3.3 Greek Toilets and Waste Management

Documentary Sources for Latrines, Waste and Waste Removal in the Greek World (Eddy Owens)

Introduction

When modern commentators consider the problems of urban life and their solutions, they invariably have a diversity of contemporary evidence available on which to base discussion and from which to draw conclusions. Unfortunately, the same is not the case in the ancient world. Documentary evidence is incomplete and archaeological remains are often only fortuitously preserved and randomly uncovered. This is especially true when considering the problems associated with waste, rubbish and drainage. Most of the documentary evidence comes from a variety of different authors - poets, playwrights, historians and lexicographers. Cumulatively, however, the evidence is not great and most of it is confined to incidental references. Furthermore, comedy provides most of the literary references and so caution has to be exercised, because often the author is trying to extract humor from an embarrassing situation or bodily function.

Besides the literary sources, laws and legal documents recorded on inscriptions and in court speeches provide a further source of evidence. Such evidence, however, is also problematic. First, like the literary evidence, legal evidence is usually incomplete and fragmentary. Secondly, the laws often relate to specific issues in a specific city or location, and it is not necessary to conclude that the same practices or regulations operated in other places. In consequence we must accept that, while generalizations might be valid, facilities and conditions varied.

Portable Vessels and 'Going Outside' in the Ancient Greek World

Several texts indicate that, when appropriate facilities were not available, individuals merely 'went outside' and used any convenient place to urinate and even defecate. In Aristophanes' *Pax*, Trygaeus observed two boys coming outside to urinate.[43] While urine would quickly disappear through absorption or evaporation, faeces potentially created numerous anti-social and health problems. Nevertheless, it is evident that both children and adults at times defecated outside. In comparing the differences in customs between the Egyptians and other peoples, Herodotus observed that the Egyptians seem to have reversed the ordinary practices of mankind, and specifically contrasted the attitude of the Egyptians, who defecated inside, but ate outside in the streets, because they believed that what was unseemly should be done in private, with those of other peoples.[44] In Aristophanes' *Nubes*, Strepsiades relates to his son, Pheidippides, how when he was young and would say 'kakka', he would immediately take him outside to defecate in order to prevent mess in the house.[45] It was not only children, who might use the street; in *Pax*, Trygaeus, whilst riding his dung-beetle, observes a man defecating in the street close to a brothel.[46]

The idea of defecating outside is a central theme in a scene from the *Ecclesiazousai* of Aristophanes.[47] Blepyros, one of the main characters of the play, awakes before dawn since he needs to defecate. Because he cannot find his own clothes and shoes, which had been taken by Praxagora, his wife, he has to dress in his wife's saffron robe and Persian slippers. At the door he looks around for a convenient place to defecate, but decides that any place is convenient in the dark, because nobody will see him. Blepyros' concern to avoid being observed while defecating has been interpreted to mean that his actions were unusual and Blepyros might even have incurred a fine if caught.[48] It is, however, clear, as the scene unfolds, that Blepyros' desire to avoid being seen stemmed not from the fact that he was defecating outside, but because he did not want to be seen dressed in his wife's clothes. When a neighbor looks out of the window of his house and sees him, he casually observes that Blepyros is defecating. Blepyros is obviously embarrassed, but the dialogue revolves around Blepyros' clothes and their color, not what he was doing. When Chremes, another character in the play, enters after attending an assembly, he shows no real surprise to see what Blapyros was doing, but is astonished to see him in women's clothes.

A law dealing with the duties of the *agoranomoi* in Peiraeus suggests that fouling the streets was a problem. The text is fragmentary and so the provisions of the law are disputed. The relevant section was originally restored to read as a prohibition against the digging of cesspits in the streets or agora of Peiraeus. As it would have been difficult to conceal such an obvious action as digging a cesspit, however, it has been plausibly suggested that the legislation aimed to prevent defecating in the streets and the agora. Alternatively, as the law records the duties of the *agoranomoi* in connection with the procession in honor of Zeus Soter and Dionysos, it is possible that the legislation was concerned specifically to prevent the fouling of the route, which the procession took.[49]

It is a commonplace that laws highlight problems, but do not necessarily offer adequate solutions to the problems. In the case of Peiraeus, the need to legislate against fouling the streets and the agora illustrates that individuals were prepared to defecate in the open and not even the most public and sacred parts of the city were excluded. Euboulos' comment that every house in Thebes had a *kopron* (place to deposit garbage and excrement) at the door, because this prevented individuals having to go a long way to find a place to defecate, especially when the need to control the bodily functions caused embarrassment, again emphasizes that it was not unusual to 'go outside'.[50] Theophrastus illustrates the potential dangers of 'going outside' at night. In his discussion of 'Stupidity' he observes how a man, who went out at night to relieve himself, returned to the wrong house and was bitten by his neighbor's dog.[51]

The whole problem of 'going outside' was to a certain extent mitigated by the fact that few Greek cities were totally built up, but included open spaces and undeveloped land. Even when the

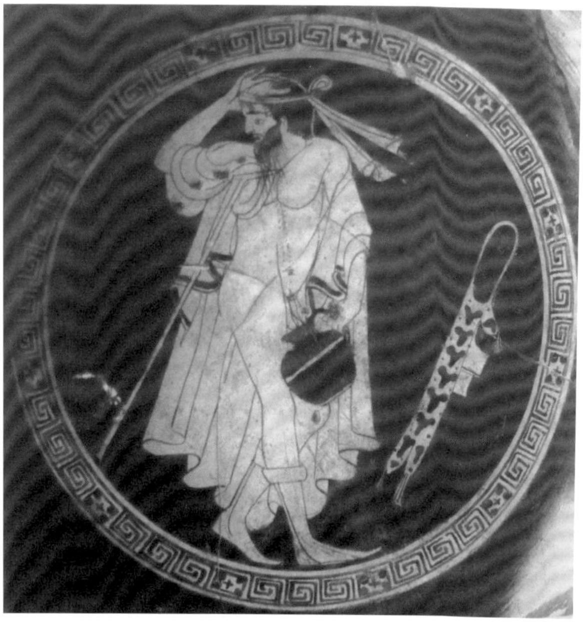

Fig. 3.7. A man urinates in a jug (Kilmer 1993, plate R528.1).

population of a city was substantial, free space remained. According to Xenophon, Athens still included undeveloped land in the 4th century BC, which he recommended should be exploited by the city authorities to generate income.[52] The text of the decree of Alexander concerning the return of exiles to Tegea indicates that the city was spacious with houses, gardens and agricultural plots.[53] In such cases it might be easy to find a 'convenient' place to defecate.

Portable vessels were certainly employed. In reality, any receptacle could be used (*fig. 3.7*),[54] and indeed, in Aristophanes' *Pax* Trygaeus even utilised a breastplate as a means of insulting the arms-seller in the play.[55] Athenaeus specifically credits the invention of chamber pots to the Sybarites, who used to take them to feasts.[56] In Greek there were several words for specific vessels used as 'potties' and bedpans. They include *amis*, *skaphion* and *skōramis*, whilst a *lasana* (also called *diphros* or *diphriskos*) usually referred to the stand on which chamber pots were placed.[57] Aristophanes distinguishes the *amis* as a vessel used exclusively by men.[58] The discovery of such vessels, which are partly enclosed at the top, indicates that only men could conveniently use them (*fig. 3.8*),[59] whilst depictions on several vases of the classical period show women standing astride open vessels (*fig. 3.9*).[60] A specialized child's seat with commode is also known to have been in use as early as the

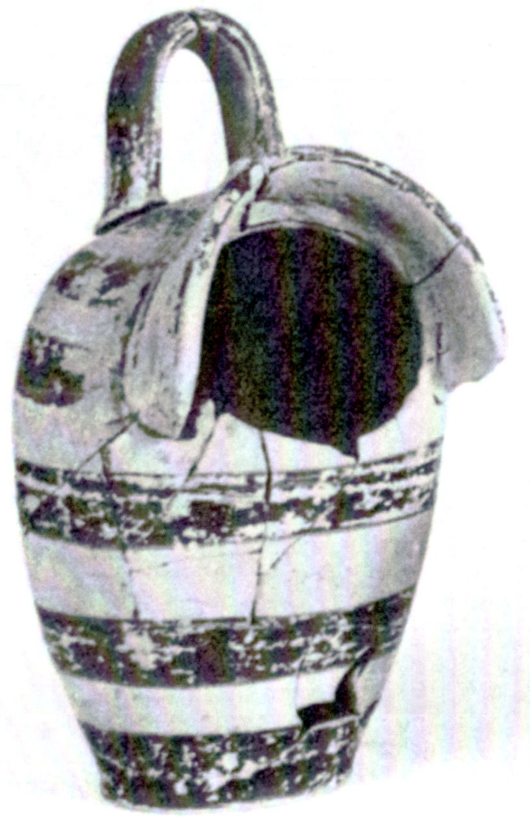

Fig. 3.8. Amis *(Sparkes/Talcott 1958, fig. 22).*

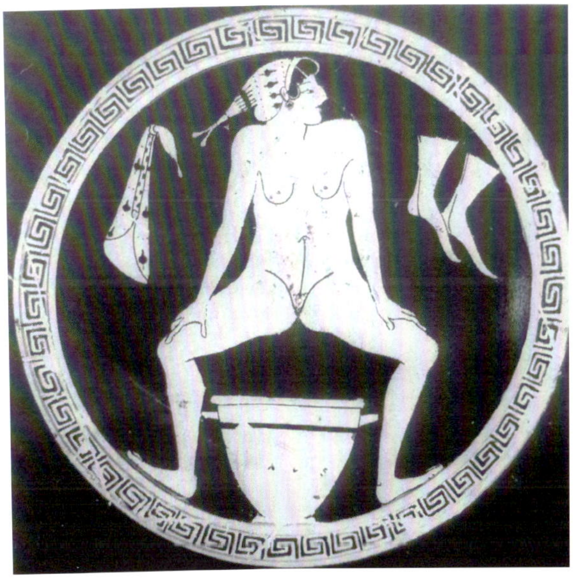

Fig. 3.9. A woman urinates over a bowl (Kilmer 1993, plate R531).

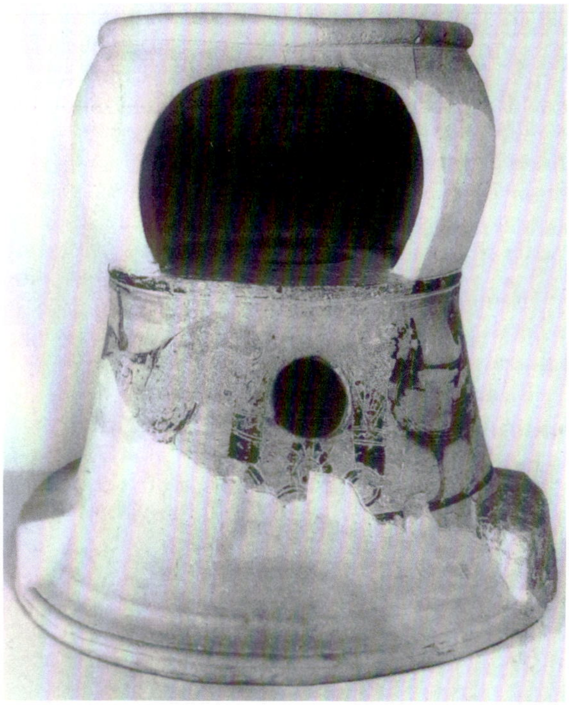

Fig. 3.10. Child's commode (Lynch/Papadopoulos 2006, fig. 1a).

second quarter of the 6th century BC (*fig. 3.10*).[61] Households might have a slave, known as the *lasanophoros*, whose specific duty was to look after the portable facility.[62]

All such vessels required emptying. At Pergamon there were statutory dumps into which householders were required to deposit their sewage.[63] It is possible that the *epistatai kopronon*, whom Demosthenes derogatively mentioned in connection with certain Athenian generals, might also have been responsible for similar dumps at Athens.[64] The fact that an inscription mentions a *kopron* to help locate a mortgaged property in Piraeus suggests that facility was sufficiently large to be used as a 'local landmark' for other properties in the district.[65]

Whatever official facilities might have been available into which to deposit sewage, householders must always have been tempted merely to empty such vessels in the street or any other convenient location. A law of 485/484 BC at Athens forbade the dumping of animal dung in the Hecatompedon on the Acropolis.[66] Similar legislation was introduced in other cities. The dumping of ash and *kopros* in the sanctuaries of Leto and Dionysos on the island of Delos was forbidden,[67] and laws were enacted at Epidauros[68] and on the island of Paros to prevent similar transgressions.[69] If temples and sanctuaries were not immune from the indiscriminate dumping of *kopros*, it seems unlikely that few locations in a city were. There were potential hazards in thoughtlessly emptying vessels onto the street. A papyrus from Egypt deals with a complaint by a passer-by, whose clothes were soiled when a woman carelessly threw urine onto the street.[70] According to Juvenal, the contents of a bowl indiscriminately emptied from an upper window were only one of numerous hazards, which pedestrians, who ventured on to the streets of Rome at night, faced.[71]

Latrines, Outhouses, Cesspits, Dung Heaps

The word *kopron* is commonly used in connection with facilities for the collection and storage of waste, animal manure and human faeces. Other words include *aphodos*, *apopatatos*, *aphedron*, *boleon*, *thakos*, *ipnos*, *kopria* and *laura*.[72] Unfortunately, none of the surviving evidence illustrates the character of, or any differences between, the installations. It is evident, however, that some of the words are derived from bodily actions, the waste itself, or are employed euphemistically or colloquially. Sometimes, in the context of specific passages, it is possible to speculate that installations were probably meant to be public, but ultimately there is no certainty. Thus, when an old woman in Aristophanes' *Ecclesiazousai* wants to take a youth home for sex in compliance with the newly introduced marriage laws, he makes an excuse that he wants to go to the *aphodos* first, to which she replies that he can defecate inside her house instead.[73] In the context of the passage, the *aphodos* can be regarded as a public facility. Antiphon implies that an *apopatatos* was a public installation. He comments that no matter how rich a man is, when he enters an *apopatos* he will see that everybody is the same.[74] Both *kopron* and *laura* are probably used in the context of public installations in Aristophanes' *Pax*.[75]

In domestic contexts, houses had private facilities. In *Thesmophoriazousai*, Mnesilochos went down at night to meet her lover on the pretext of going to the *kopron*.[76] That she lubricated the hinges of the door to sneak outside in order that her husband would not hear the door opening indicates that the *kopron* was inside the house, and Euboulos' observation that houses at Thebes had *koprones* close to the door has already been noted. In Odysseus' house a dung heap, admittedly for animal dung, was located at the door.[77] Private latrines might also be located in the street outside houses. The archaeological evidence from numerous sites confirms a location for latrines and cesspits usually close to the door or in the courtyard.[78] The location of *koprones* so close to a property could be dangerous and so at Gortyn on Crete a law forbade the location of ovens and dung heaps within a certain distance of a house wall.[79] While this law might possibly be concerned with hygiene, it is also equally probable that it was introduced to prevent damage to neighboring property, if such an installation was located too close to a property.

Waste and Waste Removal

It would, initially, seem that pollution was a potentially serious problem in the cities of ancient Greece. Laws at both Athens and Pergamon, however, indicate that the state intervened to ensure the cleanliness of the city. It was the duty of the *astynomoi* or their assistants, the *amphidarchoi*, or the *agoranomoi* to ensure that streets remained clean. At Thebes the responsibility for ensuring that the streets were free from dung and waste was undertaken by a minor official called a *telmarchos*, a position once held by Epaminondas.[80] Legislation, however, placed the onus for maintenance of a decent standard of cleanliness on individual property owners. It was the duty of the city officials to enforce the law and compel property owners to maintain streets and remove waste. At Thasos the individual who leased the land associated with the 'Gardens of Heracles' had responsibility for the removal of sewage.[81] The law at Pergamon required property owners to clean the streets outside their properties and up to a certain distance either side. There were statutory dumps either provided by the state or by individuals in which *kopros* and other forms of waste could be deposited. Householders at Pergamon were grouped into associations and were required by law to employ contractors periodically to empty the dumps.[82]

That *kopros* had an economic importance also reduced the problems associated with the removal of waste from the cities of the Greek world. *Koprones*, whether public or private, were not exclusively used only for human excrement. All sorts of domestic waste were probably thrown into the *kopron* and this would have provided a valuable source of fertilizer. An inscription from Delos records the payment to a certain Nicias for removing pigeon dropping from roofs of buildings and *kopros* from the agora.[83] Presumably, Nicias was not only paid to remove the waste, but he also recycled it, thus increasing his profit.

Human fertilizer has long been used in agriculture and continues in use into the present day. The contents of the dung heap at the door of Odysseus' house were used as fertilizer. The importance of the contents of a *kopron* as fertilizer ameliorated the problem of pollution in towns and cities. Many towns remained essentially rural, and either agriculture was the primary occupation of many city dwellers or householders owned and exploited a market garden or small allotment within the city. The exile decree of Alexander from Tegea, mentioned above, indicates that the city was a spacious rural market town, with houses interspersed with gardens and agricultural plots of land. In such conditions the contents of a *kopron* would have provided a valuable source of fertilizer for crops which were grown inside the city.

Besides its uses by private individuals as manure, it is likely that the waste from cities was also exploited commercially. Several mortgage *horoi* record the sale of *koprones* with houses, which suggests that the installations were sufficiently large to be included in the sale, and so were a source of profit to their owners. Not only might they have charged for their use, but also, as the dumps would have had to be emptied periodically, their contents could be sold. The astynomic law from Pergamon mentions that private contractors were hired by the associations of householders to empty the statutory dumps periodically. Both Aristophanes and Aristotle mention that in Athens such contractors, or at least their employees, were known as *koprologoi*. These were summoned when necessary to remove dung and deposit it outside the city limits. In Aristophanes' *Pax* two of Trygaeus' servants call the *koprologoi* to help remove the foul-smelling dung, with which they had been feeding his dung-beetle, while Aristotle states that it was the duty of the city's *astynomoi* to ensure that the *koprologoi* deposited the waste at least ten stades from the city.[84] Almost certainly, the *koprologoi* operated as private entrepreneurs, collecting the contents of *koprones*, recycling it as fertilizer, and removing the remains from the city. A similar system probably operated in Thebes. If Athens, Pergamon and probably Thebes are typical, it can be assumed that most Greek cities had an organized system of waste removal, which was based on legislation, the notion of personal responsibility and private enterprise.

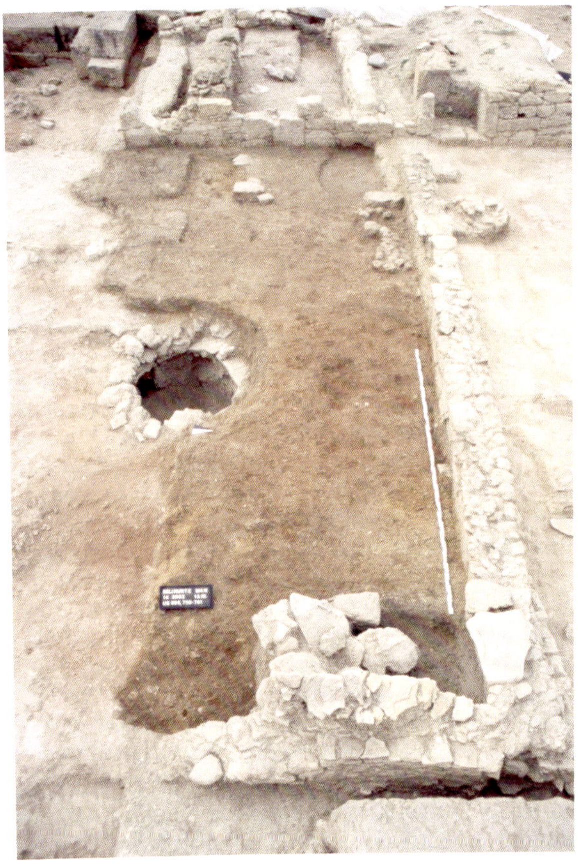

Fig. 3.11. Selinous, eastside of the Agora, House 3, kopron *in the courtyard (right bottom of photo) (photo A. Thomsen).*

Archaeological Evidence of Cesspits, Sewers and Latrines from the 6th to the 4th Century BC (Gabriel Zuchtriegel)

Already in the 6th century BC some Greek cities had more than five-thousand inhabitants, possibly even more than ten-thousand,[85] but latrines and sewage systems as we know them from the imperial period are lacking in the Archaic and Classical periods. Archaeological remains of pipes for fresh water, drains for rainwater (i.e. at Rhodes, Corinth, Akragas, Metapontum, and elsewhere), and other plumbing fixtures prove, however, that the absence of latrines and sewers is not due to a lack of technical knowledge and capacity.[86] Although single households could eventually have proper pipes running into public drains in order to get rid of their sewage, as observed for example in Athens at the so called Great Drain,[87] the reason that most did not have any need for such fixtures can be attributed to two main reasons. First, depositing sewage and manure in cesspits, on dung hills, or on the streets was obviously not

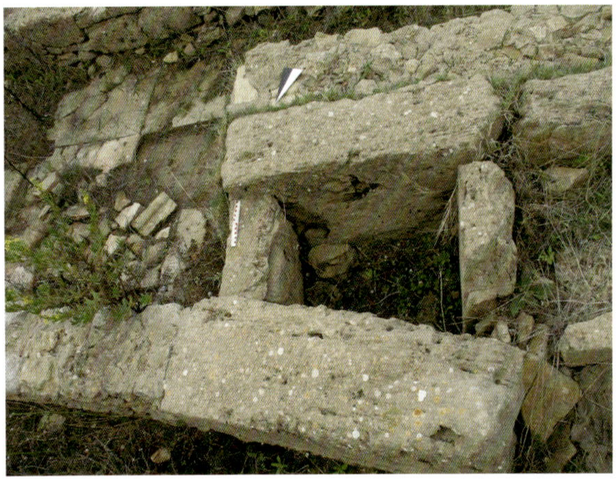

Fig. 3.12. Selinous, Northeast Quarter, probable kopron *in the* ambitus *(photo G. Zuchtriegel).*

considered an aesthetic or hygienic problem,[88] and second, the agricultural activities of many inhabitants created a demand for sewage as compost, which was collected and recycled.

Cesspits (*koprones*) of the 6th to the 4th Century BC

The earliest structures within settlements that can be related to the handling and removal of garbage, faeces and sewage, are cesspits. After the 4th century BC they disappear from urban settlements. The terminus *kopron* for cesspits, meaning deposits and compost heaps for faeces and other manure, is taken from ancient literature.[89] The word κοπρός, from which κοπρών derives, can mean faeces and garbage, but also manure. If a pit is lined with bricks and can neither be a cistern (i.e. because it could not hold water) nor a storage room or cellar, and if the filling is distinctly organic, this structure can be interpreted as a *kopron*.

Koprones have been found in the following sites. During the recent excavations at the Agora in Selinous (Sicily), a cesspit was found in House 3, in the courtyard next to the *pastas* (*fig. 3.11*). The rectangular pit measures 0.8 x 1.3 m and is situated in the north-eastern angle of the courtyard. It was lined with bricks. An enclosure preserved to a height of approximately 0.5 m might have served as a seat or in order to protect the structure from rain and/or to give privacy to the person utilizing it. From the *pastas*, where several fireplaces have been found, one could use a small opening in the wall to pour out or throw away kitchen waste or other refuse directly into the pit. The structure is attributable to the 6th century BC.[90] A similar structure (1.0 m x 0.78 m) has been identified in House 1 in the Agora Quarter, in a courtyard towards the rear of the house. It contained organic materials and dates to the second half of the 6th/beginning of the 5th century BC.

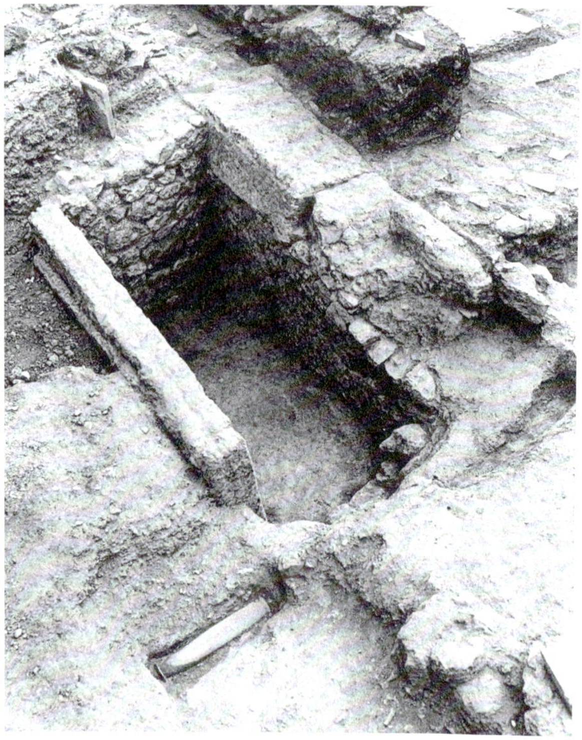

Fig. 3.13. Athens, Northern Slope of the Areopagos, south-eastern habitation, kopron *in front of the door (from Thompson 1959, pl. 21a).*

A pit lined with blocks of stone (ca 1.0 x 1.0 m), situated next to the small alcove (*peristasis* in Greek or *ambitus* in Latin)[91] and below a stairway in a house in the so called Northeast Quarter, excavated in the 1970s,[92] might also have been a *kopron* (*fig. 3.12*). The pit, with a small area in front of it paved with terracotta tiles, was accessible from the back part of the house and from the alcove. This area of the house was probably also utilized for other household activities. The *insula* dates to the 5th century BC and was later abandoned.[93]

In Athens two pits lined with bricks were found in the quarter at the northern slope of the Areopagos (0.82 x 1.3 m, deep 0.60 m; 1.10 x 1.70 m, deep 1.15 m). The base of the pits was not paved, and during excavation it could be observed that the lower layers were of a dark color. The material from the pits dates to the 5th century BC. The first one mentioned is situated in the courtyard of the 'north-eastern habitation' of the *insula*, immediately in front of a doorway. The second one is situated on the street in front of the entrance of the 'south-eastern habitation' (*fig. 3.13*).[94]

Another pit, rectangular but not lined with bricks or any other building materials (0.75 x 1.30 m, deep 0.50 m), has been found at the northern foot of the Areopagos on the side of a street, next to a wall. It was finally filled in around 480 BC.[95]

From 4th-century Athens we have another two cesspits lined with bricks in the 'Industrial District', house A and B (house A: 1.95 x 0.40 m, depth unknown, house B: dimensions unknown - for both there are no existing plans). The context within the houses is not clear (courtyard?).[96]

The excavations in Euesperides in Libya brought to light two cesspits from the 5th century.[97]

A pit in Stymphalos (Peloponnese) in the Lower City is attributable to the 5th century. The structure in question ('wall 30') according to the description is a 'rectangular area lined with bricks'; approximately 3.0 x 5.0 m. It is situated in a courtyard next to a well.[98]

Several cesspits of the Classical period are known from Halieis on the Peloponnese, studied by Bradley Ault (Houses 7, A, D). The pits measure between 1.0 and 2.5 m in length and between 1.0 and 1.5 m in depth. They are all lined with bricks and were filled not only with organic material, but also with a lot of pottery fragments. They were all situated in the courtyard.[99]

In the palace of Burunçuk/Larisa there is a *kopron* from around 450 BC, constructed during the Persian occupation of the area. It is situated right on the outside of a small room, to which it is connected by a drain.[100]

In cities like Selinous, Stymphalos, Athens or Halieis not all houses had *koprones*. Apparently some households organized waste disposal by other means (dung heaps etc.). A *kopron* situated on the street could have been used by several households. The apparent absence of cesspits might in many cases also be due to excavation techniques. In sum, our knowledge remains fragmentary.[101]

Drains, Latrines and Sewers of the 4th Century BC

Cesspits are, in the context of urban spaces, a phenomenon of the 6th to the 4th century BC. In the 4th century, however, a new development takes place: the installation of drains, by which waste, faeces, and/or sewage could be flushed from the inside of the houses into the open (alcoves or streets) where it ended in aboveground drains or in the gutter. Only in few cases can these drains be related to actual latrines or cesspits; more often we can just say that they provided the possibility to get rid of anything liquid or semi-liquid, be it the contents of a chamber pot, kitchen-waste or anything else.

Drains or latrines with drains leading into the open have been found in the following sites. In Dystos, in house J: entering the courtyard, one had on the right side the *oikos* and other rooms; and on the left, two little rooms, in one of which were found two toilet seats made of stone. The seats are built into the wall, with a concave backrest carved into the square stones behind the seats. The drains of these toilets end on the outside of the wall under a large stone. The construction of the house can be dated to the 4th century BC as a result of analyzing the building technique of the structure. The latrines cannot be a later alteration, as the stone used for the seats is part of the masonry.[102]

In Thasos, in house b of Îlot I, a little room (no 4) trapezoidal in shape and measuring only a little more than 4 m² in size, was found with some kind of basin, from which sewage could be flushed into the street (4th century BC). This quite simple installation consists of a stone slab that was inclined towards a drain. A similar installation was found in room 1 of house a.[103]

In Olynthus, in the part of the city inhabited between 432 and 349 BC, different kinds of drain arrangements can be observed. In the first place, terracotta basins were interpreted by Robinson as 'urinal and toilet seats',[104] but more likely represent sewage fixtures. The only example that is completely preserved was not found in its original context (*fig. 3.14*).[105] Another, however, of which only the exit-pipe remains still *in situ*, is inserted into a wall at ground level leading from the inside of the house into the street (*fig. 3.15*).[106] The diameter of the exit-pipe measures 0.08 m. Other fragments of basins of this kind have been found in the House of Zoilos[107] and in a stoa in area A IV.[108] In the House of Zoilos there is also a stone slab like the one in Thasos, inclined towards a little drain in the wall which ends on the street. The slab measures approximately 0.5 x 0.5 m. The room ('room o') where it is located is situated next to the entrance and is rather small: 1.9 x 1.7 m.[109]

On the other hand, in some Olynthian houses the drainage of the courtyards was led through a room out to the street. Considering that this drainage system was not covered, it could thus be used to pour out liquids and flush them outside. The rooms in question are situated next to the

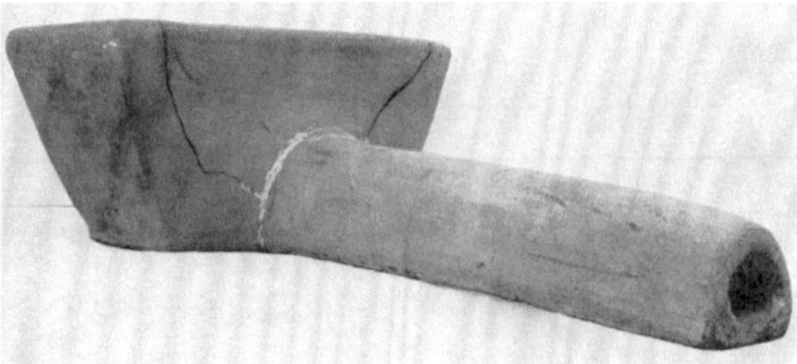

Fig. 3.14. Olynthos, House E II10, terracotta basin (from Robinson 1946, pl. 157).

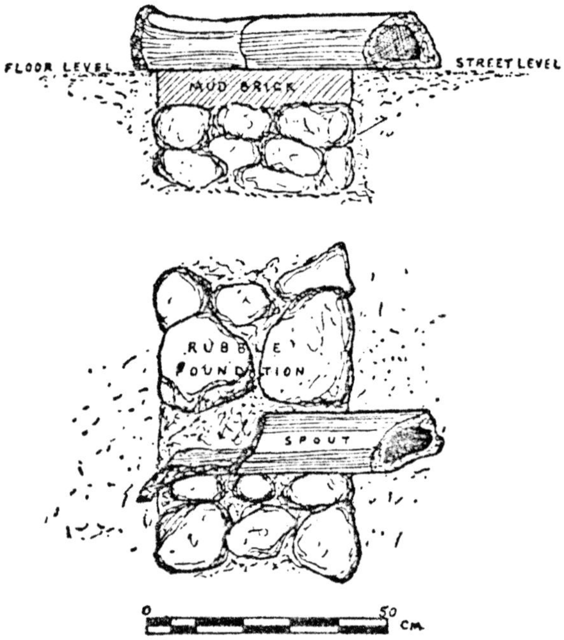

Fig. 3.15. Olynthos, House A VII 9, terracotta pipe (from Robinson/Graham 1938, fig. 16).

entrance, and Wolfram Hoepfner and Ludwig Schwandner suppose that they were some kind of 'stable and *kopron* (...) where domestic manure for the suburban garden was collected'.[110] Such rooms have been found for example in the houses A VI 5,[111] A VIII 4 (room m; *fig. 3.16*),[112] and A VIII 6.[113]

In Olynthus, both waste water and rainwater flow off mainly in open drains along the streets and in the alcoves between the houses.[114]

An almost totally intact terracotta toilet seat, open at the bottom and hollowed out on one side to collect urine, was found in one of the alcoves, which might be the location where it had also been used ('primary refuse').[115]

A drain into the open has also been found in Orraon (north-western Greece). It belongs to the

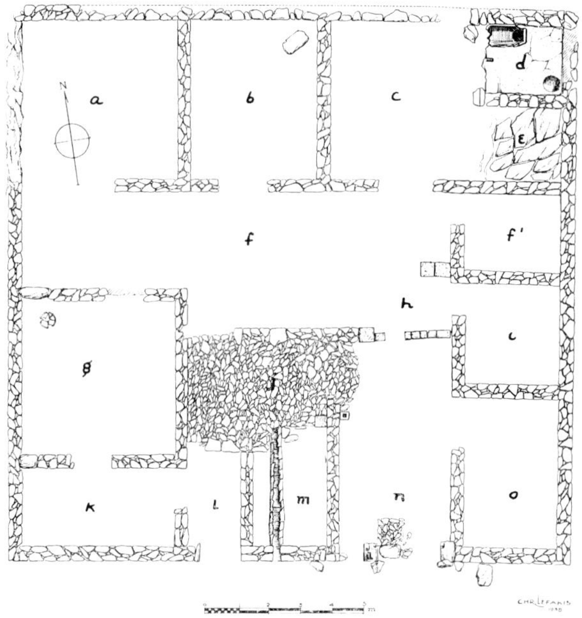

Fig. 3.16. Olynthos, House A VIII 4, drain in room m *(from Robinson 1946, pl. 14).*

second half of the 4th century BC. The drainage of the court was split and sent in two separate channels, one of them running through the *oikos* with fireplace, the other one through room e, a stable or storage room.[116] If the only intended purpose of this drainage system was to carry off rainwater one channel would have been sufficient. Additionally, in the *oikos* there seems to be some kind of basin, connected to the drain.

In House II at Eretria there is a drain leading from a small room through the wall into the street; it has been interpreted as a latrine. The structure dates to the end of the 4th/beginning of the 3rd century BC.[117] In some houses in Euesperides, there seem to have been drains that ended in the streets, too.[118]

Whatever was poured out or flushed from these installations ended up in the streets. The scope of the facilities mentioned here, therefore, cannot have been to improve the cleanliness of the streets. Rather, they facilitated daily life in the dwellings themselves. Further, if drains lead into the streets or into the open, we have to assume that sewage could be deposited there by other means as well. As some households flushed sewage directly into the streets using drains, probably many others as well were allowed to do so without using plumbing (by carrying the sewage to these areas using vessels, chamber pots and so on). Consequently

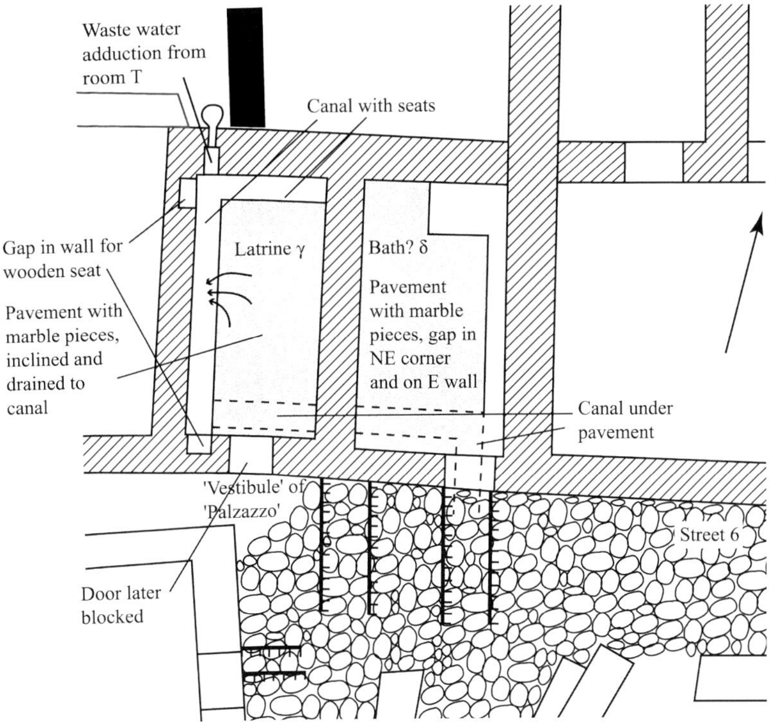

Fig. 3.17. Thera, 'Palazzo', Latrine γ, plan (M. Trümper after Thera III, fig. 136).

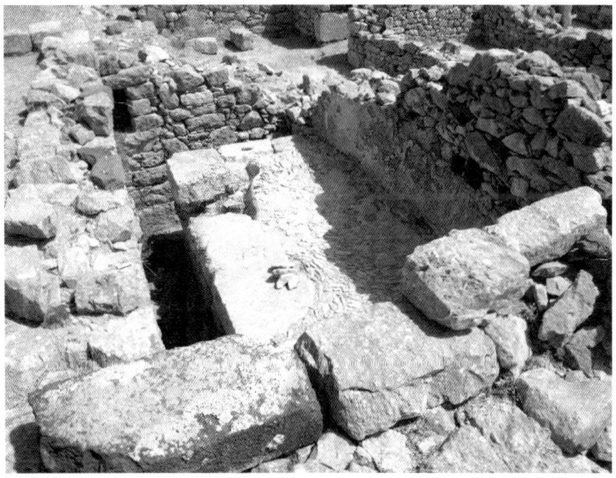

Fig. 3.18. Thera, 'Palazzo', Latrine, view from northwest (photo M. Trümper).

in cities like Olynthus streets and alcoves were regularly exposed to pollution; an impression that is confirmed by literary evidence speaking about defecating and urinating in the streets.[119]

A change came when sewers and drainage channels were covered and connected to drains and latrines inside houses. These developments began in the 4th century BC (cf. Monika Trümper, below).

Some subterranean drains from Thasos, running along the side of the street (whereas the later ones run in the middle of the streets), date as early as to the 4th century BC.[120]

In Athens we have evidence of drains from houses, leading to public drains, for example in the valley between Acropolis and Pnyx[121] or in the Kerameikos.[122] Apart from the fact that we cannot be sure about the dating - 4th century or later? - we do not know what the latrines or sewers inside the houses looked like.

In Priene the subterranean canalization was part of the original city plan from the middle of the 4th century BC, but in the beginning it probably served merely to carry off rainwater, and only later were latrines connected to it.[123]

Hellenistic Latrines (Monika Trümper)

In the Hellenistic period, latrines developed as separate rooms in private and public contexts all over the Mediterranean. These latrines have many similarities, both in layout and socio-cultural significance, with the equivalents of the Roman imperial period which suggests that a continuous development of toilet culture was initiated by the Hellenistic *koine*. The latrine was not yet, however, a standard feature of any building type or functional context. Only a few building types were provided with the novel feature and in its distribution and popularity remarkable regional differences can be observed. After a brief discussion of the most common characteristics of Hel-

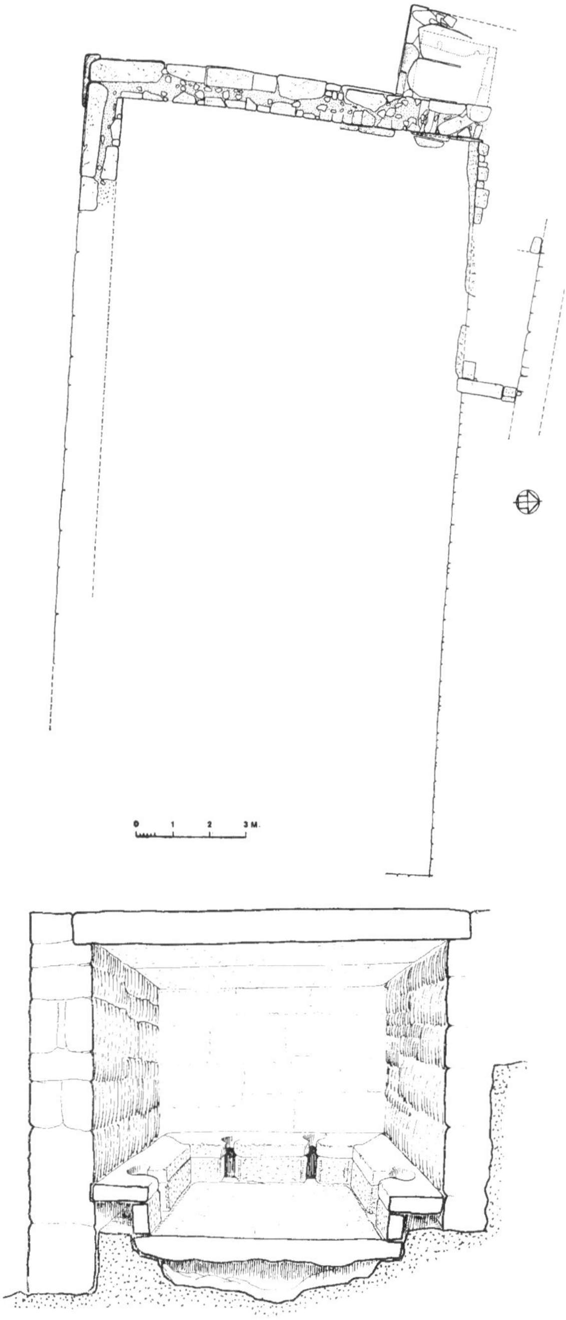

Fig. 3.19. Mina/Amorgos, Gymnasium, latrine, plan and reconstruction (Marangou 1986, 227-228 figs 3-4).

lenistic latrines, a short overview is offered of the geographical and quantitative distribution of latrines in the Mediterranean, with focus on its eastern half. This is followed by a case study, Delos, which best allows for a more detailed analysis of key features such as the distribution of latrines according to building types, location and accessibility within the building, capacity, water supply, and socio-cultural significance.

Hellenistic latrines were commonly provided with a waterproof canal of 0.30-0.50 m width and 0.30-1.00 m depth[124] along at least one wall of the room (*figs 3.17-3.27*). The canal most often evacuated directly into the adjoining street or terrain and sometimes also into a drain that traversed other rooms before exiting the building. It was either open or covered with wooden or stone seats.[125] The rooms were equipped with various types of water-proofing: simple pavement types (various stones, cement with marble or terracotta pieces) and hydraulic stucco. Except for small lamp niches and a few larger niches that might have housed statuettes, signs of a more lavish decoration are lacking. The methods of flushing and draining the canals were not standardized, but depended on local conditions such as the availability of water, the organization of drainage within buildings, and the existence of an urban sewer-system.

An analysis of the distribution of latrines in Hellenistic domestic architecture shows that they were conspicuously absent in palaces and many settlements in which a sizeable group of houses was excavated. No latrines have hitherto securely been identified in the domestic architecture of sites such as Pella, Pergamon, Monte Iato, and Solunto which all have yielded lavish large houses. Of the thirteen houses in Morgantina, only two large lavish ones were provided with latrines in the 3rd century BC. These latrines seem not to have been connected to an urban sewer system, although a sophisticated drainage system was found in the city's agora and smaller drains surfaced in various places of the city.[126] Of the five large houses in Eretria only two were provided with rudimentary toilet-installations in the 4th and 2nd centuries BC, respectively. While some streets of Eretria were equipped with subterranean canals from the 2nd century BC onwards, the latrines were not linked to these or to cesspits attested in other areas of the city, but were simply evacuated onto the adjoining street.[127] Only one single latrine was identified in the 70 houses of Priene, although the city had subterranean canalization from the 4th century BC onwards.[128] Of the almost 100 houses in Delos, however, 69 of all different sizes were provided with latrines that evacuated into the extensive urban sewer system (*figs 3.20-27*).[129] Neither geographical-topographical, political or economic reasons, nor even the existence of well-developed public sewer systems can convincingly

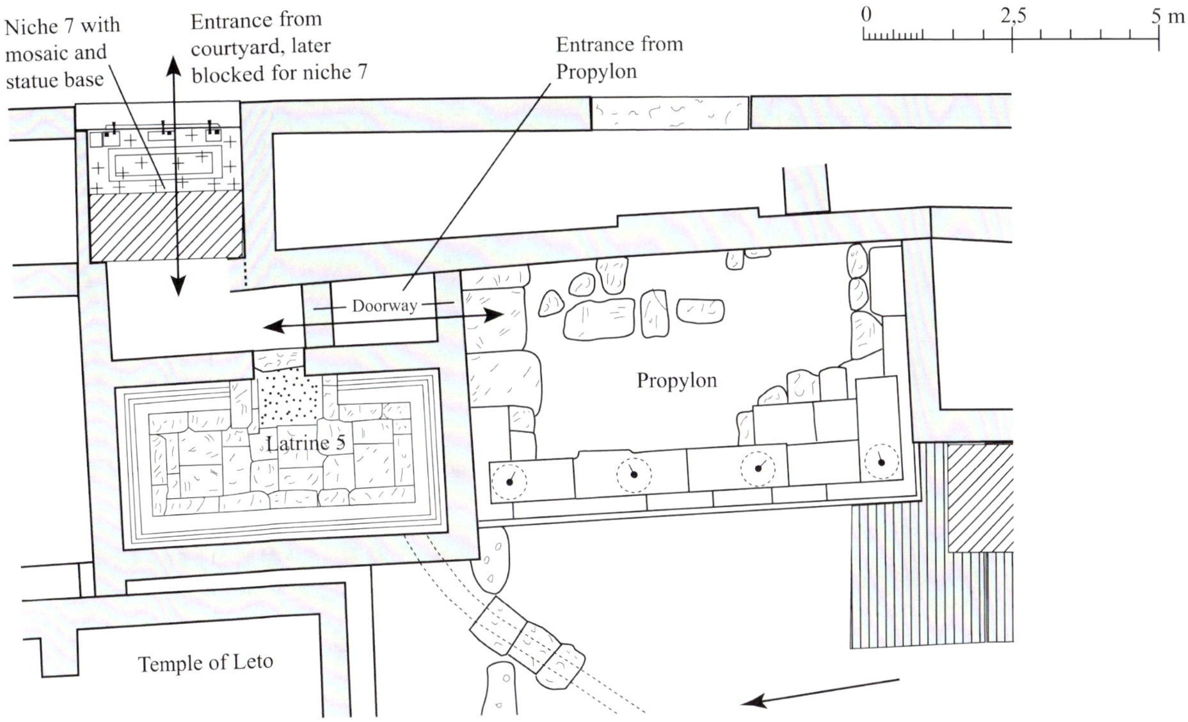

Fig. 3.20. Delos, Agora of the Italians, latrine 5, plan (M. Trümper after EAD XIX *fig. 2).*

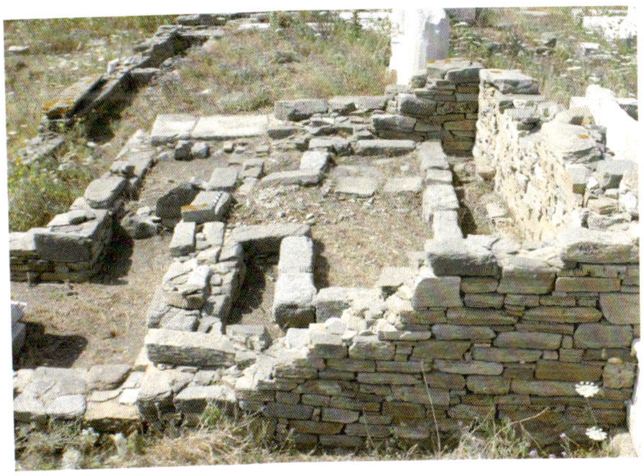

Fig. 3.21. Delos, Agora of the Italians, latrine 5, view from north (photo M. Trümper).

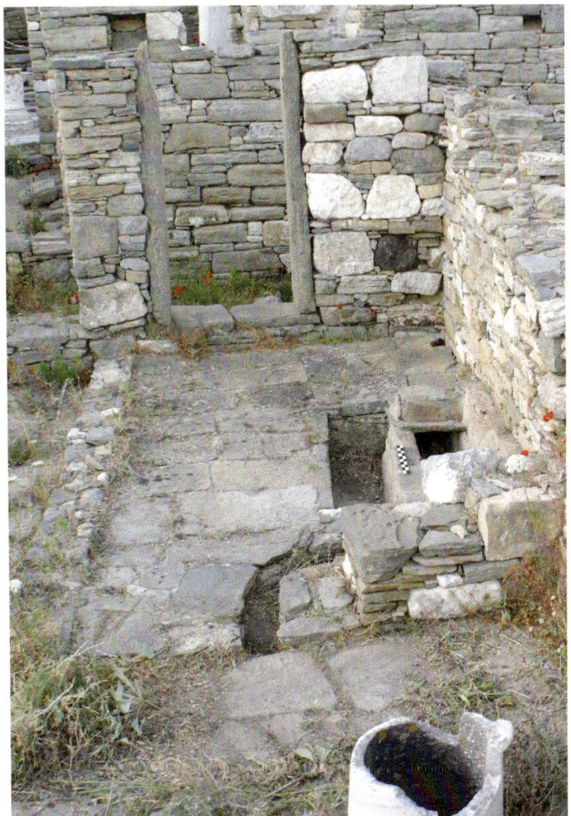

Fig. 3.22. Delos, Quarter of the theater, insula VI, house D (85 m²), latrine in vestibule with 2 parallel canals, overview from north (photo M. Trümper).

be held responsible for this remarkable distribution-pattern. Chronology might have been a crucial factor, as the numerous Delian latrines all belong to the period after 167/166 BC and therefore to the latest examples of Hellenistic latrines.

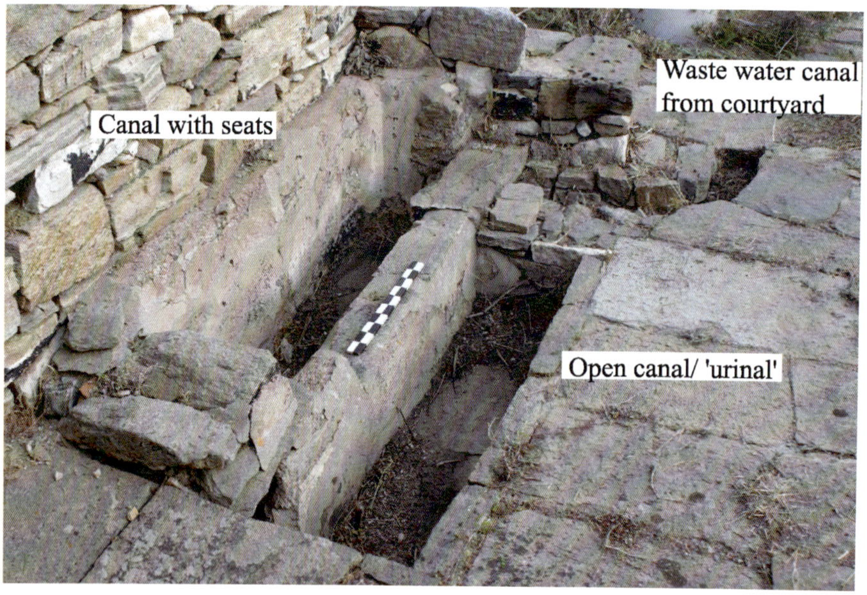

Fig. 3.23. Delos, Quarter of the theater, insula VI, house D (85 m²), latrine in vestibule with 2 parallel canals, detail from south (photo M. Trümper).

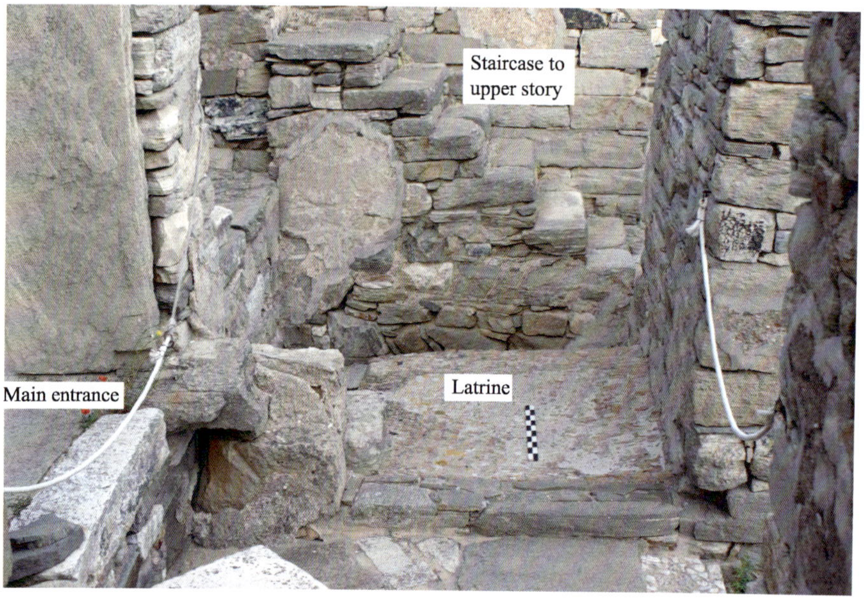

Fig. 3.24. Delos, Quarter of the theater, insula IV, house B (246 m²), latrine b with 2 canals, overview from east, (photo M. Trümper).

The main reason seems, however, to have been different local socio-cultural customs and preferences which were, interestingly, not necessarily linked to a general improvement of sanitary facilities. While most of the houses in Monte Iato have lavish bath-suites, but no latrines, only twelve Delian houses had - predominantly simple - bathrooms.

A similarly inhomogeneous picture emerges for public latrines which are not regularly found in building types where they could have been expected when compared to the Roman imperial period. Examples have been identified in very few *palaestrae* (*fig. 3.19*),[130] bath buildings,[131] hostelries and semi-public clubhouses[132] and again, the main evidence comes from Delos. Thera is considered the only Hellenistic city with independent, truly publicly accessible latrines that were connected to the public subterranean canalization. Currently, six latrines can be identified, of which only two or three were certainly accessible from public space, while the others opened onto vestibules and were therefore not necessarily public (*figs 3.17-18*).[133] Since none can be safely dated to either the Hellenistic or the Roman imperial period and at least two were later additions to the original

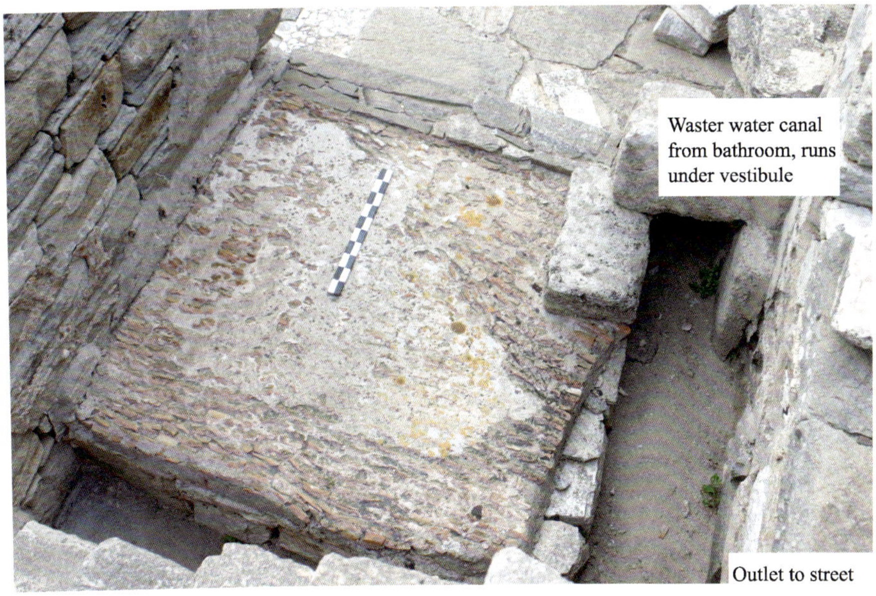

Fig. 3.25. Delos, Quarter of the theater, insula IV, house B (246 m²), latrine b with 2 canals, detail from west (photo M. Trümper).

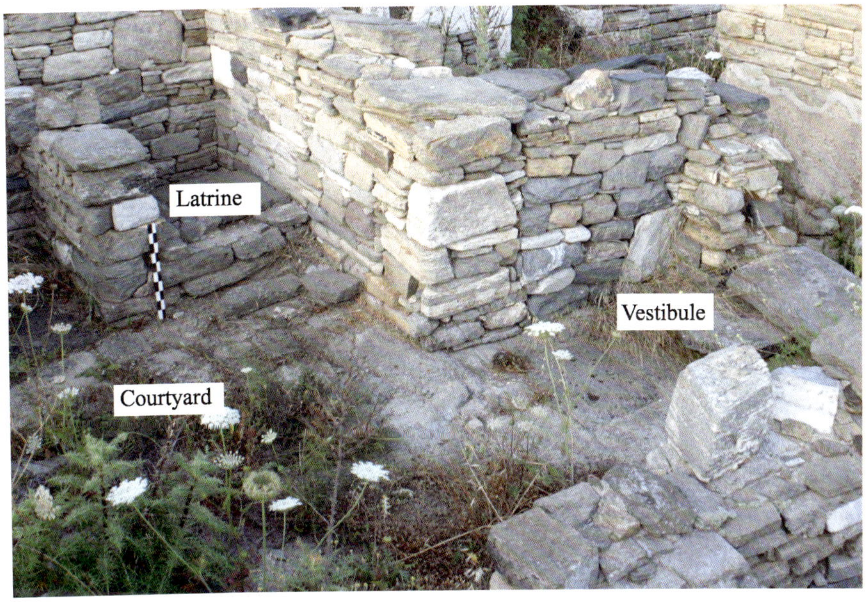

Fig. 3.26. Delos, Quarter of the theater, insula III, house C (65 m²), latrine with one canal in courtyard, from northeast (photo M. Trümper).

plan, it must remain open whether the independent public latrine was already an achievement of the Hellenistic period. In general, public latrines were still a relatively rare feature in the Hellenistic eastern Mediterranean and their installation was obviously determined by local practices and traditions, as in the case of private latrines.[134]

Latrines in Delos

With 82 latrines in 77 different buildings, Delos provides by far the best evidence currently available for the Hellenistic period.[135] All belong to the period between 167/166 BC and the mid 1st century BC, when the island was a booming cosmopolitan trade center. Delos is characterized by a semi-arid climate with rainfall as the only source of freshwater that had to be carefully collected and sparingly utilized. Among the 77 buildings with latrines are five clubhouses, one hostelry,[136] the Sea-Palaestra,[137] the so-called Agora of the Italians (a lavish Garden-Porticus-complex; *figs 3.20-21*),[138] a public bath (originally a house),[139] and 68 (or 69) houses (*figs 3.22-27*). The latter include a broad size-range from the smallest, most modest houses (50-65 m²) to the largest,

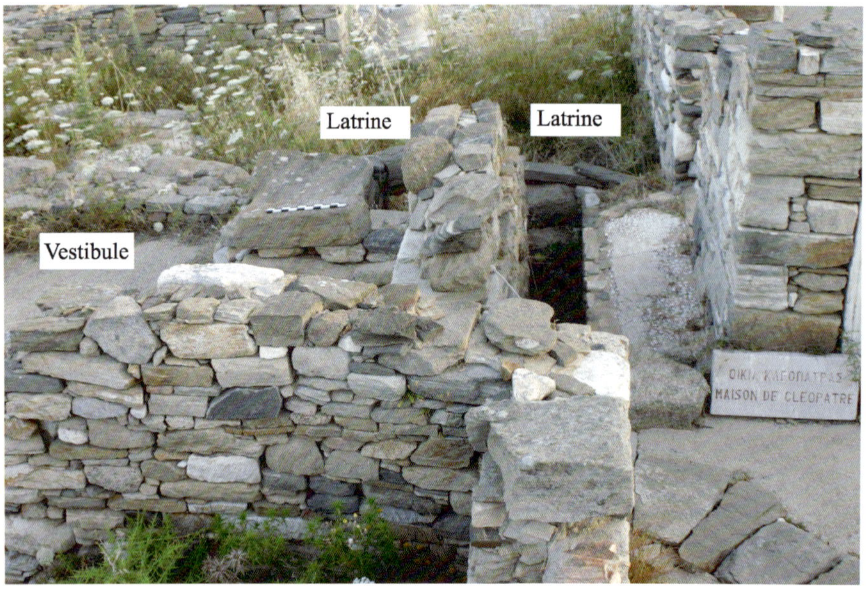

Fig. 3.27. Delos, Quarter of the theater, insula III, house I (house of Cleopatra, 405 m^2), latrine p with one canal and house J (228 m^2), latrine with one canal in vestibule, from south (photo M. Trümper).

most lavish examples (ca 600-800 m^2). By contrast, latrines are conspicuously absent in some of the largest and richest houses and also in many public buildings such as the so-called Gymnasium, the three Agorai and the numerous sanctuaries of the island.

The majority of domestic latrines (54) were situated next to the entrance or vestibule and even in the vestibule and thus fully visible and accessible to anybody entering the house (*figs 3.22-27*).[140] This location was primarily motivated by its vicinity to the street sewer and by the general layout of houses that had service sections in the front part, next to the street. In the largest and richest houses, the clubhouses, and the public buildings, however, latrines never opened directly onto the entrance or vestibule; they were instead situated in remote parts of the buildings and service sections or were accessible by separate corridors and anterooms. The choice of the location of latrines was obviously first dictated by practical requirements, but wherever possible also by the wish to keep unpleasant smells and sights away from the main entrance area. Since access to all private and public latrines was always from within the buildings that could all be locked, no latrine was truly publicly accessible. Nothing indicates that domestic latrines located next to the entrance were open to passers-by on a regular basis.[141]

The size of latrines varies from about 1.10 (*fig. 3.26*) to 16 m^2 (*figs 3.20-21*) and is mostly in reasonable relation to the size of the buildings. 34 latrines have a canal along one single wall of the room, the length of which ranges from 0.80 to 3.30 m (*figs 3.26-27*). For toilets of the Roman Imperial period, the length of canals is usually considered indicative of the number of seats, calculated with an average width of 0.50-0.60 m. According to this, the Delian latrines with one canal offered one to six seats and the majority offered space for at least two. Most latrines were even provided with canals on several walls: two (40; *figs 3.24-25*), three (6), or all four (2; *figs 3.20-21*) with a maximum total length of 16 m (24-30 seats). No seats are preserved, but they can be reconstructed in most cases due to gaps in walls or built-up pillars in the canals that held wooden boards with holes. In many latrines with several canals, however, evidence of seats is missing for one of the canals. This suggests that these latrines included a deliberate differentiation between open canals that might have served as urinals and covered canals that provided seats. Although this reduces the presumably high number of spaces in many latrines, most latrines - even those in very small houses - still seem to have been conceived for collective use, and there are even examples in private houses that offered seats for some nine to eleven persons at a time. Even households of middle-sized and small houses were obviously large enough to require collective latrines. Furthermore, the location and size of domestic latrines suggest that they were used by all household members alike.

Several supplies and devices were used to flush the latrine canals: canals or pipes leading waste or rain water to the latrine from the courtyard, a room where water was used (bath, kitchen, service etc.), the upper floor, or the roof; a street sewer leading through the latrine; or water carried by hand to the latrine which could have been waste water, but also fresh water from nearby wells, cisterns, or reservoirs. Almost half of all latrines lack access to any running water and therefore seem to have been fed solely by hand; among these astonishingly is what was also the largest latrine in Delos, the public latrine 5 of the Agora of the Italians (*figs 3.20-21*). About 33 % of all latrines were provided with one external flush water source among which the courtyard sewer figured most prominently; 15 % had two and only 6 % had three external sources. Since flushing by external sources was highly unreliable, that is to say irregular and not always sufficient in quantity, they were probably only used in addition to the predominant supply by hand. Given the relative paucity of fresh water in Delos, it is questionable whether latrines could always be flushed on a regular basis at all, particularly in dry seasons. The availability of water will also have affected the urban sewer system, whose year-round functionality and efficiency was strongly doubted.[142] But even if sewers were often obstructed, streets will still mostly have been visually free of feces and other solid waste, if not of their smell.

55 (or even more), by far the majority of latrines, in private and public premises alike, were installed subsequently, most often as part of an enlarging and embellishing remodeling process. It is highly suggestive, but cannot be derived from the evidence, that this phenomenon was linked to aspects like an improvement of water supply or the urban sewer system. The increasing number of latrines testifies, however, to the high value and even prestige of a latrine, and most likely also to a change in social practices and standards. A separate room for defecation combined with a well-organized disposal of waste will certainly have improved the lifestyle of home-owners and rendered the visit to public buildings more agreeable. In addition, in this international trade port, houses had an increasingly important public function; when the home-owners received business partners and entertained guests, a latrine was undoubtedly convenient and probably also considered a status symbol. Dynamics of local society might have induced owners of small houses, who rarely had occasions to receive outsiders, also to participate in the enhanced urban lifestyle and install a latrine, even if this had to be located right in the courtyard or in the vestibule.

Despite the significant presence and power of Italians and Romans in the international trade port of Delos, the introduction of latrines cannot safely be associated with them, nor can it be concluded that Italians and Romans imported the latrine from the eastern to the western Mediterranean. The latrine was an invention of the Hellenistic *koine*, and its design, standards, and popularity still varied enormously from city to city.

Notes

1 Seul un article déjà ancien, consacré aux installations sanitaires attestées en Égypte, tente de dresser une liste des «latrines» égyptiennes: Honigsberg 1940.

2 Ricke 1932 présente les caractéristiques du plan «amarnien» et de l'équipement domestique qui s'y trouvait, notamment l'*Abortsitz* (34-35).

3 Borchardt 1912, 19 et fig. 12-15. Les sièges de briques découverts présentent de légères variantes qui les différencient plus ou moins les uns des autres, mais insuffisamment pour procéder à une catégorisation.

4 Voir par exemple Peet/Wooley 1923, 29-30 (maison O49.24) et Borchardt/Ricke 1980, 24 (maison Q46.1). Si l'on se fonde sur la documentation publiée, aucun fragment de ces récipients n'a été découvert *in situ*. Il n'est donc pas possible de déterminer le type de vaisselle utilisé.

5 Frankfort/Pendlebury 1933, 47 et pl. XLII.3 (objet n° 30/ 182) ; Freed et al. 1999, 253, fig. 165. Il me faut signaler qu'en figure 3.2, les mesures suivies de la mention * ne sont qu'approximatives et ont été déduites des proportions générales de l'objet (il en est de même pour le siège présenté en figure 3.1). P. Honigsberg (1940, 16-17) signale à juste titre un objet comparable, mais de terre cuite, dans le Village d'artisans de Deir el-Médina (Bruyère 1939, 223-224 et fig. 112).

6 Voir par exemple Borchardt/Ricke 1980, plan 30 (maison P47.7), plan 57 (maison O48.1) et plan 58 (maison O48.4).

7 Voir par exemple Borchardt/Ricke 1980, plan 107 (maison O50.2) et plan 110 (maison N51.3).

8 Voir par exemple Borchardt/Ricke 1980, plan 33 (maison P47.23) et plan 69 (maison J49.2).

9 Quibell 1923, 11-13, 29, 31 et pl. XXX-XXXI. Il faut néanmoins rester prudent quant à cette identification, J.E. Quibell n'ayant pas publié de relevé des structures mises au jour et aucune vérification ne pouvant actuellement être entreprise (ces tombes s'étant réensablées).

10 Dans la même pièce (Borchardt/Ricke 1980, plan 27 (maison P47.2) et plan 23 (maison P47.19)) ou dans une pièce annexe communiquant avec la salle d'eau (Borchardt/Ricke 1980, plan 87 (maison P49.4) et Borchardt 1916, fig. 26 (maison U36.54)).

11 Pour le tabouret percé de la tombe de Kha à Deir el-Médina, voir Schiaparelli 1927, 117-118 (Je tiens à remercier ici le Musée de Turin, en particulier le Dr. Sara Caramello, qui a eu l'amabilité de faire ouvrir la vitrine pour prendre les mesures de ce siège). Pour celui de la tombe de Khnoummose (n° 253) à Gourna et ses dimensions, voir Pillet 1952, 90-91.

12 Pour des photographies de ces sièges d'accouchement, voir notamment Pillet 1952, 91-93 (qui est d'ailleurs partisan de cette interprétation) et Blackman 2000, 63, fig. 28.

13 Échantillon correspondant aux maisons publiées par les équipes de l'*Egypt Exploration Found* (Peet/Wooley 1923; Frankfort/Pendlebury 1933 ; Pendlebury 1951) et de la *Deutsche Orient-Gesellschaft* (Borchardt/Ricke 1980; Borchardt 1916 ; Ricke 1932). Bien entendu, la représentativité de mon échantillon est approximative puisqu'elle dépend aussi du hasard de la conservation des vestiges.

14 À propos des installations sanitaires et de leurs diverses déclinaisons, voir Gräzer 2009.

15 Totalement absentes des maisons jugées de bas niveau (1a, 1b et 1c), des latrines sont attestées de façon sporadique dans celles de «moyen niveau» (types 1d et 2c) et se systématisent dans celles de «haut niveau» (type 3e): Tietze 1985, 65-71.

16 Dans la campagne égyptienne du début du 20e siècle, on procédait encore à la toilette corporelle à l'aide d'une aiguière et d'un bassin de cuivre. A l'époque pharaonique, il en était probablement de même dans beaucoup d'habitations qui ne disposaient pas d'une plaque de douche (Gräzer 2009).

17 Von Pilgrim 1996, 216-217: fouille de la maison H70. Selon lui, les habitants de l'île utilisaient peut-être aussi les rives à cette fin.

18 Signalons à titre d'information qu'au Moyen Empire, les rues principales de certaines zones urbaines, planifiées par le pouvoir royal, étaient dotées d'un caniveau central à ciel ouvert débouchant à l'extérieur de l'enceinte: notamment la ville de pyramide de Kahoun (Petrie 1891, 8) et la forteresse de Bouhen (Emery 1979, 35 et fig. 19-20).

19 Voir Dixon 1972.

20 Le recyclage des excréments de ruminants est encore largement pratiqué de nos jours à la campagne pour alimenter le feu (au sujet de la *gella* (galette de fumier), voir Rizqallah/Rizqallah 1978, 11).

21 Sur ces deux animaux, voir par exemple Yoyotte/Vernus 2005, 511-512, 556-560.

22 Hauschteck 2004. Von Pilgrim proposait déjà l'hypothèse de la coprophagie des chèvres, présentes en grand nombre à Éléphantine, pour expliquer l'absence d'excréments humains dans la zone urbaine: Von Pilgrim 1996, 217, n. 645.

23 Sur l'identification de ces structures comme enclos pour les truies gestantes et sur le comportement du porc en général, voir Shaw 1984 (en particulier 49-53). En temps normal, les porcs devaient très probablement déambuler librement aux abords des zones habitées: sur le porc comme animal du «gebel», voir Yoyotte/Vernus 2005, 558.

24 Sur l'analyse des restes de fèces humaines et de porcs découverts dans ces enclos et les critères de leurs identifications respectives, voir Shaw 1984, 47-49, 56 et 57-59.

25 Sur l'identification de ces latrines, et sur un lien entre ces représentations détaillées de l'équipement domestique et la politique «loyaliste» du roi Akhenaton, voir Traunecker 1988, 80, 92-93.

26 Hérodote, 2.35, mentionne la pudeur manifestée par les Égyptiens à ce sujet.

27 *wsšt* (*Wb* I, 358, 1-3). Même si l'urine est généralement évoquée en parallèle des fèces, sa gestion n'a pas dû poser les mêmes problèmes aux Égyptiens. Répandue à l'extérieur, sur le sol, l'urine devait très vite devenir inoffensive en s'évaporant. On sait d'ailleurs que la solution pour se débarrasser des eaux usées issues de la douche consistait à les déverser simplement à l'extérieur de la maison.

28 *ḥwꜣꜣt* (*Wb* III, 51, 1), *ḥs* (*Wb* III, 164, 4) et *ḥtp-kꜣ* (*Wb* III, 195, 1). Ma traduction des deux derniers termes se base sur Kadish 1978-1979, 204, n. 4. L'emploi de termes euphémiques traduit probablement la volonté de conjurer, en le niant, le danger impliqué par ces matières.

29 Pour un point rapide sur la notion d'*excreta* et les dangers qu'elle implique, voir Gräzer 2009; sur les notions de pureté et de purification, voir Meeks 1976.

30 L'usage d'eau plutôt que de papier ou de tissu est encore la solution privilégiée actuellement en Égypte pour ses avantages sanitaires.

31 Pour une traduction de ce texte, voir Lichtheim 1975, 184-192. Sur la «portée sociale du négligé et de la saleté», voir Meeks 1976, col. 439-440.

32 Il faut signaler l'ambivalence en Égypte de certains métiers, à la fois dépréciés pour leur contact avec la saleté et estimés pour l'intimité qu'ils impliquaient avec le maître de maison: voir le cas du laveur (Hall 1986, 48-56).

33 Sur les nombreux passages «scatophages» de la littérature funéraire égyptienne, voir Kadish 1978-1979. Une fois encore, la négation d'un contact avec les excréments doit probablement être comprise comme un moyen d'en conjurer les effets: à propos de la «toilette éthique» du défunt, voir Meeks 1976, col. 445. Signalons également l'existence d'un démon-portier de l'au-delà, le «mangeur d'excréments» (*wnm-ḥwꜣꜣt*), qui a longtemps incarné un danger redoutable pour le défunt: voir Pantalacci 1983.

34 À propos de l'au-delà comme «monde inversé», voir Hornung 1968, 15.

35 En plus des latrines «grandeur nature» identifiées dans les tombes précédemment mentionnées, P. Honigsberg identifie un siège de latrines dans un modèle funéraire de terre cuite daté du Moyen Empire (Petrie 1907, 20): Honigsberg 1940, 10 et fig. 9.

36 Cahill et al. 1991, 64-65.

37 The Ophel (also called 'City of David') is the name of the narrow promontory beyond the southern edge of Jerusalem's Temple Mount.

38 One was found by the Parker expedition, one excavated by Kathleen Kenyon and one by R.A.S. Macalister. See Cahill et al. 1991, 65; Chapman 1991, 4-8.

39 Cahill et al 1991, 67-69.

40 Mustard: cabbage, turnips, radishes, mustard, Carrot: parsley, caraway, coriander, cumin, dill, Mint: hyssop, thyme, sage, marjoram, mint, Composite: lettuce, endive, artichokes, chicory.

41 Bennett 1974, 8-9.

42 Hirschfeld 1995, 66-67, fig. 42; Magness 1998, 38.

43 Aristophanes, *Pax* 1265-1266.

44 Herodotus, 2.35.2; Lloyd 1976, 150.

45 Aristophanes, *Nubes* 1384-1385.

46 Aristophanes, *Pax* 164.

47 Aristophanes, *Ecclesiazousai* 311-326.

48 Vatin 1976, 557.

49 Owens 1983, 45-46.

50 Euboulos, 62 = Athenaeus, *Deipnosophistae* 11.460e.

51 Theophrastus, *Characters* 14.5.

52 Xenophon, *Poroi* 2.6.

53 Tod 1948, II, 294-301, no 202.

54 Kilmer 1993, plate R528.1.

55 Aristophanes, *Pax* 1228.

56 Athenaeus, *Deipnosophistae* 12.17.

57 Henderson 1975, 191.

58 Aristophanes, *Thesmorphoriazousai* 633.

59 Sparkes/Talcott 1958, fig. 22.

60 Kilmer, 1993, plate R531.

61 Thompson 1971, figs. 39, 40; Lynch/Papadopoulos 2006, 1-32.

62 *LSJ*, s.v.

63 Dittenberger, *OGIS*. 483. ll.79-84.

64 Demosthenes, 25. 49.

65 *IG* II^2 2496.

66 IG I^2 4.

67 Solokowski 1962, 107, no 53.

68 Sokolowski 1962, 59, no 24.

69 *IG* XII.5. 107.

70 Guéraud 1931, 191-193.

71 Juvenal, *Satires* 3. 273-279.

72 *LSJ*, s.v.

73 Aristophanes, *Ecclesiazousai* 1059.

74 Antiphon, Fr. 40. 5.

75 Aristophanes, *Pax* 99, 158

76 Aristophanes, *Thesmorphoriazousai* 483-485.

77 Homer, *Odyssey* 17.296-298.

78 See below, p. 38.

79 *Inscriptiones Creticae* IV 73A. 7-10.

80 Plutarch, *Moralia* 811 B.

81 *IG* XII. 8. 265; Vatin 1976 560-564.

82 Dittenberger, *OGIS*. 483. 79-84.

83 *IG* XI. 287. 62-63.

84 Aristophanes, *Pax* 9; Aristotle, *Ath. Pol.* 50.2; Owens 1983, 48-50.

85 Kolb 1984, 75-84.

86 Wilson 2000a, 164-165.

87 Courtesy of Eddie Owens.

88 In later times, however, domestic architecture and urban infrastructure became more and more a subject of aesthetic discourse: Heracl. *Crit.* 1.1; 1.21; Strabo 14.1.37; see also: Kolb 1984, 122-123; Lauter 1986, 90; Wörrle/Zanker 1995, V.

89 Ault 1994a, 198.

90 Mertens 2006, 179, fig. 316; Selinunt-Database at Rome: I iv 2003 US 459; Selinuntarchiv at Rome G 79/13-21.

91 Mertens 2006, 179.

92 Rallo 1977, 720-728, pl. 163.

93 Mertens 2005.

94 Thompson 1959, 101-102, pl. 16-17, pl. 21; Travlos 1971, 342; Hoepfner 1999, 241.

95 See previous note.

96 Young 1951, 194-195, 201, pl. 66 d; Thompson 1959, 102 note 26.

97 Courtesy of Andrew Wilson.

98 Williams 1996, 95-96; Williams et al. 1997, 25, 36, fig. 1; Ault 2005, 65.

99 Ault 1994a, 197-199; 1994b, 218-230; 1999, 549-559; Ault in Hoepfner 1999, 541-542; Ault 2005, 62-65.

100 Boehlau/Schefold 1940, 30-34, fig. 5, pl. 44; Lawrence 1957, 239, fig. 134; Owens 1983, 47.

101 Because of the scarcity of structures regional diversity as addressed for example in Eubulus (*Cecr.* fragm. 53 = Athenaeus 10.417) can not be specified in the archaeological record so far.

102 Hoepfner 1999, 353-366.

103 Grandjean 1988, 111, 177-178, 417-419, pl. 65, 88, supplement no 1.

104 Robinson 1946, 179.

105 Robinson/Graham 1938, 205; Robinson 1946, 178-182, pl. 156-157; Martin 1957, 71; Hoepfner/Schwandner 1994, fig. 75.

106 Robinson/Graham 1938, 205-206, fig. 16.

107 Robinson 1946, 163, pl. 133.

108 Robinson/Graham 1938, 205; Robinson 1946, 93.

109 Robinson 1946, 165, pl. 133, 135,2.

110 Hoepfner/Schwandner 1994, 97.

111 Robinson/Graham 1938, 104-105, pl. 98.

112 Robinson 1946, 23, pl. 14.

113 Robinson 1946, 23.

114 See Robinson 1946, pl. 41,2, 52, 62-63, 73, 98, 110, 113, 124, 195-196.

115 Robinson/Graham 1938, 205 n. 90; Crouch 1993, 176.

116 Dakaris 1986, 119-141, fig. 4-7, pl. 37b; Hoepfner 1999, 395-411. The drain in the *oikos* was possibly installed subsequently: Hoepfner 1999, 408.

117 *Eretria* X, 108-109, 139-140, fig. 164, 170.

118 Wilson 2000a, 166.

119 For example Herodotus 2.35; Aristophanes, *Eccl.* 331-326; *Nubes* 1382-1390; *Pax* 9, 98-101, 157-166, 1265-1267. See also the section by E. Owens in this book.

120 Grandjean 1988, 429-230.

121 Dörpfeld 1901, pl. 38.

122 Tölle-Kastenbein 1990, 170.

123 Courtesy of Henning Fahlbusch (Lübeck); see also: Wiegand/Schrader 1904, 74-75, 294, fig. 312, pl. 21; Martin 1957, 70.
I would like to thank the following persons for their support and advice: Franziska Lang, Dieter Mertens, Heinz-Jürgen Beste and Sinja Rist. I owe a special thanks to John Heine and Ann Olga Koloski-Ostrow for corrections to this text.

124 Average sizes are only available for Delos: *EAD* VIII, 184.

125 So far, stone seats are only preserved in one instance, the latrine of the gymnasium in Mina/Amorgos (fig. 3.19): Marangou 1986b, figs. 3.4 pl. 93-96; Marangou 1987; Antoniou 2007, 160 fig. 6: latrine and gymnasium were built contemporaneously at the end of the 4th century BC; according to Neudecker 1994, 16 note 36 the date of this latrine is, however, uncertain. See now Antoniou 2010.

126 House of the Doric capital room 15, House of Ganymede room 22: Tsakirgis 1984, 62, 71-72, 382-383; Wolf 2003, 91; Crouch 1993, 193-195, 219-220, 229, fig. 16.1 shows an alleged third latrine to the east of the House of the arched cistern, but its identification, context, and date are uncertain.

127 *Eretria* VIII, 82-83; *Eretria* X, 56, 109, 140, 146, figs 51, 74, 76, 164, 170. Although both are identified as latrines in the publication, the example in house II, room a3 (and probably also the one in house IB, room C) served most likely as a simple pour-out as suggested above (G. Zuchtriegel): the canals are very shallow with at most 0.10 m in depth and rather narrow with 0.10-0.30 m in width; the one in house II is curved and runs in a distance of about 0.20-0.80 m from the north wall of the room. Cf. Trümper 2002, 634-635.

128 Wiegand/Schrader 1904, 294, fig. 312; cf. above G. Zuchtriegel note 123.

129 *EAD* VIII, 181-190; Trümper 1998, 29-30, 66. - For latrines in domestic architecture of the western Mediterranean, particularly the Vesuvian area, see the many works by G. Jansen.

130 Amorgos, see n. 125; Delos, Sea-Palaestra, after 167/166 BC: *EAD* XXV, 105-106, pl. XVII figs 109-111, pl. XXVIII.

131 Dionysias/Qasr Qarun: Schwartz/Wild 1950, 51-62; Tell el Herr: Valbelle 2007, 104-127; the date of both these Egyptian buildings (Ptolemaic or Roman Imperial period) is debated. - Delos: Trümper 1998, 277-279; 2006b.

132 Delos: Clubhouse of the Poseidoniasts of Berytos, House of the Diadumenos, 'Perfumery' in the quarter of the stadium, 'Granite-Palaestra', House of Fourni,

'Hostelry'. Trümper 2006a; Trümper 2010.

133 *Thera* V, plan 1: 1. included in no 30 ('Palazzo'), opening north off street 6; 2. opening off south of street 6; 3. in a building behind the Stoa basilike; 4. in the market-stoa south of the Agora; 5. in a house opposite the theater, west of street E; 6. in a complex west of street B. This distribution is not fully congruent with Neudecker 1994, 15 fig. 3. - *Thera* I, 250-251; *Thera* III, 157-159 fig. 141; Neudecker 1994, 14-15.

134 The Late Republican latrines in the western Mediterranean, particularly Italy, cannot be discussed in detail here; note, however, that they were also not yet a standard feature of building types such as public baths that were later commonly provided with latrines. Many Late Republican Roman baths such as the examples in Antipolis/Antibes, Baetulo/Barcelona, Cabrera del Mar, Valentia, Crotone, Musarna, and the Republican bath in Pompeii had no latrines.

135 For literature see n. 129. A detailed study of all Delian latrines, based on fieldwork, is in preparation by M. Trümper.

136 See n. 132.

137 See n. 130.

138 Trümper 2008.

139 See n. 131.

140 Only four latrines could be locked by doors at all.

141 Contra Neudecker 1994, 16; it was, amongst other things, simply not possible to see from the outside whether a building was provided with a latrine or not. For a possible truly public latrine in the Agora of the Italians see Trümper 2008, 275-277.

142 *EAD* VIII, 87-92, esp. 91-92.

Roman Sources

4.1 Das römische Latrinenwesen im Spiegel der literarischen Zeugnisse *(Günther E. Thüry)*

In einem Handbuch zur Archäologie der antiken Latrine ist es unumgänglich, auch die literarischen Zeugnisse zusammenzustellen und die darin enthaltenen Informationen zu sammeln und auszuwerten. Für römische Zeit unternimmt so der folgende Beitrag den Versuch, das Material zu einer systematischen Verwertung der griechischen und lateinischen Texte bereitzustellen. In der bisherigen Literatur sind sie zwar gelegentlich auch ausführlicher mit herangezogen worden;[1] eine systematische Sammlung der Stellen und ihrer Aussagen fehlt aber bisher.

Um die vorliegende Zusammenstellung leichter benutzbar zu machen, werden die Texte im Katalog nicht nach Autoren, Gattungen oder Chronologie, sondern nach ihrem jeweils stichwortartig angegebenen Inhalt angeordnet. Die Reihenfolge der Stichworte ist alphabetisch. Betrifft eine Stelle z.B. das Gefühl der Abscheu gegenüber der Latrine, findet sie sich unter dem Stichwort 'Abscheu gegenüber der Latrine'; gibt sie uns die Zahl der in Rom vorhandenen Latrinen bekannt, lautet das Stichwort 'Zahl der Latrinen'. Hat ein Text mehrerer solcher 'Betreffe', kehrt er unter verschiedenen Stichworten wieder.

Außer Zitaten, die sich ausdrücklich auf Latrinen beziehen, wurden in einzelnen Fällen auch solche aufgenommen, in denen es zwar um die Kanalisation geht, die aber ein Licht auch auf das Latrinenwesen werfen. Nicht berücksichtigt sind dagegen a) sonstige Stellen über die Abwasserkanäle, b) die literarischen Belege für mobiles Nachtgeschirr und c) die Zeugnisse für eine Verschmutzung von Verkehrsflächen durch das Entleeren solcher Geschirre und durch ein Notdurftverrichten im Freien.

Dem Katalog geht eine kurze Zusammenstellung der lateinischen und griechischen Bezeichnungen für die Latrine voraus.

Lateinische und griechische Bezeichnungen für 'Latrine'

Für die Latrine waren im Lateinischen folgende Begriffe üblich:[2] *forica; latrina; secessus; sella;* und spätlateinisch *necessaria.* Das Pissoir hieß *amphora; dolium; testa.* Als euphemistische Umschreibung für die Benützung des Örtchens formuliert einmal Plautus (*Curculio* 362): 'Es fragen mich meine Sklaven, wohin ich gehe; ich sage: Ich gehe dort hin, wohin die satten Leute zu gehen pflegen' (*dico me ire quo saturi solent*).

Die griechischen Worte für 'Latrine' sind:[3] *anankaia; aphedron; apopatos; aphodos; hedra; hipnos; koprodochos; lasana; lasanon;* die Latinismen *sella* und *sellarion;* und der späte Ausdruck *soteria.*

Katalog der Autorenstellen[4]

Abfall > **Entsorgung**

Abscheu gegenüber der Latrine

1
Cicero, *de natura deorum* 2.141: In Gebäuden verstecken die Architekten 'vor den Augen und der Nase der Bauherrn das, was Abwasserabflüsse notwendigerweise an irgendwie Widerwärtigem mit sich bringen'.

2
Cassius Dio 47.19: Die Caesarerben nahmen dem Ort, an dem Caesar hatte sterben müssen, die Würde einer Tagungsstätte des Senats und bauten ihn in eine Latrine um.

3
Augustin, *de libero arbitrio* 3.9.27: In einem Haus gibt es nichts, was 'von so niedriger, vollkommen würdeloser Natur ist (*tam abiectum et infimum*) wie die Latrine' (hier als *cloaca* bezeichnet).
Zur Abscheu gegenüber der Latrine vgl. auch unten die folgenden Stellen: 9, 11, 13-14, 24, 27, 31-32, 35.

Abwassergebühr > **Steuer für Latrinenbetreiber**

amphora in angiporto > **Pissoirs**

damnatio memoriae > **Entsorgung**

dolium curtum > **Pissoirs**

Dung aus Latrinen

4
Varro, *de re rustica* 1.13.4 (in einer Passage, in der es um die beste Konstruktion des Misthaufens auf dem Landgut geht): Einige Besitzer von Landgütern platzieren die Latrinen für die Sklaven (*sellas familiaricas*) über dem Misthaufen.

5
Columella 10.85: Der Gärtner müsse den Boden düngen mit 'allem, was die Latrine aus schmutzigen Rohren ergießt' (*immundis quaecunque vomit latrina cloacis*).

Eintrittsgeld > **Pacht von Latrinen**

Entsorgung von Müll in Latrinen und Kanälen und Entsorgung von Gegenständen, die der *damnatio memoriae* zum Opfer fielen

6
Livius 1.56.2: Bezeichnet die Cloaca Maxima in Rom als 'Behältnis für allen Müll der Stadt' (*receptaculum omnium purgamentorum urbis*).
7
Sueton, *Nero* 24.1: Kaiser Nero wollte den Ruhm anderer Gewinner von Wettkämpfen vergessen machen und ließ daher alle ihre 'Statuen und Bildnisse' umstürzen und 'in die Latrinen werfen' (*abicique in latrinas*). Wegen der Größe der Gegenstände kann aber hier mit *latrinae* wohl nur die Kanalisation gemeint sein.
Vgl. zum Thema auch die Funde von Haushaltsmüll in Kanälen in- und außerhalb des Latrinenbereichs sowie die Nachrichten über die *canalicolae*, die aus offenen Kanalrinnen noch brauchbare Gegenstände herausfischten.[5]

Gerüche von Latrinen und von Abwasserkanälen
8
Cicero, *de natura deorum* 2.141: In Gebäuden verstecken die Architekten 'vor ... der Nase der Bauherrn das, was Abwasserabflüsse notwendigerweise an irgendwie Widerwärtigem mit sich bringen'.
9
Columella 9.5.1: Bienenstöcke müsse der Gutsbesitzer auf einer Seite des Landhauses anlegen, auf der keine scheußlichen Gerüche - wie sie etwa von einer Latrine oder von einem Misthaufen ausgehen - auftreten können.
10
Martial 6.93.1-2: Hier wird der Körpergeruch einer Dame namens Thais mit dem Gestank eines alten Gefäßes (*testa vetus*) verglichen, das ein 'unersättlicher Tuchwalker' aufgestellt hat und das 'eben gerade mitten auf der Straße zu Bruch ging'. Gemeint ist damit eines der öffentlichen Pissoirs in Form einer Amphore, die von den Tuchwalkern als Quelle für den in ihrem Beruf benötigten Urin aufgestellt werden durften (s. unten Text 22).
11
Apuleius, *metamorphoses* 1.17: Der Text nennt jemanden, der nach Urin riecht, einen 'Gestank/Gestankverbreiter aus der schlimmsten Latrine' (*fetorem extremae latrinae*). Vgl. auch unten Text 37-38 und die Stelle bei Plinius d. J., *epistulae* 10.98-99 über den Gestank eines kloakenartig verschmutzten Flusses in Amastris in der Provinz Pontus et Bithynia.[6]

Kränze als Schmuck von Latrinen
12
Tertullian, *de corona* 13.8: Zur Zeit Tertullians würden sogar Bordelle und Latrinen mit Kränzen geschmückt (*a saeculo coronantur et lupanaria et latrinae*). Dafür ist außer magisch-religiösen Gründen auch ein praktischer (Geruchsverbesserung) denkbar.

Majestätsbeleidigung durch Mitnahme von Münzen und Ringen mit Kaiserbildern in die Latrine
13
Sueton, *Tiberius* 58: Tiberius habe den Tatbestand der Majestätsbeleidigung so definiert, daß es auch schon strafbar war, wenn man 'ein Kaiserbild, das auf einer Münze oder einem Fingerring angebracht war, in eine Latrine oder in ein Bordell mitgenommen hatte'.

Mäuse oder Ratten in der Kanalisation und Latrine
14
Anthologia Latina 196.1 Shackleton-Bailey: In einem Spottgedicht wird hier jemand als 'Kanalmaus' bzw. 'Kanalratte' (*sorex cloacae*) beschimpft. Wie auch Funde illustrieren, ist mit einer solchen Kanal- und Latrinenfauna tatsächlich zu rechnen.[7]

Müll > **Entsorgung**

Münzen > **Majestätsbeleidigung**; > **Verlorene Wertgegenstände**

Namen von Bedürfnisanstalten
15
Martial 12.77.9: Eine Bedürfnisanstalt in Rom nennt der Dichter hier *sellas Patroclianas*. Sie war also nach einem Betreiber mit dem griechischen Personennamen Patroclus, Patrocles oder Patroclianus benannt. Alle diese Namensformen sind aus Rom epigraphisch belegt.[8]

Pacht von Latrinen und von Abwasserkanälen
16
Plinius, *naturalis historia* 36.6: Ein Kanalpächter (*redemptor cloacarum*) verlangte bei einem Transport schwerer Marmorsäulen in Rom die Zusicherung, daß man für eventuell dadurch entstandene Schäden an der Kanalisation aufkommen werde.
17
Iuvenal 3.38: Der Satiriker spricht hier von Personen, die *conducunt foricas*, d.h. die 'Bedürfnisanstalten pachten'. Dazu Ludwig Friedländer im Kommentar zur Stelle: 'Sie pachten öffentliche Bedürfnisanstalten, die ohne Zweifel für Eintrittsgeld benutzt wurden, und um zugleich aus dem Verkauf der Exkremente Gewinn zu ziehen.'[9]
18
Fronto, *ad M. Antoninum de orationibus* p. 154 Van den Hout: Die Tatsache, daß man in Kanälen gelegentlich Wertgegenstände finde, sei noch kein Grund, daß 'wir Kanäle zur Reinigung pachten' (*cloacas purgandas redimemus*).
19
Digesten 22.1.17.5 (Paulus): Wenn ein Latrinenpächter (*foricarius*) dem *fiscus* seine Pacht zu spät entrichtet, erhebt der *fiscus* Verzugszinsen.

Papier > **Toiletten-'Papier'**

Pissoirs
20
Caius Titius bei Macrobius 3.16.15 = *Oratorum Romanorum fragmenta*, 4. Auflage, 51: In dieser um das Jahr 123 v. Chr. gehaltenen Rede erwähnt Titius die Einrichtung und Benützung der *amphora in angiporto*. Das sind Amphoren, die in den Gäßchen der Stadt stehen und den Passanten als Pissoirs dienen.
21
Lukrez 4.1026-1028: Wenn Schlafende träumen, sie stünden 'am Becken oder am niedrigen Faß' (*lacum propter ... ac dolia curta*) und höben dort ihr Gewand, dann geschehe es oft, auch wenn es reinliche Leute (*puri*) seien, daß sie ihre 'Flüssigkeit ergießen'.

22
Martial 6.93.1-2. Die Tuchwalker benötigten Urin in ihren Betrieben und durften die Gefäße daher offensichtlich aufstellen (s. oben Text 10).
23
Martial 12.48.7-8: 'Jeder beliebige Hund und das am Wegrand stehende Gefäß' (*iunctaque testa viae*) möge wissen, wozu sich das beste Gastmahl nun einmal verwandle.
Zur Pissoirsteuer (*urinae vectigal*) s. unten die Texte 37 und 38.

Ratten > **Mäuse**

Reinigung von Latrinen und Abwasserkanälen
24
Plautus, *Curculio* 580: Hier wird in abschätzigem Ton von einer *ancilla* gesprochen, deren Aufgabe das Putzen der Latrine ist (*ancillam meam, quae latrinam lavat*).
25
Dionysios von Halikarnassos, *antiquitates Romanae* 3.67.5: Hier werden - in Form einer Gesamtsumme - Kosten für die Reinigung und Ausbesserung der *Cloaca Maxima* erwähnt.[10]
26
Livius 1.59.9: Tarquinius Superbus habe die Römer gezwungen, Kloaken zu reinigen.
27
Trajan bei Plinius d.J., *epistulae* 10.32: Der Kaiser erwähnt hier, daß ältere Strafgefangene nach Ablauf einer längeren Strafdauer üblicherweise zu gemeinnützigen Arbeiten verwendet würden, die 'von einer Strafe nicht weit entfernt sind' (*quae non longe a poena sint*). Dazu gehöre auch die Aufgabe der Kloakenreinigung (*purgationes cloacarum*).
28
Digesten 19.1.54, *praef.* (Labeo): Spricht von der Gefährlichkeit der Praxis, daß Sklaven zu Reinigungszwecken in *cloacae* herabgelassen würden.
29
Digesten 7.1.15.1 (Ulpian): Sklaven würden zum Latrinenleeren (*stercorandis latrinis*) eingesetzt.
30
Digesten 43.23.1 (Ulpian): Im Interesse der Hygiene und der Sicherheit (*ad salubritatem civitatium et ad tutelam*) müssen Kloaken gereinigt und überhaupt in Schuß gehalten werden.
31
Firmicus Maternus, *mathesis* 4.13.6; 8.19.12; 8.20.1: Hier wird der Beruf des Reinigers von Kloaken (4.13.6) bzw. von 'Latrinen und Kloaken' (8.19.12 und 8.20.1) erwähnt.
32
Augustin, *de libero arbitrio* 3.9.27: Ein Sklave, der sich etwas zuschulden kommen ließ, war im Haushalt z. B. *mundandae cloacae dignus*, d. h. mußte die *cloaca domus* reinigen. Darunter ist hier wohl die Latrine zu verstehen.
33
Augustin, *in psalmum* 103, *sermo* 4.10: Zu denjenigen Sklaven, die im Haus die niedersten Dienste verrichten müssen, gehören die Kloakenreiniger (*ad mundandas cloacas*).
Vgl. auch oben die Stellen 17-19 über das Verpachten der Reinigung von Abwasserkanälen.

Schwamm (*spongea oder spongia*) in der Latrine
34
Seneca d. Ä., *controversiae* 7, *praef.* 3: das Wort für den Stielschwamm, das Wort *spongia*, sei für einen Redner ein unanständiges Wort.
35
Seneca d. J., *epistulae* 70.20: Bei einem Kampf der Bestiarier trat einer der zum Kampf gezwungenen Germanen bei der Vorbereitung der Vormittagsvorstellung aus; und auf der Latrine stieß er sich den Holzgriff eines Stielschwamms, der dort 'zur Reinigung der Beschmutzung aufgestellt ist' (*lignum id, quod ad emundanda obscena adhaerente spongia positum est*), ganz in die Kehle hinunter und erstickte sich so selbst. Seneca würdigt dieses mutige Beispiel eines selbstbestimmten Todes trotz der an sich würdelosen Tatwaffe.[11]
36
Martial 12.48.7: 'Der unglückliche Schwamm, am schuldigen Stäbchen befestigt' (*infelix damnatae spongea virgae*) möge wissen, wozu sich das beste Gastmahl nun einmal verwandle; und ebenso mögen es die Hunde und die Pissoirs am Weg wissen.
Im Griechischen hieß übrigens der zu den verschiedensten Zwecken verwendete Stockschwamm allgemein *xylospongos* bzw. *xylospongion*. Speziell für den Latrinenschwamm ist das Wort nicht literarisch, aber in der Form *xylosphongium* durch ein Graffito aus Ostia überliefert.[12]
Die genaue Verwendungsweise des Latrinenschwammes schildern uns die literarischen Texte nicht.

Steuer für Latrinenbetreiber und Abwassergebühr
37
Sueton, *Vespasianus* 23.3: Vespasian habe ein *urinae vectigal*, also eine 'Pissoirsteuer' eingeführt. Als ihn sein Sohn Titus dafür tadelte, habe er ihm Geld aus dem ersten Zahlungseingang der neuen Steuer unter die Nase gehalten und ihn gefragt, ob er etwas Unangenehmes rieche. Titus habe das verneint; und Vespasian habe gesagt: 'und doch kommt dieses Geld vom Urin' (*atqui e lotio est*).
38
Cassius Dio 65.14.5: Dio berichtet hier die gleiche Begebenheit. Als Vespasian seinem Sohn die Münzen gezeigt habe, habe er gesagt: 'Schau, mein Sohn, ob die irgendwie riechen!'
Keine der beiden Stellen 37 und 38 überliefert also wörtlich das bekannte *non olet* (das im Lateinischen übrigens auch eine allgemeine Redewendung mit dem Sinn: 'man merkt ihm nichts an' ist).
39-40
Digesten 7.1.27.3 (Ulpian); Digesten 30.39.5 (Ulpian): Für die Nutzung der Kanalisation mußte eine Abwassergebühr (*cloacarium*) gezahlt werden.

testa > **Pissoirs**

Toiletten-'Papier'
41
Catull 36.1 und 36.20: Der erste und der letzte Vers dieses Gedichtes nennt das von Catull nicht geschätzte epische Werk des Volusius 'die Annalen des Volusius, dieses Scheißpapier' (*annales Volusi, cacata charta*). Da

ja *cacatus* sonst kein lateinisches Schimpfwort war, läßt das vermuten, daß es auch bereits ein Toiletten-'Papier' gab.[13]

Unterhaltung in der Latrine

42

Martial 3.44.11: Martial verspottet hier einen Dichterling, der selbst noch dem Latrinenbesucher (*cacanti*) seine Werke vorlese.

43-44

Martial 5.44.6 und 11.77: Ein Grund für einen Aufenthalt in der Latrine ist danach, dort jemanden zu treffen, der einen zum Essen einlädt.

45

Sueton, *Lucanus*: In einer öffentlichen Bedürfnisanstalt habe sich der Dichter Lucanus, der Nero haßte, mit einem kräftigen Laut den Bauch entleert und dazu aus einem Gedicht des Kaisers den Vers rezitiert: 'Unter der Erde, so könnte man meinen, habe es gedonnert.' Unter den anderen Abortbenutzern, die sich sogar an diesem Ort vor dem langen Arm des Kaisers fürchteten, habe das despektierliche Zitat aus den Werken des Kaisers eine Massenflucht (*magna consessorum fuga*) ausgelöst.

Verlorene Wertgegenstände in Latrinen und Abwasserkanälen

46

Seneca d.J., *epistulae* 87.16: In den Besitz mancher Menschen gelange Geld nicht anders als 'ein Denar auch einmal in eine Kloake fällt' (*quomodo denarius in cloacam cadit*).

47

Fronto, *ad M. Antoninum de orationibus* p. 154 Van den Hout: 'Auch Silberplättchen findet man mitunter in Kloaken' (*etiam lamminae interdum argentiolae in cloacis inveniuntur*). Aber das sei noch kein Grund, Kanäle zur Reinigung zu pachten.

48

Digesten 9.2.27.21 (Ulpian): Die Stelle untersucht die juristischen Folgen davon, daß jemand einer anderen Person Münzen aus der Hand schlägt und daß diese Münzen dabei in einen Latrinen- oder Abwasserkanal (*in cloacam*) fallen.

Versteck Verfolgter in Latrinen

49

Scriptores Historiae Augustae, Heliogabalus 17.1-2: Kaiser Elagabal hatte sich vor seinen Mördern in einer Latrine versteckt. Er wurde dort aber gefunden, getötet und durch die Stadt geschleift. Man versuchte dann, ihn durch einen Kanalschacht zu werfen (so auch nochmals *ibidem* 33.7). Als das nicht gelang, versenkte man seine Leiche im Tiber.

Daß in Bürgerkriegen, bei Putschen oder bei Christenverfolgungen mitunter Leichen in die Kloaken geworfen wurden, erfahren wir auch an anderen Stellen (Cicero, *pro Sestio* 77; *Scriptores Historiae Augustae, Gordiani tres* 13.8; *Corpus Glossariorum Latinorum* 5, p. 584 (über Märtyrer, mit dem Zusatz *causa despectionis*); vgl. auch Augustin, *in psalmum* 36, *sermo* 2.20).

Zahl der Latrinen in der Stadt Rom

50

Notitia urbis regionum 14, p.105.11 Nordh: Es gebe in der Stadt (sc., im Rom des 4. Jhs. n.C.) 144 öffentliche Bedürfnisanstalten.

51

Curiosum urbis Romae, p. 105, 11-12 Nordh: gleichlautende Information.

52

Zacharias, *Historia ecclesiastica* 10.16, p.133 Brooks: Es gebe in Rom (sc., im 5. Jh. n.C.) 254 öffentliche Bedürfnisanstalten.

53

Itinerarium Einsidlense, Corpus Christianorum, Series Latina 175, p. 342-343: die Honorianische Mauer in Rom enthalte 116 Latrinen (*necessariae*). Gedacht waren sie gewiß für den Gebrauch durch die Mauerbesatzung.[14]

Stellenindex

Sueton, *Nero* 24.1: 7
Sueton, *Tiberius* 58: 13
Sueton, *Vespasianus* 23.3: 37
Tertullian, *de corona* 13.8: 12
C. Titius bei Macrobius 3.16.15 = *Oratorum Romanorum fragmenta*, 4. Auflage, 51: 20
Trajan bei Plinius d.J., *epistulae* 10.32: 27
Varro, *res rusticae* 1.13.4: 4
Zacharias, *Historia ecclesiastica* 10.16, p.133 Brooks: 52

4.2 Jewish and Christian Texts on Ancient Latrines *(Stefanie Hoss)*

Jewish Texts

In the Jewish tradition, defecation is considered ritually impure.[15] This concept is already described in Deuteronomy (23:12-14), where the Jewish people are commanded to defecate in a specified place outside the camp and cover up their excrement. Excrement is not defined as dirty or unhealthy, but as ritually impure.[16] As a result latrines were considered impure places.

In addition to this, the Jewish attitude towards nakedness was markedly different from Hellenistic-Roman ideas. In all cultures, nakedness not only describes the state of being without clothes, it also has many socio-cultural implications.[17] In Jewish culture, nakedness was a sign of shame, poverty and vulnerability and even used on purpose to shame a person.[18] Somebody who is naked is at least ridiculous in Judaism; at worst he or she loses his or her 'honour'.

But Jews had different attitudes to nakedness, especially between the sexes. For men nakedness was defined as exposing the genital organs, which was an offence in the presence of God,[19] whose prohibition is already mentioned in Exodus (20:26, 28:42-43). Male nakedness was also seen in connection with social hierarchy:[20] seeing the 'nakedness' of male social superiors (e.g. Ham seeing the nakedness of his father Noah) was a humiliation for the superior and a forbidden, punishable act for the inferior. To expose oneself before a man of socially higher standing was a clear sign of disrespect. Satlow proves that a connection exists here, since the relations between a man and his social superior were understood in a similar way to those between man and God.[21] This concept was not applied to nonsacral and nonhierachical contexts, as working naked on the fields or going into the bathhouse naked causes only mild criticism from the Rabbis.[22]

For women nakedness was not seen in connection with social status, but exclusively interpreted in the context of its effect on men. The very definition of nakedness was stricter for women too. In order not to be considered 'naked', a woman had to cover her whole body (including her hair, if she was married).

While the attitude towards female nakedness did not differ greatly from other peoples round the Mediterranean, the avoidance of male nakedness is typical for the Near East, and, in my opinion, also existed in the non-Jewish populace of Palestine and the surrounding regions.

Both these religious taboos - the concern with ritual purity and the avoidance of nakedness - seem to have contributed to the scarcity of Roman public latrines in Palestine (see contribution Kamash, p. 185).

Considering these circumstances, latrines are mentioned quite often in the Rabbinical Jewish literature of the Late Roman period. These writings were collected in two great groups of writings originating in different places, one being compiled between the 3rd and 6th century AD under Roman and Byzantine rule in Palestine,[23] the other in the 5th century AD in Babylonia under Sassanid rule.

It is traditionally assumed, that many statements in these compilations were handed down through an oral tradition reaching back into the time before the destruction of the Second Temple. Modern scholarship, however, has proven that no distinguishing criteria can be deduced from 'neutral' textual indicators, such as composition or form, to differentiate the older passages of the texts from newer ones.[24] Consequently the Rabbinic corpus can only be regarded as a product of the time of its final editorship and its editors. For matters pertaining to the situation in Palestine (especially in material culture), statements from the Babylonian Talmud must be excluded, except when a similar quotation can be found in the Palestinian Talmud.[25]

According to the Palestinian Talmud, latrines were common in urban houses, but chamber pots are also mentioned several times. One of these passages suggested that the pot was placed under the bed.[26] Another passage indicated that shards, pebbles or grass could be used as cleaning devices.[27]

One passage in the Palestinian Talmud describes a toilet that is reported to have stood in the priest's court at the Temple destroyed in 71 AD:

> 'There was [...] a latrine of dignity and that was its dignity: if he found it locked, he knew that some one was there; if open he knew that no one was there.'[28]

Wilfand states that this latrine is an exception in several ways: Its name already designates it as a 'special' latrine ('latrine of dignity'), and in addition, it was used by 'special' people, the priests, who had to follow stricter rules than normal individuals because they came into direct contact with God.[29]

Most passages in the Palestinian Talmud give no hint as to the design of the latrine and are either concerned with health issues (when and how to relieve oneself) or with religious matters. Examples of the latter are the question if one may hang a *mezuzah*[30] on the door of a latrine or bring *tefillin* (*phylacteries*[31]) into it. The answer to both is negative, because both *mezuzahs* and *tefillin* contain strips of paper with God's name on them, which may not be defiled by bringing them into ritually unclean places. Greetings, which also contain God's name, may not be spoken in the latrine and religious law may not be discussed there, since it could also contain God's name.[32]

Two different names (both euphemisms) are used in connection with latrines in the Talmud, one meaning *'the house of the chair'* the other *'the house of the water'*.[33] While the former only indicates that one sat while relieving oneself, the latter seems to indicate a Roman-style toilet with running water. According to Wilfand, the latter name is rare and mostly used in connection with Roman baths.[34]

The same connection with the Roman bathhouse is made in one of the minor tractates of the Talmud concerned with correct deportment, manners and behavior: 'In the latrine-room the one who enters must not hurry the one who is sitting there, and the same [should happen] in a bathhouse.'[35] While it is possible that a latrine with several seats is meant here, it is also conceivable that the person on a single latrine should not be hurried by the next visitor.

The following passage also speaks of two people in a toilet, even though it is not clear form this passage if the toilet was meant to be used by two people or was a single toilet:

> 'Said Rabbi Aqiba: "I followed Rabbi Joshua to observe his habits." They said to him: "What did you see?" He said to them: "I saw him sitting with his side facing west. He did not uncover himself until he sat down. He did not sit down until he had rubbed the place [anus]."'[36]

We also learn form this passage that one defecated sitting down and as covered as possible. If we consider that most people at that time were wearing a tunic (or tunic-like garment), almost full cover is possible, reducing the problem of nakedness.

Another example allowing us to conclude that Rabbis sometimes frequented toilets together is an exception (or contradiction) to the rule on discussion religious law in the latrine mentioned earlier:

> 'Rabbi Jacob the son of Idi in the Name of Rabbi Joshua the son of Levi: "It is permissible to ask questions about the [religious] laws of the bathhouse in the bathhouse itself, laws of the latrine in the latrine itself."'[37]

This passage implies that the latrine was designed for several people, or an exchange of questions and answers about 'the law' could not have taken place. In addition to that, this passage again demonstrates the connection of the latrine with the Roman bathhouse.

Another passage tells an amusing story designated to demonstrate the power of God, but also the brutality of Roman soldiers:[38]

> 'Rabbi Eleazar went to a privy and sat down. A Roman soldier came and made him get up and sat down in his place. [Eleazar] said to himself: "He pushed no one in the world aside but me. It is not possible for me to leave here, until I find out what this is all about." There was a snake [other translations: a scorpion] in the privy and it came out and gave [the Roman] a bite in his anus. [...]'

Rabbi Eleazar then thanked God for his deliverance.

While this story does not tell us where the latrine was situated, it can be deduced from the text itself that is was both public (or the soldier would not have just walked in uncommented) and a latrine with more than one seat (or the Rabbi would not have commented that the soldier chose him instead of others to move from his place).

In conclusion we can say that while public group latrines were not often mentioned in the Palestinian Talmud, but when they were - as with the designation 'house of water' - a connection with a Roman bathhouse is likely. As most Roman-style latrines in Palestine were found in bath-complexes, this fits with the archaeological evidence.

Christian Texts

The Christian literature of Late Antiquity is comprised of historical writings, the *vitae sanctorum* (descriptions of saint's lives), sermons and the *canones* (church rules). Latrines are mentioned relatively rarely in the Christian texts. Except for one passage, the design of the latrines is not mentioned. In this text, a polemic against the worship of statues, Clement of Alexandria states (ca 150-211/216) that 'the Romans, although they ascribe their greatest successes to Fortuna, and believe her to be the greatest deity, they carry her statue to the privy and erect it there, thus assigning her a fit temple.'[39] As mentioned elsewhere (see here Jansen, pp. 167-170), some Roman latrines had statues of gods placed in them and Fortuna/Tyche was indeed the most frequent deity in latrines.

In a moralizing critique of the luxurious life, which mirrors similar subjects of earlier Roman writers (see here Wilson, pp. 95-97) and reappears in the Christian literature of Late Antiquity, the owners of chamber pots made from precious materials (glass, silver, gold) are ridiculed.[40] In contrast to this, it was considered a gesture of special humility for a monk to clean the latrine.[41]

Holy men like Symeon the Fool or Jacobos the Hermit defecated publicly to demonstrate their disregard for worldly things, but their behavior only proved that they were acting abnormally.[42]

Stories taking place in a latrine are often used to discredit others, for instance heretics or Jews. Socrates Scholasticus of Constantinople (born ca 380 AD) in a description of the death of Arius (founder of the heretic Arianism) recounts:

> 'As he [Arius] approached the place called Constantine's Forum, where the column of porphyry is erected, a terror arising from the remorse of conscience [presumably because of his heresy] seized Arius, and with the terror a violent relaxation of the bowels: he therefore enquired whether there was a convenient place near, and being directed to the back of Constantine's Forum, he hastened thither. Soon after faintness came over him, and together with the evacuations his bowels protruded, followed by a copious hemorrhage, and the descent of the smaller intestines: moreover portions of his spleen and liver were brought off in the effusion of blood, so that he almost immediately died. The scene of this catastrophe still is shown at Constantinople, as I have said, behind the shambles in the colonnade: and by persons going by pointing the finger at the place, there is a perpetual remembrance preserved of this extraordinary kind of death.'[43]

While the description is rather vague - 'a convenient place' may describe a toilet proper but also an informal place for people to relieve themselves - the location at the back of the forum makes it quite likely that we are dealing with a toilet here. Several toilets have been excavated around the Mediterranean situated in close proximity to the forums of the cities (cf. Jerash/Gerasa in Jordan and Timgad, pp. 106-108).

The Christian attitude towards public group latrines seems not to have differed greatly from the Jewish attitude. But contrary to the Jews, who as a settled community had to deal with the new phenomenon of public group latrines coming into their country, Christianity was born into a society in which these institutions were generally accepted. Many of the newly baptised Christians had been used to visiting the public latrines and saw nothing indecent in it. Because of the necessity to set themselves off against the groups surrounding them, the Christians had to find their position towards this custom and try to define morality without confining their brothers and sisters in faith too much.

Notes

1 So vor allem von Becker/Göll 1881, 279-281; Drexel 1979, 310-311; Thédenat 1904, 987-991.

2 Thédenat 1904, 987 und Sprachlexika.

3 Thédenat 1904, 987 und Sprachlexika. S. hier S. 26, 28.

4 Zumal die Sammlung des Materials unter Zeitdruck durchgeführt werden mußte, kann für die Vollständigkeit der Stellen keine Garantie übernommen werden.

5 Über beides Thüry 2001, 12-13 und 56.

6 Dazu Thüry 2001, 46-47.

7 Thüry 2001, 13.

8 Solin 1982, 136 und 511. - Zur Lage der *sellae Patroclianae* Neudecker 1994, 98.

9 Zur Frage einer Benützungsgebühr für Latrinen Thüry 2001, 12.

10 Aufgenommen bei Szaivert/Wolters 2005, 187.

11 Der Kontext der Stelle mißverstanden bei Neudecker 1994, 17.

12 Calza 1939, 101; *Année épigraphique* 1941, 5.

13 So mit Scobie 1986, 411. Andere Sichtweisen z.B. bei Kroll (zur Stelle), der *cacata charta* mit 'beschmiertes Papier' (im Sinn von: mit wertlosem Zeug beschriebenes Papier) übersetzen möchte; oder bei Neudecker 1994, 22.

14 Vgl. Scobie 1986, 417.

15 To write this contribution, I greatly benefited from reading the then not yet published article of Y. Wilfand (Wilfand 2009).

16 Purity is an important concept in Judaism and must be observed in areas of the body, clothes, food and food-containers. Although different rational explanations for individual regulations were suggested, so far there is still no convincing rational explanation for the whole system underlying the regulations. Various scholars have over the centuries suggested that the ritual purity regulations are primitive hygienic measures, but the texts clearly show that purity and impurity must be understood symbolically, that they are not connected to actual cleanliness or uncleanliness. The most interesting attempts of explaining the phenomenon originate in anthropological research, especially that of Douglas (1966). She could show that ritual purity was defined by the Jews as normality and wholeness. Their opposite is the sphere of death and the unnatural. The concepts of ritual purity and impurity derive not from

objective physical reality, but from a cultural understanding of society. The body is regarded as a symbol of the whole society and thus is the locus where ritual purity gets manifested. The concern about what enters or leaves the body is a concern about the borders of society (see Wright, 1992, 739 and Neusner 1973).

17 Satlow 1997, 429, see also Vogel 2000, 452-455.

18 Vulnerability: Genesis 9:18-27; Shaming: Isaiah 20:4, Amos 2:16, Habakkuk 2:15.

19 This sanctum or presence could be created by uttering of God's name in a prayer or by reading God's word.

20 The following after: Satlow 1997, 440-442.

21 Satlow 1997, 440.

22 Satlow 1997, 453-454.

23 Mishnah (compiled around 200 AD), the Tosefta (around 300 AD), the Talmud Yerushalmi or Palestinian Talmud (around 400 AD), and the Midrashim (5th-6th centuries AD).

24 Avery-Peck 1995, 181.

25 Efron 1987, 143-147.

26 After Heszer 1998, 445 (y Ber. 3:5, 6d).

27 yT *Shabbat* 82a (11c 2-20).

28 *m Tamid* 1:1 after Wilfand 2009.

29 Wilfand 2009.

30 The amulet-like *mezuzah* on the doorpost is a container with several biblical quotations written on parchment.

31 Leather straps with small rectangular capsules containing biblical verses written on parchment. They are now mostly worn (by adult male Jews) during prayer, but they used to be worn the whole day. bT *Shab* 62a.

32 yT *Shabbat* 40b (3,4/6). Similar precautions are required by the Koran for Muslims entering a toilet. The code governing these practices is known as Qadaahul Haaja.

33 Wilfand 2009.

34 Wilfand 2009.

35 Derekh Eretz Rabba, 10.

36 yT, *Berakhot*., 14c (9:5).

37 yT *Shabbat* 6a (3:4), after Wilfand 2009 and Neusner 1991, 135.

38 After Heszer 1998, 445 (y *Shab* 6:10, 8c).

39 Clem. Alex., *Protrepticus* 4. After Butterworth 1919, 115.

40 For instance Clement of Alexandria (*Paid.* 2,3,39), John Chrysostom (*Col. Hom.* 7,5 [PG 62, 349]) and Gregory of Naizanz, (*or.* 38, 5 [SC358, 112]). See also Brashear/Breitenbach 2006, Sp. 805.

41 Brashear/Breitenbach 2006, Sp. 802.

42 Brashear/Breitenbach 2006, Sp. 802.

43 Socrat., *Schol. Church History* 1.5.

Design, Architecture and Decoration of Toilets

5.1 Design and Architecture *(Ann Olga Koloski-Ostrow)*

Toilets (both public and private) were not an isolated phenomenon appearing exclusively in the Roman period, but stand in a long tradition going back to the 3rd millennium BC (Mesopotamia and Egypt),[1] and the development and dating of such provisions can be traced by the conformity of their designs and similarities in technical characteristics.[2] This earliest evidence for sanitary facilities will not be explored in this section, but it should be stated that from the 3rd and especially the 2nd centuries BC, public toilets begin to appear in Athens, Delos, Olynthus, and Priene.[3]

Some of our best evidence for the growing emergence of public toilet installations, in fact, comes from the Hellenistic world of Delos,[4] where a number of publicly accessible latrines have been discovered. In addition to larger, completely public facilities, several private houses on Delos were fitted with toilets near their vestibules, which could therefore be accessed by passers-by as well as inhabitants of the house. While it is also beyond the limits of this inquiry to study these and other Hellenistic toilets in any detail, their existence sets an important precedent for Roman Italy. Many Roman merchants would have traveled to Greece and observed such amenities in these trading ports and during their business dealings in the various *agorai*, even though they were probably unpleasant and crowded to use.[5] Still, these latrines would have offered the Romans a 'vision' of a potentially cleaner, more convenient city.

Even though Roman eyes had certainly seen them by the 2nd century BC, and perhaps much earlier, such facilities clearly did not cause a revolution in Roman urban hygiene. It is possible, though, that they at least provided the spark that eventually brought the public latrine into closer proximity to the Roman *macellum*, as we clearly see instituted both at Pompeii and at Puteoli (*fig. 5.1*).

No such public facilities are known in Italian cities of the late Republic, although their lack does not necessarily argue fairly against their existence. Richard Neudecker remarks that such structures might have been made of wood that has not survived.[6] Furthermore, the presence of latrines in Roman comedy proves at the very least that they were an understandable concept to the Romans, although it does not prove their existence in the real urban landscape.[7] We do hear that as early as 161 BC simple urinals were available in the Roman Forum.[8] Once latrines were a fixture in the Roman marketplace, the groundwork was set to utilize them in other settings in the city, with an increasing realization of their potential to help control the loathsome human by-products of moving bowels and urinating. However modest our evidence for Greek disposal of feces and urine from the fourth century to about the 1st century BC may be, it is nevertheless sufficient to prove that the idea for toilets, public or private, was not a Roman invention in itself.

Before we consider the design and architecture of Roman toilets more fully, some initial disclaimers are in order. We shall not here provide a catalogue of every public and private Roman toilet and latrine in all areas of the empire, nor shall we cover all periods of Roman history. While facilities of the late Republic and early and later Empire provide the main evidence, this is not the

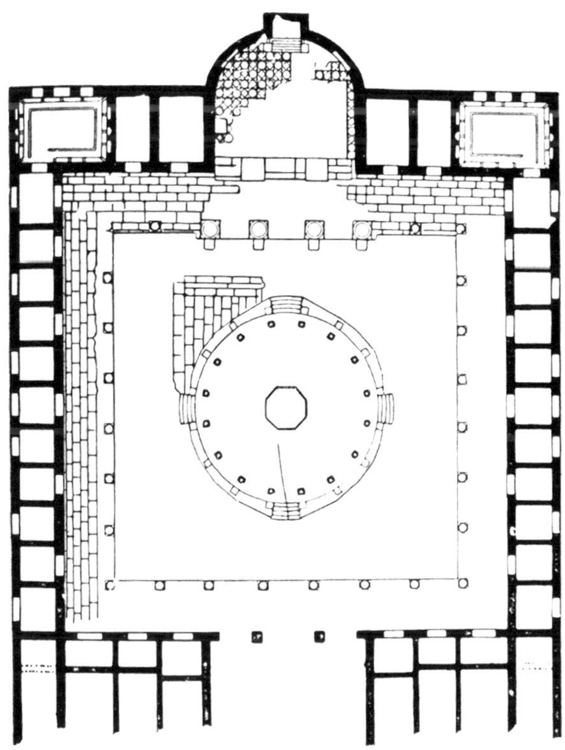

Fig. 5.1. Puteoli, macellum *plan (from Boëthius/Ward-Perkins 1976, 298 fig. 114).*

place for broader questions pertaining to later periods regarding health and sanitation, water use, or the underlying social and political motivations behind latrine architecture, especially when it survives in urban settings. Other important issues must also, of necessity, be omitted here: Why did public latrines get built in the first place in Roman Italy and elsewhere? Why did toilets change over time, if they did change? Who built and maintained them? What social function(s) did they serve? And so on.

Many of these important questions will be addressed in other chapters in this volume or elsewhere.[9] Here we survey a small sample of archaeological remains and rely only on a few relevant literary references in order to offer a very basic overview of latrine architecture and design over the wide expanse of the Roman period. Other potentially valuable types of evidence (epigraphy, numismatics - although no toilets have been recorded on coins that I know of - papyri, and legal texts) also must remain outside the parameters set here.

We should first say a word about latrine terminology as it appears in Latin texts. The word 'latrine' derives from Latin *latrina*, itself a contraction of *lavatrina*, which originally encompassed both a bathing facility as well as a toilet.[10] We can speculate that from the 3rd century BC, when *bal(i)neum* began to denote separate private bath buildings, the word *latrina* came to specify a toilet. The oldest common words for a toilet in Latin are *latrina* and its collateral forms, *lavatrina* and *latrinum*, which we find in Plautus and Varro, the former writing in the late 3rd to early 2nd century BC and the latter writing in the late 2nd to 1st century BC.[11] Toilet synonyms, *secessus* (privy or private) and *sella* (chair), were used by the Romans for toilets within houses, as opposed to toilets accessible to the general public.

Forica, on the other hand, was a special word reserved for a large multi-seat lavatory with an arrangement in an open plan.[12] *Foricae* are generally found near fora, theaters, sometimes in apartment blocks, and either in or near public baths. (More about the location of public toilets is discussed in chapter 8.1, pp. 113-114) In the literary evidence from the time of Plautus to the 2nd century AD, the Latin words, *latrina* and *forica*, both referring to a toilet, seem relatively clear-cut concerning whether their designation is for a public or private toilet. The most obvious distinction in the archaeological remains seems to be one of size and public location. By the 4th and 5th centuries AD, on the other hand, the precise meaning of Latin words denoting Roman toilets (and here we refer specifically to *foricae*) can get quite blurry.[13] Interestingly, the actual archaeological remains of toilets, even of the best preserved toilets from the imperial period, are much more difficult to pin down in terms of their public or private nature as we try to 'read' them in their architectural landscape.

We can say with some certainly that Roman public sanitary facilities really began to flourish in a wide variety of settings in and outside of cities probably from the 2nd century BC onwards, although the quality of the ruins varies considerably from site to site and in different time periods (*fig. 5.2*). The myth propagated in modern Latin classes that multi-seat Roman public toilets were everywhere, as ubiquitous as Roman baths, and available for everyone in ancient Roman cities at frequent intervals, is significantly overstated.

Now that we have established the philological differences in terminology, perhaps a simple description of the basic elements of Roman public and private toilets is in order. Most public toilets were accessible from the street by way of a door (an ordinary hinged door, in at least one case, possibly a revolving door, or a double door arrangement

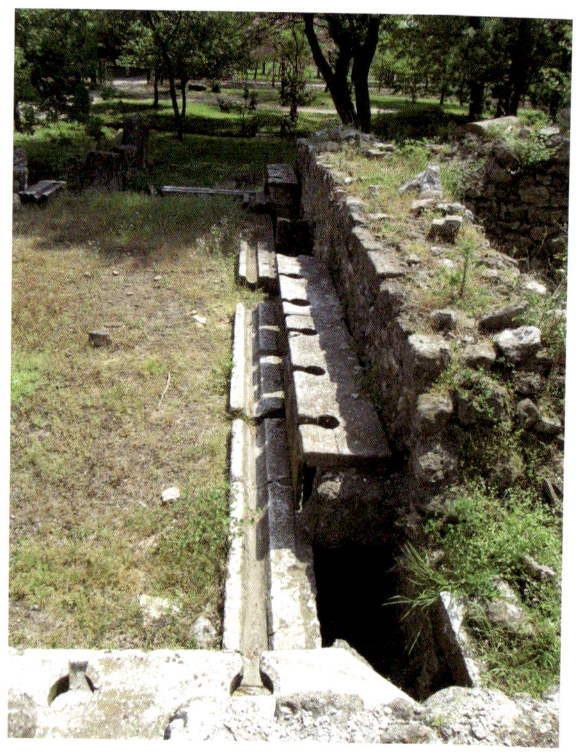

Fig. 5.2. Dion (Greece), public latrine (photo A.O. Koloski-Ostrow).

that was splayed to protect the privacy of those inside or to keep the outside public from seeing the activities inside). Mostly, public toilets are simple in design - square or rectangular rooms or buildings made of *opus caementicium* and faced with stucco and rather plainly decorated walls (white or zebra stripes are common). The bench into which the toilet seats were cut could be made of marble, other types of stone, or wood. Generally the toilet seat bench rested on stone struts that jutted at intervals from the walls of the latrine. A common height from floor to bench seat was ca 50 cm. The seat holes could be between 15.5 cm and 20 cm wide, and the distance between seats ranged from ca 20 to 65 cm apart, depending on the toilet. Sometimes the seats were constructed in a kind of key pattern whereby the hold extended below the seat in the wall of the bench, presumably to facilitate cleaning the toilets. Usually a small, shallow gutter ran along the floor underneath the seats, perhaps for rinsing sponge sticks or for spit. (These features are discussed at more length in chapter 7.4, pp. 99-105) The seating bench is generally located over a sewer trench measuring between 1 and 3 m deep. Flushing the sewer trench in the latrine was treated in different ways - often by waste water from some nearby bath or other industrial complex. One or two windows, usually high on the walls of the latrine, brought in some light and fresh air.

Private toilets, on the other hand, in Pompeian atrium houses, for example, were usually single - at most double - seat affairs, often tucked into small corners off the kitchen or under stairways. Terracotta tiles were positioned to form a significant slope in the floor at either side of the toilet hole to facilitate disposal and cleaning. While most of the single seats - presumably because they were made of wood - are missing in Pompeii and Herculaneum, we can often see their impressions in the concrete walls around the toilet in order to make accurate reconstructions. These small private toilets often have no windows and for access, only one small doorway - closed by a door, a curtain, or no covering. Unlike *foricae*, private toilets are cesspits, not emptying into city sewers.

About 250 ancient public toilets[14] have been recorded in the Mediterranean world colonized by Greeks and Romans. While there was no need for the expertise of Rome's greatest architects to build them - or the small private toilets in Roman houses and villas - Antonella Merletto and others have noted many differences in plan and design of the public toilets according to the tastes and styles required of different geographical areas and historical periods. Merletto herself suggests six distinctive designs for public toilets: 1) peristyle latrines (latrine seating usually built around three of four sides of an open-to-the-sky colonnaded courtyard or peristyle); 2) square or rectangular latrines (the most common type and simplest to build, covered with a slanted roof with windows acting as vents); 3) semicircular latrines (very similar to the peristyle type with one side colonnaded and the latrine seats placed along a semicircular wall behind the column screen); 4) irregular latrines (usually using spare rooms of the building in which they are located); 5) geometrical latrines (identifiable by geometric shapes such as a hexagon, circle, octagon, trapezoid, or more complex designs); 6) latrines with undefined plans (either because of poor or incomplete excavation or because they are not clearly readable). Some of these designs only exist in certain geographical regions. The peristyle type, for example, was totally nonexistent in the Northern and Western provinces where the temperatures were far too cold for buildings with no ceilings.

Neudecker's magisterial publication on imperial luxury latrines (built in the 2nd century AD and later) considers their complex development and decline in six Roman cities: Rome, Ostia, Timgad, Cuicul, Corinth, and Ephesus, all chosen for the quality of their remains. With a rich selection of plans,[15] he showed the variety of shapes for these luxury latrines and the overall elegance that could be achieved within them - brick and mortar buildings fitted with mosaic floors and marble fixtures, sculptural decorations, toilet seats, and floor channels. He proposed that urban administrations in imperial cities of the 2nd century AD and later expended more and more care and money upon the making of these new 'luxury' latrines not just from some new desire to beautify toilet architecture and therefore cityscapes, but because of new social forces favoring a regimentation to promote order. Neudecker unraveled the Roman ideology whereby cleanliness developed as a symbol of social hierarchy. He directly connected the presence of luxury latrines in Roman urban settings to new ideas about health and sanitation in specific medical and philosophical texts. He argued that the previously 'unmentionable' public latrine rather suddenly played a major role in changing the physical environment of Roman cities in the 2nd century and later.[16]

If the *domini*, the Roman elite, preferred their chamber pots[17] for their own excretions, what did public toilets, the *foricae*, and other types of public

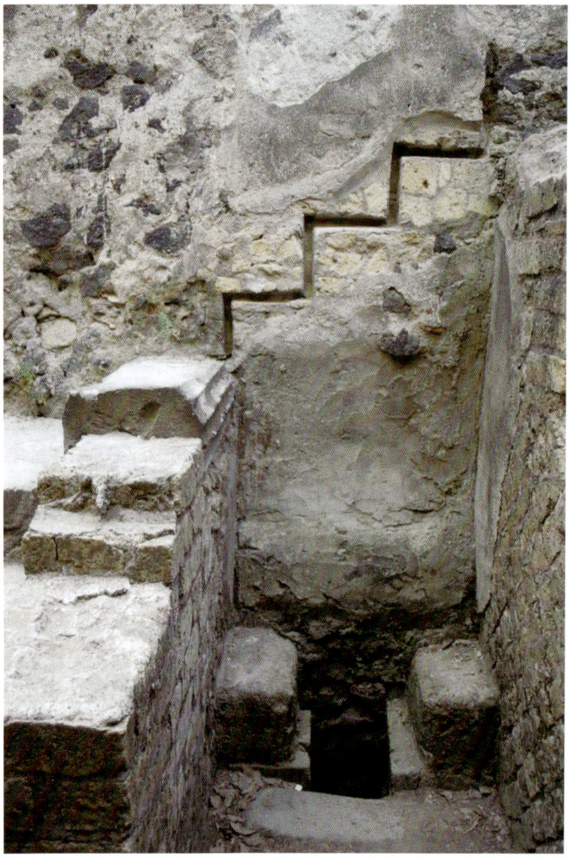

Fig. 5.3. Herculaneum, House of the Gran Portale (V 35), toilet (photo A.O. Koloski-Ostrow).

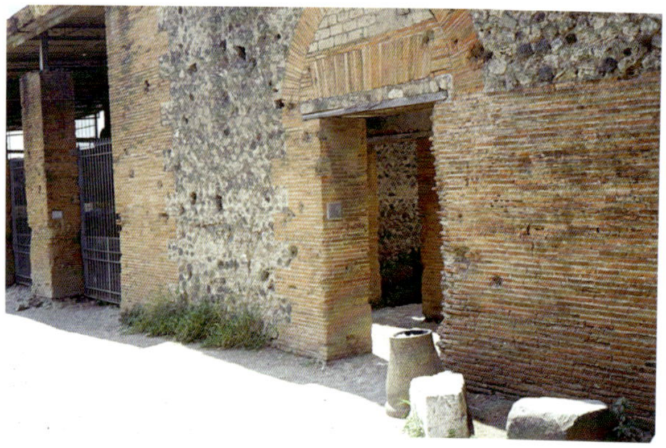

Fig. 5.4. Pompeii, forum, public latrine (VII 7, 28), splayed entrance (photo A.O. Koloski-Ostrow).

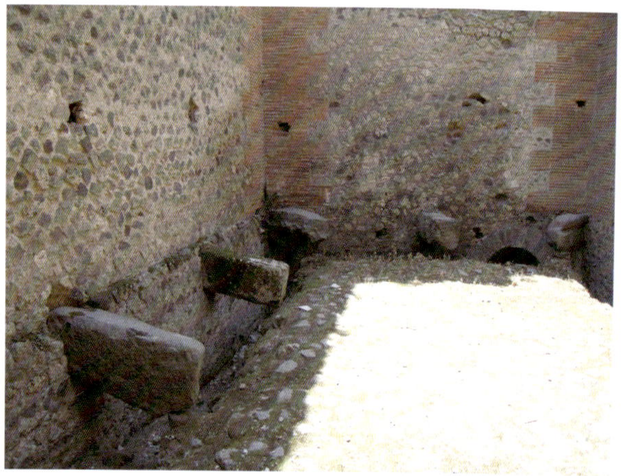

Fig. 5.5. Pompeii, forum, public latrine (VII 7, 28), general interior, NW corner with sewer opening and struts for seating (photo A.O. Koloski-Ostrow).

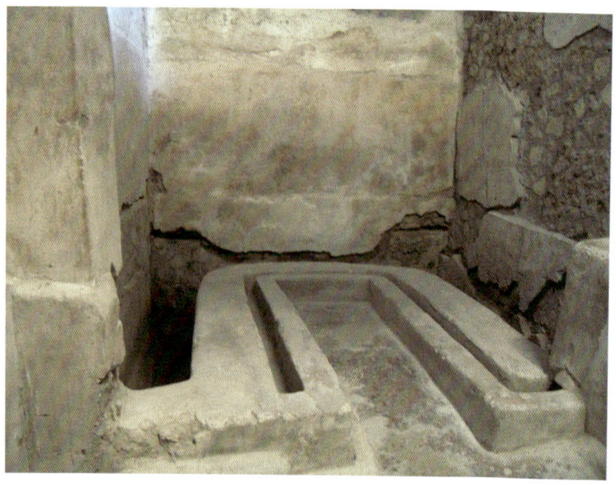

Fig. 5.6. Villa at Oplontis, multi-seat latrine (photo A.O. Koloski-Ostrow).

facilities within a Roman city look like before the age of the luxury latrine? In towns like Herculaneum and Pompeii, we find single-seat, essentially cesspit toilets in almost every private house (*fig. 5.3*).[18] Their architecture, of course, is closely merged with the architecture of the atrium houses in which they sit. But there were also multi-seat, plain, public latrines, facilities without elegant appointments, in a wide variety of public settings: inside theater buildings; in amphitheaters; or as free-standing structures near fora. These latter latrines were built in brick or stone faced concrete masonry from the middle of the 1st century BC (*figs 5.4-5*).[19] The *forica* near the forum of Pompeii, for example, which was probably not in service yet when Vesuvius blew its stack in 79 AD, is rectangular in plan, efficient in design, presents a window high in the west wall, and has a double-door arrangement that is splayed to prevent anyone in the forum from looking inside.

Sometimes, as in Pompeii, we can find one-seat public latrines built into niches along the streets.[20]

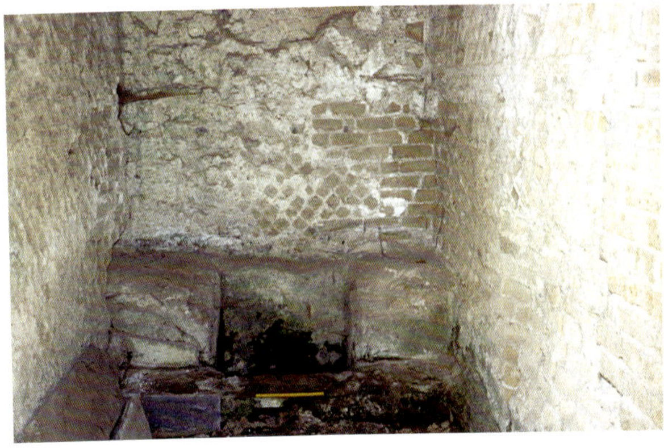

Fig. 5.7. Hadrian's villa near Tivoli, Canopus, one-seat toilet (photo A.O. Koloski-Ostrow).

These, of course, again merge with the architectural composition of the structures to which they are attached. In aristocratic country villas, multi-seater latrines could be used along with more private one-seater affairs (*fig. 5.6*).[21]

At Hadrian's Villa at Tivoli, constructed in the 2nd century AD, we find that elegantly appointed 'imperial' single-seat toilets were also constructed (*fig. 5.7*). The point is that different groups of people visiting or living at Hadrian's Villa or other private villas would definitely be afforded different types of toilets with different levels of privacy, depending on which toilets were made available to them. If Romans had the means to afford it and had the space, it does seem that the single-seat toilet was their preferred venue for this aspect of their personal hygiene.[22]

Toilets were built by people at all levels of Roman society in all types of buildings, public and private. The public, multi-seat latrines were very likely financed and built by city administrators or even private benefactors. Unfortunately, the evidence of inscriptions is lacking, probably because no one wanted close association with a toilet.

While the impact of public toilets on Roman society should not be put on a par with the impact of the amphitheater or of hypocaust heating systems in public baths, toilets do carry particularly powerful weight when applied to broader questions about Roman sanitation. For better or worse they should get a lot of credit for eliminating filth and for improving cleanliness and health, although to date such assessments are generally based on generations of hearsay rather than on scientific study. They have been more or less ignored altogether in the scholarship of Roman architecture, an omission that is indeed troubling.[23] Roman toilets need to be studied, not in isolation, but along with urban infrastructures, such as sewers, aqueducts, and the water supply systems that serviced them.

5.2. Decorations on Roman Toilets
(Eric M. Moormann)

Roman house toilets are normally seen as gloomy and dirty spaces. Some of them, however, were decorated with mosaics on the floors and paintings on the walls and ceilings. Sometimes toilets even had precious plaques of marble and marble adornments in the form of sculptures and reliefs. We do not have much concrete proof of toilet accessories like lamps and jugs of water.Wall and ceiling decorations give us a clue as to the chronology of latrines, but in most cases they are too generic to allow us to pinpoint to a certain date.

Floors, Wall and Ceilings: Ways of Decoration

Most floors of toilets have very simple coverings. Many of them are in *cocciopesto* or are covered with tiles. Sometimes we see marble veneer or even mosaic in *opus sectile* or *opus tessellatum*. A marble threshold may enhance the idea of luxury.[24] Apart from plain white floors at Ostia and in Hadrian's villa at Tivoli, mosaics consist of geometric patterns, e.g. in the Baths of Varius at Ephesus (*fig. 5.8*; cf. table). In the latrine of the Baths next to S. Giovanni in Laterano in Rome there was a grid of crossing bands; on the crossings circles in black surrounded the now white crossing sections.

Figural motifs can either be inserted into the grid in the shape of small panels filled with single objects like fish or birds (Apamea), or occupy the entire central space in front of the seats. The

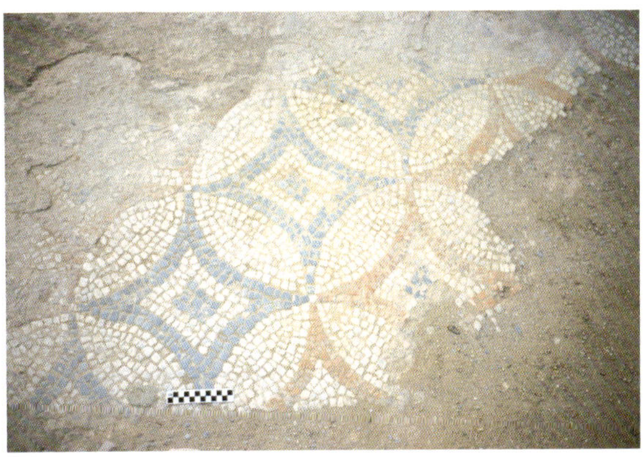

Fig. 5.8. Ephesus, toilet next to Varius baths, mosaic floor (photo G.C.M. Jansen).

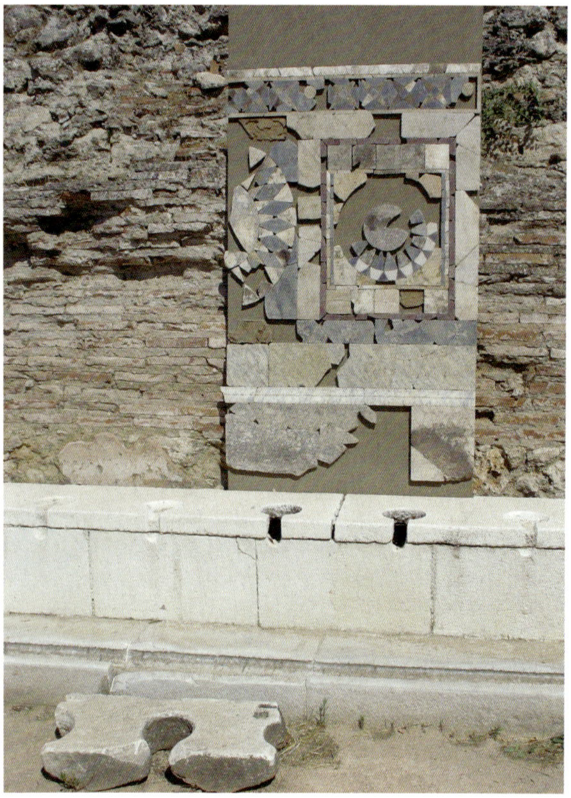

Fig. 5.9. Magnesia near Meander, public toilet with marble revetment (photo G. Wiplinger).

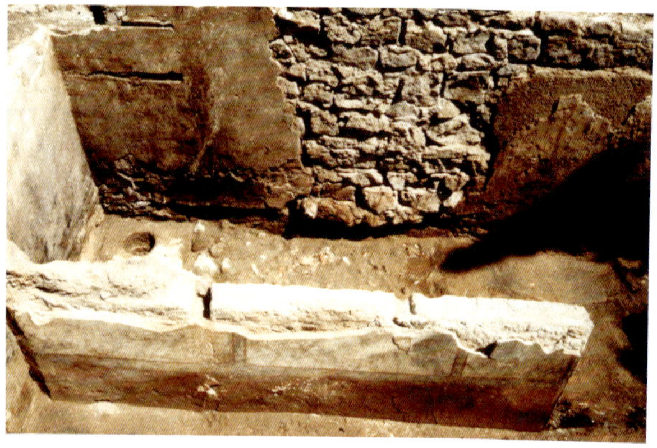

Fig. 5.10. Frejus (France), House in Place Jules-Formigé, toilet with marble imitation (photo A. Barbet).

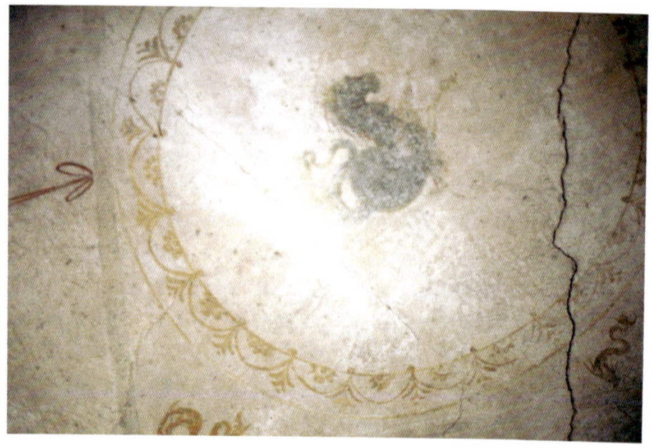

Fig. 5.11. Pompeii, House of the Silver Wedding (V 2, i), toilet ceiling (photo G.C.M. Jansen).

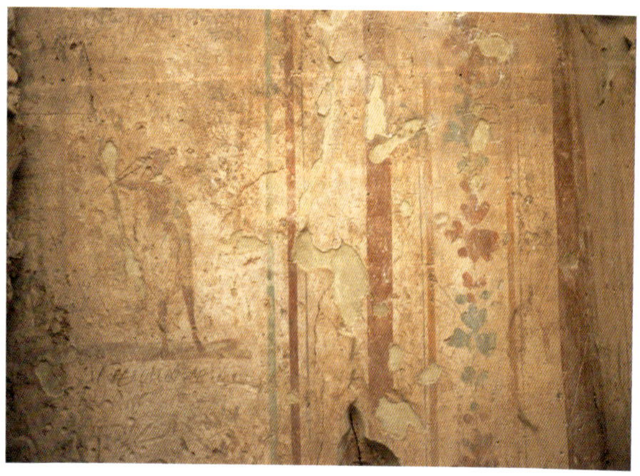

Fig. 5.12. Ephesus, Terrace House 2, 2, toilet SR 29, painting of caricature philosopher (photo G.C.M. Jansen).

visitors to the toilets in the Baths of Itálica (Spain) and Timgad (Algeria) could look and laugh at pygmies in a Nilotic landscape. Such themes are discussed below.

As to the walls, we observe either painted decorations or marble veneer; in the latter case, the toilets clearly belong to the class of the *Prachtlatrinen*, an appropriate term for luxurious toilets coined by Richard Neudecker (*fig. 5.9*).

Painted decorations are mainly subdivided into two horizontal layers: a dado and a register filled with panels of which lines often are the only remains.[25] The dado can either be monochrome or have a 'zebra pattern'; the latter has been seen as an imitation of marble veneer, especially a white marble with grey veins known as *bardiglio*, but there is no clear consensus about this matter.[26] Gemma Jansen has proposed that the dark paintings on the lower parts of the walls had the practical function of blotting out the dirt.[27] As a matter of fact, bright dados are rare, but we cannot say that this is specifically more so for the toilets than for other rooms, whether luxurious or for practical functions. In contrast, if marble veneer is used in the *Prachtlatrinen*, it is white and shining instead of black.[28] This may be true for painted marblings as well, like that at Fréjus (*fig. 5.10*).

Ceiling or vault decorations are rarely preserved and will be discussed from the following locations: House of the Silver Wedding at Pompeii (*fig. 5.11*); Domus Tiberiana in Rome.

Among the oldest examples of paintings in Roman toilets we know of are some instances at Pompeii. A First Style painting is preserved in House I 20, 4, but these murals belong to a room decoration of the late 2nd century BC originally with the function of a *cubiculum* that was converted into a toilet in the last decades of Pompeii's life. This change is also observable in the House of the Ceii at Pompeii, where *cubiculum* I, with Augustan decorations, was converted into a kitchen with a latrine next to it. The simple panel decoration has remained visible and contains vignettes in the shape of monochrome yellow landscapes and wreaths, which have nothing to do with the last function of the room.

An elegant tiny red architectural scheme, with apse-like entablatures on the north and south walls, adorns the toilet of the House of the Silver Wedding. In the center of the toilet's ceiling is a hippocamp surrounded by a circle-shaped embroidery border and a lozenge with four dolphins in its corners. Flower garlands adorn the toilet of the House of the Dioscuri.

Panel decorations remained in use until late antiquity. Among the latest examples is the public latrine, a forica,[29] on the Janiculum Hill in Rome, opposite the church of San Pietro in Montorio. The panels in red and green stripes are adorned with simple foliate motifs and vignettes in the shape of a Medusa head and a goat. Vegetal candelabra are among other items.[30] In Hanghaus II at Ephesus we have the toilet with philosophers within frames (*fig. 5.12*).

Figural themes

A trident, a shrimp and fish adorn the floor of a partly excavated large latrine in the Baths of Vedius at Ephesus, explored in 2004. The animals swim and 'float' on a white background within a double frame. The black-and-white mosaic found forms a tiny fragment of the floor of some 81 m^2 that can be dated to the years 147-149 AD and belongs to the complex erected by Marcus Claudius Publius Vedius Antoninus Phaedrus Sabinianus, who seems to have introduced the rather Roman fashion of black-and-white mosaic in his hometown.[31] In the public latrine of Apamea from the middle of the 2nd century AD, fish are combined with birds. At Kos we see dolphins in a sort of *emblema* framed by marble slabs.

The Baths of Neptune at Ostia have mosaics with pygmies as is the case in toilets at Timgad, Dar Buc Ammeira, and Itálica, and - in a painted version - at Bolsena. At Ostia, the dog-like crocodile is apparently attacking a dwarf on the right which is almost entirely vanished. The theme is difficult to explain, unless we think of the notion of apotropaic power of such representations that provoked laughter (see chapter 12, pp. 165-167): the users of the latrines are in a vulnerable position. Veronika Scheibelreiter has suggested that the Nile as a metaphor of water might make sense in this setting, an idea that is attractive. The notion that Egypt represents luxury, *truphe*, also cannot be discarded.[32]

The 4th-century villa of Piazza Armerina has three toilets, one of which (room 14b) has a rather simple mosaic of a geometrical pattern and may have been used by the personnel of the complex.[33] Latrine 2 is a private multi-seater with a white floor on which animals are running in a circle (*fig. 5.13*). We can distinguish two birds, a cat, a donkey and a horse that follow each other as in a *decursio*. The animals run in the direction of the exit, so that the users could contemplate the image. In contrast, the *cantharus* with a large vine in yellow on a black ground in latrine 59 is turned toward the direction of the entrance (*fig. 5.14*). All three toilets have a fake marble veneer on the walls. Whereas the two first items date to the period of the construction (around 330 AD), the last one seems to belong to a phase of new ownership some decades later.

As to painted images, the following cases can be singled out. The public latrines at Bolsena with copious seating must have had marble toilet benches and marble veneer on the walls. Above this rich decoration two painted zones were applied: on top two superposed vegetal scrolls and under them a frieze on green ground with the pygmies mentioned (*fig. 5.15*) and parts of mythological scenes, interpreted as Polyphemus and Galatea and Hippolytus fallen from his chariot. It remains a puzzling question why these two *amours fatales* would be appropriate for a toilet. As the remains are rather scanty, one should be cautious with these readings; the presence of a laughter-provoking caricature is again possible, but attempting an interpretation of certain myths may be fruitless. If we consider the tale from Ovid, however, which highlights the hairy body of Polyphemus, as well as the marine setting of both stories, perhaps the myth's appropriateness becomes more clear.[34] Perhaps the point of correspondence between the myth of Hippolytus and the place-

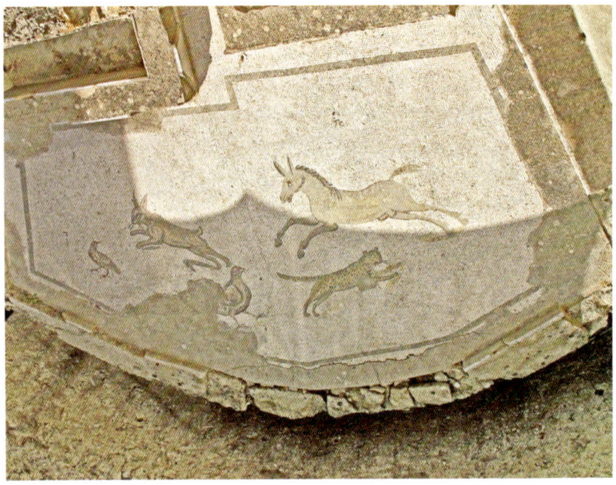

Fig. 5.13. Piazza Armerina, latrine 2, detail of the mosaic floor (photo M. Dolmans).

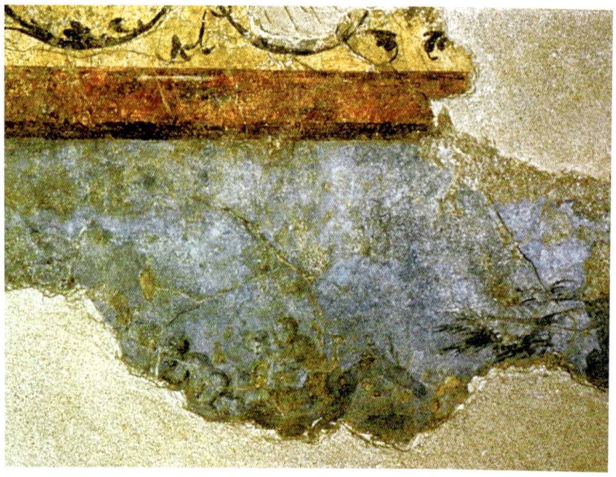

Fig. 5.15. Bolsena, insula 1, public toilet with pygmee painting (photo A. Barbet).

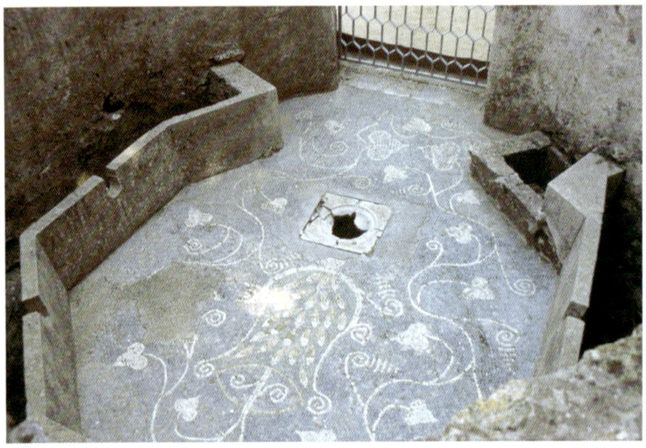

Fig. 5.14. Piazza Armerina, latrine 59, mosaic floor (photo G.C.M. Jansen).

ment of this theme in a latrine was his purity. The hairiness of the monster Cyclops might refer to the bottoms of the men seated in the toilet and of the ugliness they exposed, whereas Hippolytus forms a strong contrast with his beauty and purity.

At Pompeii, five instances of Fortuna are known (cf. G.C.M. Jansen in chapter 12.1, pp. 167-170). The famous Pompeian image of Fortuna next to a defecating man flanked by two snakes has been illustrated in many books and articles since its discovery in 1880. It adorned the toilet of IX 7, 22 and is marked by the inscription *Cacator, cave malu(m)* (see here *fig.12.5*). Fortuna, sporting her rudder and cornucopia - her usual attire, shown in the other images as well - is standing next to him while he is flanked by two snakes in the function of *agathodaimones*.[35] The Fortuna in the Barracks of the Firemen's barracks at Ostia can be added to the Pompeian instances (*figs 12.8-9*). The goddess clearly protects the users of the toilets from the evil eye and the bad smell.[36]

The latrine in sector 12, under room 71 of the Domus Tiberiana on the Palatine, has on the preserved south and west walls, above the now lost wooden benches, a yellow dado with red veins (imitation of *giallo antico*?) followed by a white surface. On the long wall three gladiators are preserved: *thrax*, man in heavy armory, and a *lanista*, trainer. The gladiator on the right is accompanied by the inscription, a *ianuarius*. The legs of two more gladiators are preserved on the short wall. The vault bears a stray pattern of flowers, small twigs, and birds on a white ground. This latrine probably dates to the Vespasian period and was likely used by the personnel.[37] All the men had names and represent well-known fighters in their day. They served as role models for the users of the toilets, who belonged to the same social ranks as the heroes of the amphitheater. These gladiators had obtained some fame serving in the emperor's games and were now even depicted.[38] Other gladiator representations have been found in 1989 in a 3rd-century toilet at Poitiers (see A-M. Jouquand-Thomas and J. Seigne, case study, chapter 6, p. 89).

A long series of athletes and pairs of boxers were painted in an arcade of the two walls of a large latrine in the Baths at S. Romain-en-Gal: the north wall has five panels, the west wall has twelve, whereas the south wall had three scenes, all rather stiff and statuesque. On the top of this is a suggestion of a colonnade in which sculptural groups are exposed - like the portico surrounding a *palaestra* - the painters designed a rich entablature, with metopes and triglyphs and a horizontal *sima*. In connection with the baths the themes suggest the notion of a healthy body, made better by good training. Interestingly, the last image on the south wall, next to the exit, seems to show the arbiter who invites the users to do sports.[39]

According to Neudecker, the gladiatorial games make a reference to digestion, and he suggests that the vigorous exercise of these fighters was healthy and good for promoting defecation.[40]

The eight-to-nine-seater toilet of Hanghaus 2, 2 at Ephesus contains a panel decoration on a white ground above the seats. In the center of each panel a philosopher is rendered as a caricature, wearing a sort of *exomis* (short tunic of workmen) and having an ugly and bald head (*fig. 5.12*). Each man is facing a column supporting a sundial. Whereas the text above the man on the west wall is lost, we read next to the others the following in rather large characters ca 2.5 cm tall: north - τὴν ὥραν ἢ τὸν θάνατον ('the hour or the death') and (south) - τρεῖς ἐξ ἐννναῖα ('three out of nine'). The latter refers to the number of seats and the minimum as well as maximum numbers of participants in a dinner party, going from the number of Graces to the number of Muses. The first text is about good, regular digestion. I think that these texts say, with gross exaggeration, that if a man does not have regular digestion, he will die. Volker Michael Strocka dated them in his fundamental publication to AD 400-410, but his timeframe has been revised now, and the pictures must have been executed in the second quarter of the 3rd century. They belong to a set of paintings by a specific workshop that produced murals at different levels, depending on the status of the rooms, so that the differences cannot be explained as stylistic features, but as variations of the same stylistic language. In this case at Ephesus, we have the simplest decorative scheme, including only a few colors on a white ground.[41]

To the same period a similar set is dated, viz. the persons in a panel decoration adorning a toilet in the House of the Rape of Europa at Kos. Here the white dado is enlivened with tendrils, whereas the main zone has panels. One of the vignettes shows a man bearing a sundial on a pole over his shoulders, accompanied by a text (see below). The two other figures, probably similar, have been lost. The sundial apparently is a device seen as typical for these images, although it is an instrument connected with the early natural philosophers as well.[42] It might refer both to the regularity of defecation and its timeless character alike: we all have to cope with the 'problem' every day and hope to have regular bowels.

Texts

Sometimes images are accompanied by texts. The defecating man in house IX 7, 22 at Pompeii (*fig. 12.5*) is accompanied by *cacator, cave malu(m)*: 'shitter, beware of danger!' The cult niche in the latrine of the Baths of the Guardians in Ostia (*fig. 12.9*) bears the inscription *Fortunae sanct(um)*: 'dedicated to Fortune'.

An important example of texts is that of the Ephesus toilet described above. Ephesus yielded some more inscriptions in a latrine next of the Bath of Constantine, found during one of the first campaigns of the Austrian excavations. It is said that the letters of these hexametric verses were written with care on simple stucco decorations, viz. '*einfachen Stuckmalereien*', whose nature remains unknown, but we may think of panels.

[no 1]
λὰξ ποδὶ κινήσας καὶ πὺξ χερὶ μακρὸν ἀείρας
καὶ βήξας κραδίηθεν, ὅλον δέ τε σῶμα δονήσας
ἐξ ὀνύχων χέζων φρένα τέρπεο μήδε σε γάστηρ
μήποτε λυπήσειεν ἐμόν ποτε δῶμα μόλοντα.

Kicking afoot and raising fists high ahand
And coughing your heart out and shaking your whole body
Take full pleasure in shitting your brains out, and may your stomach
Never give you pain whenever you come to my house.[43]

[no 2]
ἀν μὴ γελῶμεν τόν βὶον τὸν δραπιτήν
πίνοντες ἢ τρυφῶντες ἢ λελουμένοι
ὀδυνὴν ἑαυτοῖς προξενοῦμεν πάντοτε
ἀναξίους ὁρῶντες εὐτυχεστέρους.

If we don't laugh during our whole fleeting life,
drinking or luxuriating or getting ourselves bathed,
we will in every way gain pain for ourselves
as we watch the undeserving [being] happier [than we are].

These epigrams are similar to various literary epigrams, the latter is almost identical to a poem by Palladas.[44] The first text is addressed to someone who is having great difficulty defecating, straining, and contorting himself in the public lavatory. It expresses the hope that he may relief himself easily when invited to dinner at my place. The second epigram is Epicurean advice to take good care of your own living situation. Both texts are comparable to the sentences in the Baths of the Seven Sages at Ostia (see below).

The latrine at Kos has the following:

[no 3]
τὰς δώδεκα ὥρας
ἁπάσας ὅλας τρέχω

'I run for all twelve whole hours put together.'[45]

It accompanies the caricature of a man carrying a sundial on his left shoulder. The caricature is similar to those in Ephesus. Perhaps the sundial itself is speaking to us and is referring to the need of regular defecation, apparently happening at least once a day.

Clearly, the philosophers have become a sort of simple medical doctor or one of the Seven Sages, uttering futile warnings or advice most people did not need at all. The quasi-intellectual atmosphere had to provoke laughter (cf. chapter 12), like that stimulated by pygmies in other latrines. A merry mood would offer some relaxation to those visiting these dark corners of the house or the baths. Strikingly, few images of urinating or defecating people - not even of pygmies - are preserved in the toilets apart from the *cacator* at Pompeii.

Conclusions

These few examples of decorations in Roman toilets do not provide an image that differs considerably from walls and floors we know in other domestic contexts. They are chronologically and stylistically similar. The sober use of color and the frequency of simple schemes make clear that the mosaics and paintings belong to the simplest modes of decoration. The marble veneer in various *Prachtlatrinen* corresponds with the custom to install a marble revetment in public buildings and houses from the late first century onwards.

There seem not to be specific devices to make these decorations more suitable for the rooms they adorn. Sometimes the lower sections of the walls are covered with a sort of damp-regulating red mortar with elements of pottery in it that absorb the fluids. The tiles on the floors of small toilets have the same function. Paintings do not have a film to protect them from the acidic effects of urine, and they were apparently so cheap that they could easily be replaced by new ones.

The figural motifs decorating floors and walls could be seen best when you entered the room. The decorations covering the walls above the seats would only make sense if one could contemplate them before or after defecation. A person who came in for the first time would have felt a certain curiosity about the meaning of these depictions, and we cannot but speculate about them. In the case of the large toilet room of the Baths of Neptune at Ostia, however, people could study the pygmies while seated at the toilet. As the user entered the toilet room, all the images on the floor were upside down since the tops of the images were just inside the door. Once one was seated on the toilet, the images could be viewed and appreciated from the proper perspective.

Some of the figural motifs indeed might have had a particular meaning. As we saw, the images are not specific in the sense of depicting the activities of a latrine-goer, but they can often be related to the health of people who have good bowel movements. The theme of the gladiators seems to be a private association of particular users. It is not clear whether the rather banal motifs of flowers, twigs, and animals, like fish and fowl, really refer to sanitation and water, and so to the toilets, or not. In other contexts they are ubiquitous as well.

The mosaics and paintings, in sum, match the decorations in all other rooms of private and public buildings of the same age they were made. In other words, toilet decorations do not form a special branch of folkart.

Furniture in Toilets

Small toilets will have been very simple and, as far as we know, did not contain luxurious marble seats and armrests. Such armrests can be seen in Pozzuoli, Timgad, and Ephesus, where dolphins form the upper part of the armrests.[46] In some large latrines statues and lavish architectural features enhanced the atmosphere. The large latrine in the Macellum - traditionally called the Serapeum - at Pozzuoli, studied as early as the 18th century and now stripped of all precious elements, must have been an excellent example of such a rich furniture.[47] A toilet in Hanghaus 1, 1 at Ephesus contained the statue of a *mingens*, not in a mythological guise like Herakles (see chapter 12), but a man who comes from a symposium. It was found in the fill of latrine L, but seems to have stood in the niche encountered by the excavators during the first phase of existence, thrown away at a later time.

APPENDIX: LIST OF TOILETS WITH PAINTINGS AND/OR MOSAICS

PLACE	DESCRIPTION	a	BIBLIOGRAPHY
Apamea, latrine	Mosaic with geometric pattern in red, blue and yellow on white; fish and partridges. Middle second century AD.	P	Schmidt-Colinet 1986, 142, pl. XLVIII.1; Neudecker 1994, 60, 157; Scheibelreiter 2005, 72-73.
Bolsena, insula 1, public latrine	Black mosaic floor. Marble veneer; paintings (Nile, mythology [?] and scrolls). 30-40 AD. Fig. 5.13.	P	Hallier/Humbert/Pomey 1982, 55-71; Barbet 1982; Neudecker 1994, 60, 158; Cappel 1994, 34, 104 cat. W6; Versluys 2002, 41 n. 107; Clarke 2007, 80.
Carthage, Bath of Antoninus	Floor in Chemtou marble. Marble basin. Stuccowork on exterior walls. 145-162.	P	Lézine 1968, 33-34, 44; Neudecker 1994, 85-86, 158.
Dar Buc Ammeira/ Zliten, villa, latrine	Mosaic floor with pygmies. second century AD.	P	Cappel 1994, 44, 119-120, cat. M21.[b]
Dion, latrine next to large baths	Mosaic floor with birds. Second century AD.	P	Pandermalis 1997, 37.
Ephesus			
House II, H 2/SR 29	Panel decoration with caricatures of philosophers; inscriptions. Figs 5.12, 12.18.	PR	Strocka 1977, 87-90, figs. 180-184; Zimmermann 2002, 113.
Lower Agora, toilet	Red lines on a white ground.		*Forschungen in Ephesos* 1923, 17.
Terrace of Domitian, toilet	Panel decoration with black and red bands.		Unpublished (information G. Jansen).
Baths of the Harbor (or of Constantine)	Painted text on east wall within a frame of festoons. Fourth century AD.	P	R. Heberdey, *OeJh* 1 (1898) Beiblatt, 75; Weisshäuptl 1902; Strocka 1977, 88-89; Börker/Merkelbach 1979, no. 456; Neudecker 1994, 38, 130-131, 159.
Baths of Varius under Baths of Scholastikia	Geometric pattern mosaic in red, blue and white. C. 100 AD.	P[c]	F. Miltner, *OeJh* 43 (1956-1958) Beiblatt, 20; Neudecker 1994, 129-130, 159; Scheibelreiter 2005, 73.
Baths of Vedius, room A	Black/white mosaic with fish. Walls: marble. Vault: paintings. Dolphin seats. Inscriptions on columns. AD 147-149. Fig. 5.8.	P	Börker/Merkelbach 1979, 170 no. 454; Neudecker 1994, 128-129, 159; Scheibelreiter 2005.
Fréjus, House in Place Jules-Formigé	Marble imitation. Middle first century AD. Fig. 5.14.	PR	Barbet 2008, 76.
Herculaneum			
III 10, upper floor	White speckled ground with red frames. Fourth Style.	PR	Jansen 1993, 33 n. 2 [mistakenly II 9].
IV 14, *taberna vasaria*	White ground w. red frames. Fourth Style.	PR	Jansen 1993, 33 n. 2.
IV 21, House of the Stags	White ground w. red frames. Fourth Style.	PR	Jansen 1993, 33 n. 2.
Insula Orientalis I, 1, House of the Gem, rm 17	Graffito: *hic cacavit bene in latrina* signed by Apollinaris, doctor of Titus.	PR	*CIL* Suppl. 3.4, no. 10619; Neudecker 1994, 34.
Itálica, Casa de la exedra, latrine	Mosaic with pygmies. 200 AD.	P	Cappel 1994, 44, 121, cat. M27; Versluys 2002, 206-207 cat. 105.
Kos			
House of the Rape of Europa	Panel decoration with caricatures; Greek text. Severan.	PR	M. Morricone, *BdA* 35 (1950) 238, fig. 65; Strocka 1977, 89; Sirano 2005, 152-153, figs 14a-c; Bonini 2006, 97, 301, fig. 74.
Forica	Floor mosaic with dolphins. Marble on floors and walls; Painted vault. Nymphaeum. Third century and changes before 365.	P	Neudecker 1994, 51-52, 160, figs. 21-22; Merletto 2000, 298-299, fig. 2; Scheibel-reiter 2005, 72; here Merletto, p. 64.
Magnesia ad Meandrum, pluri-seater	Marble veneer with geometric patterns. Fig. 5.9.	P	Neudecker 1994, 161; Gülbay 2006, 462, fig. 6.
Minturno	Marble veneer with geometric patterns.		Unpublished.
Naples, Baths in Fuorigrotta	Mosaic with dolphins. Wall paintings. Second century AD.	P	Neudecker 1994, 161.
Ostia			
III x, 1, Apartment Building of the Charioteers	Black/white mosaic. White ground with foliate motifs.	PR?	Jansen 1993, 30.

Ostia (continued)			
II iv, 2, Baths of Neptune, room 7	Black/white mosaic with pygmies. Wall paintings with gardens and marble incrustations. 143 AD.	P	Baccini Leotardi 1978, 17, fig. 8; Jansen 1993, 30; Neudecker 1994, 108, 161-162; Cappel 1994, 116, cat. M9; Versluys 2002, 43-44 cat. 001, fig. 2;[d] Scheibelreiter 2005, 73 note 45; Clarke 2007, 78-80, figs 32-33.
Baths of the Philosopher	Marble floor, Trajanic. Fountain niche with red paint. Around 250 AD.	P	Boersma 1985, 124, 392-393, fig. 558; Neudecker 1994, 162.
Baths of the Swimmer, rooms III.10 and VII	III.10: Floor in *bipedales*. Basin. VII: white mosaic in *opus tessellatum* with black band; red panels on yellow ground. 90-155/160 AD.	P	Carandini 1973, 22-23, pl. LXXV; 26-31, 91, pls. III-X, LXXVII-LXXVIII; Neudecker 1994, 162.
Baths of Six Columns	*Opus sectile* floor. Paintings of plants.	P	Neudecker 1994, 162.
Firemen's Barracks II V, 1	Yellow ground. Niche for cult. Inscription. Figs 12.8-12.10.	P	Strocka 1977, 89; Neudecker 1994, 108, 162; Clarke 2003, 175.
Piazza Armerina, villa, rooms 2, 14b, 59	2: mosaic with animals. 14b: mosaic with geometric pattern. 59: mosaic with cantharus and wine leaves. Walls of all rooms imitation of marble veneer. Figs 5.13-5.14.	PR	2: Carandini 1981, 157-158, pl. XVIII.42. 14b: Carandini 1981, 115-116, pl. III.10. 59: Carandini 1981, 291-292, pl. XLIII.88.
Poitiers, public toilet	Gladiator scenes. Third century.	P	Here Jouquand-Thomas/Seigne, p. 89.
Pompeii			
I 6, 15, House of Ceii, room i	White panels. Transition Second to Third Style.	PR	Michel 1990, 26-30, figs. 143, 146, 148-150; *PPM* I (1990), 434-437; Jansen 1993, 33 n. 4.
I 7, 1.20, House of Paquius Proculus, rooms 14 and 36	Cocciopesto floors. No murals left.	PR	Ehrhardt 1998, 112-113, figs. 467-468; 76-77, figs. 323-325.
I 11, 10, Caupona of Euxinus, room 7	Cocciopesto floor. Outside: painted *lararium* over isodome masonry; inside white. Fourth Style.	PR	*PPM* II (1990), 580-581; Jansen 1993, 33 n. 2.
I 12, 11, House of the Painters, room 7[e]	Dado with zebra pattern; upper part lost. Fourth Style.	PR	*PPM* II (1990), 807 (S.C. Nappo); Goulet 2001-2002, 85-86, figs. 76-77; Laken 2003, 181.
I 20, 4, room 7 (transformed cubiculum)	Cocciopesto floor with white tesserae. First Style stucco masonry over dado w. lozenges.	PR	*PPM* II (1990), 1076-1077; Jansen 1993, 33 n. 4.
II 4, 3, Praedia of Iulia Felix, rooms 37 and 89b	37: white panels with Fortuna on north wall. 89b: dado with zebra pattern, upper part lost. Fourth Style. Fig. 12.6.	SP	37: *PPM* III (1991), 216-219; Jansen 1993, 33 n. 2, 5. 89b: Goulet 2001-2002, 70, figs. 31-32; Laken 2003, 181.
V 1, 18, rooms z and z'	All lost. z: unclear. z' (upstairs): Fortuna with donkey. Fourth Style.	PR	*PPM* III (1991), 539-540; Fröhlich 1991, 40; Jansen 1993, 33 n. 2, 5.
V 1, 30-31, rooms 2 and 2'	2: wall paper pattern of Fourth Style. 2' (upstairs): paintings lost.	PR	*PPM* III (1991), 625-627; Jansen 1993, 31, figs. 1-2; 33 n. 2; Pirson 1999, 90-91, figs. 88-89.
V 2, h, House of *Cenaculum*, room o	Corner of kitchen p, lararium painting. Fourth Style.	PR	Strocka 1977, 89 note 296; Jansen 1993, 33 n. 4; Ehrhardt 2004, 184-185, figs. 788-791.
V 2, i, House of Silver Wedding, room s'	Aediculae on white, red bands in corners. Ceiling decoration. Neronian age. Fig. 5.10.	PR	*PPM* III (1991), 728-729; Jansen 1993, 33 n. 4; Ehrhardt 2004, 158-160, 225-226, 262, figs. 86-87, 648-660.
V 4, 9, room b	Fortuna in red frame on white ground. Fourth Style.	PR	A. Sogliano, *NSc* 1899, 345, fig. 7; Strocka 1977, 89; *PPM* III (1991), 1059.
VI 9, 6, House of the Dioscuri, room 52	*Opus spicatum* floor. Red dado with panels, white middle and upper zones, garlands. Fourth Style.	PR	*PPM* IV (1993), 954-955; Jansen 1993, 33 n. 4.
VI 16, 7, 38, House of the Golden Cupids, rooms K and X	K: red finishing. X: red cocciopesto on walls. First century AD.	PR	Seiler 1992, 52, 68-69; Jansen 1993, 33 n. 4; *PPM* V (1994), 799.
VII 1, 8, Stabian Baths, room O	Dado with zebra pattern, white upper zone and vault. Fourth Style.	P	Jansen 1993, 33 n. 2; Neudecker 1994, 163; *PPM* VI (1999), 179; Goulet 2001-2002, 63-64, figs. 14-17; Laken 2003, 182.
VII 16, a, Suburban Baths	Fortuna next to altar on white ground. Text (unreadable). Fourth Style. Fig. 12.7.	PR	L. Jaobelli, *RStPomp* 1 (1987) 153-154, fig. 17; Fröhlich 1991, 40, 301 cat. L114, pl. 50.3; Jansen 1993, 33 n. 2, 5; Clarke 2007, 80.

Pompeii (continued)			
IX 7, 22, rooms g/h	South wall of entrance corridor: Fortuna and *cacator* (MN 112285). Inscription. Fourth Style. Fig. 12.5.	PR	Strocka 1977, 89; Fröhlich 1991, 40, 59-60, 296-297 cat. L106, pl. 10.1; Jansen 1993, 33 n. 2, 5; Neudecker 1994, 24, 55-56, fig. 5; *PPM* IX (1999), 869; Clarke 2003, 175; 2007, 78-80, fig. 34.
Rome			
Crypta Balbi, latrine	Mosaic. Panel decoration on walls. Late first-early second century AD.	P	Neudecker 1994, 98-99, 164; Manacorda 2001, 28, fig. 22.
Largo Argentina, *forica*, north apse	Fictitious marble incrustation. Domitian or later restorations.	P	Neudecker 1994, 95-96, 163-164, figs. 47-48.
via Garibaldi, *forica*	Black/white mosaic. Severan painting over Trajanic layer.	P	Chini 1995; 1997; Liedtke 2003, 156-157.
Domus Flavia or Augustana, room L	Red dado and white upper zone above seats. Vespasian.	PR	G. Carettoni, *NSc* 1949, 66, fig. 21; Tomei 1991, 57, fig. 4; Neudecker 1994, 69, 99.
Domus Tiberiana, under room 71	Gladiators. Inscription. Vespasian.	PR	Tomei 1991; Neudecker 1994, 43, 58-59, 105; Krause 2004, 51, figs. 80-81.
Baths of Maxentius, *forica*	Marble revetment (mortar remains). Maxentius or Constantine.	P	Herrmann 1976, 416-417, pl. 144.1; Neudecker 1994, 164.
Baths next to S. Giovanni in Laterano	B/w mosaic, with geometric pattern. Dolphins in seats. Severan age.	P	Pellicioni 1973, 78, fig. 115, pl. IV.1; Neudecker 1994, 100-101, 164.
House of Domitia Lucilla	Fortuna. 2nd century.	P	Here p. 168, with reference; p. 193 n. 64.
Rottenburg, latrine	Red dado, white panel decoration with garlands and vegetal motifs in upper zone.	P	Neudecker 1994, 40, 68, 135, 165; Heiligmann 2003, 52-53; here S. Hoss, p. 67.
Salamis	Mosaic floor.	P	Neudecker 1994, 85.
S. Romain-en-Gal, Baths of the Gladiators, latrine	White panels with athletes; architectural motifs in upper zone. Ca. 200 AD.	P	Neudecker 1994, 58 [location Vienne]; Leblanc 1995; Barbet 2008, 266-267, figs. 414-416.
Thamusida, Baths of the River, room 2	Panel paintings. Late Antonine period.	P	Rebuffat 1970, 52-57; Neudecker 1994, 166.
Thugga, Bath of Cyclops, latrine	Mosaic floor.	P	Neudecker 1994, 166-167.
Timgad, Southern Baths, latrine	Mosaic with Nilotic scene. Ca. AD 250. Now Museum of Timgad, inv. 37.	P	Neudecker 1994, 60, 117, 165-166, fig. 30; Cappel 1994, 44, 120, cat. M24; Versluys 2002, 177-178, cat. 085, fig. 109; Scheibelreiter 2005, 73 note 45; Clarke 2007, 80.
Tivoli, Villa Hadriana	Marble veneer and opus sectile. Time of Hadrian.	PR/SP	Jansen 2007; Blanco 2007.

[a] PR: private. P: public. SP: semi-public. This is not an easy distinction
[b] The room has been seen as a nymphaeum by K. Dunbabin. See Cappel 1994.
[c] Combined with a brothel, according to an inscription (text in Börker/Merkelbach 1979, no. 455, who do not accept this interpretation). See esp. Neudecker 1994, 129 n. 401. The latrine was re-decorated in the time of Scholastikia in the fourth century.
[d] Versluys doubts Becatti's interpretation. He believes that the latrine is a complete reconstruction by Becatti. 100-150 AD.
[e] S.C. Nappo calls it an 'ambiente di servizio'.

Case Study: The Latrine near the Western Baths in Kos *(Antonella Merletto)*

After the earthquake of 1933, the Western Baths of Kos in the district called *Ieni Capù* became part of the excavation program under the direction of Luigi Morricone in 1936. The public latrine (*forica*), located to the east of the *cardo maximus*, was excavated during various campaigns between spring 1937 and 1938. Its restoration was completed by 1939.[53] The latrine is located to the east of the *frigidarium* of the Western Baths and separated from the other buildings by the *cardo*. It was easily accessible to customers walking along the *cardo* from any direction. The latrine was built between two existing structures: a portico in tufa to the north and the stairs to the Acropolis to the south, both with the same alignment and whose initial structure dates to the Hellenistic period (*fig. 5.16*).[54] Photographs taken during the excavation show that the latrine was also conveniently positioned for reuse of water coming from the Western Baths and for water disposal under the *cardo*, as the city was provided with a very efficient sewage disposal system.

From photographic evidence, it is also clear that the presence of two Medieval limestone kilns[55] that were found at the topmost level of the excavation made it more difficult to detect the original shape and phases of the building. These kilns were probably installed within the building in order to burn the great quantity of marble found in the area.

The latrine building had a square[56] central courtyard surrounded by three corridors, was fronted by a porch, and had its entrance on the western side. The western side of the courtyard had a two-tiered *nymphaeum* with niches and basins, while on the other three sides *ambulacra* housed the marble seating and drainage channels of the monumental latrine with its capacity of ca 90 seats (*fig 5.18*). The façade had three arches made of reused blocks of stone, marble, and *prasinòpetra*. These materials were used only for a height of 18 feet while the remaining elevation was in *opus caementicium*. Immediately behind the entrance is a small rectangular room, probably used by the contractor or a guard who sat there to receive payment for use of the facility.

The open-air courtyard was surrounded on three sides by an arcade, where an extremely unusual *pulvinus* carried by a marble Ionic order, supported brick arches, coupled by major arches that sustained the wall. The fourth side has a wall with two levels, each with three niches, probably where statues were placed to decorate the building. The lower level also had water features that collected into three basins forming a decoration to the front of the wall and taking up part of the floor space of the open courtyard. Photographs of the reconstruction show that during the excavation, only the lower level was found *in situ*. Archaeologists decided there was a second level and built it exactly the same as the existing one.[57] The paving consisted of marble slabs along the corridors and mosaic panels in the central courtyard.[58] In the center of the courtyard was a small well, probably with a small fountain, which today has completely disappeared. This well acted as an *impluvium* and, as the mosaics have a slight inclination towards the center of the courtyard, also collected the water from the overflow of the *nymphaeum* basins and slop water when the floors were washed. The corridors were vaulted, and polychrome marbles were used lavishly everywhere. The upper sections of the walls were stuccoed and painted with architectural scenes.

The restoration of the building and other parts of the Western Bath Complex, including the *cardo*, has greatly limited the possible analysis, not only of the original construction, but also of the water system of the latrine.[59] What can be ascertained is the direction of the water flow in the channel in front of the seats. Other elements eventually came to light that confirmed the latrine identification (*fig. 5.17*).[60]

Parts of three marble latrine seats and *prasinòpetra* blocks used as seat struts were found, although the depth and inclination of the sewer can no longer be established. The study of the remaining architectural elements and of the different alterations allows us to distinguish four main building phases from the first half of the 3rd century to the 5th century, when the building experienced a change of function.[61] At the end of the 5th century AD, the small well and mosaic floor were built in the entrance room, probably connected to the Christian Basilicas. The excavation photographs show a thick level of soil between the use as room connected to the Baths and the last evidence of use: the two kilns, probably dating after the Arab invasions.

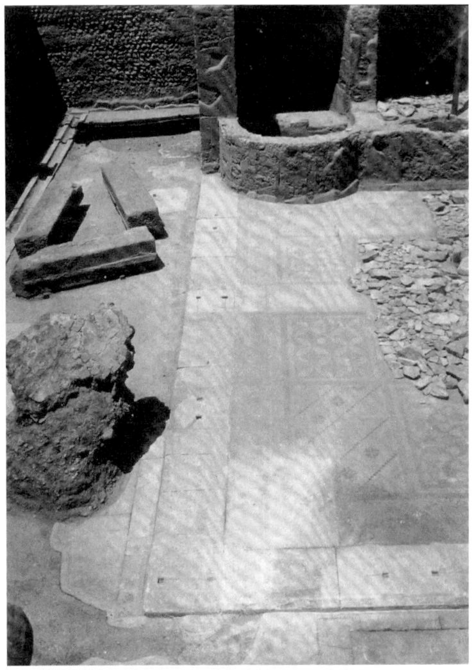

Fig. 5.17. Kos, S.A.I.A. archive photo of detail of public latrine near the Western Baths of Kos at the end of excavations.

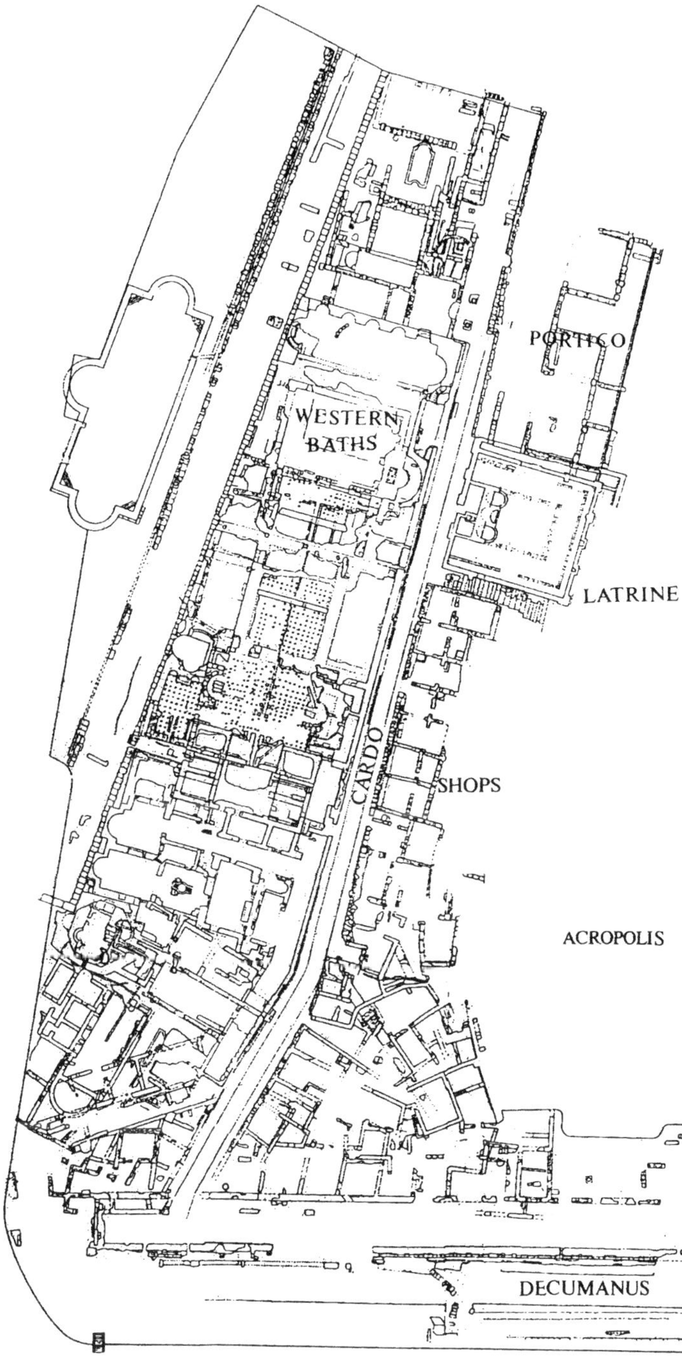
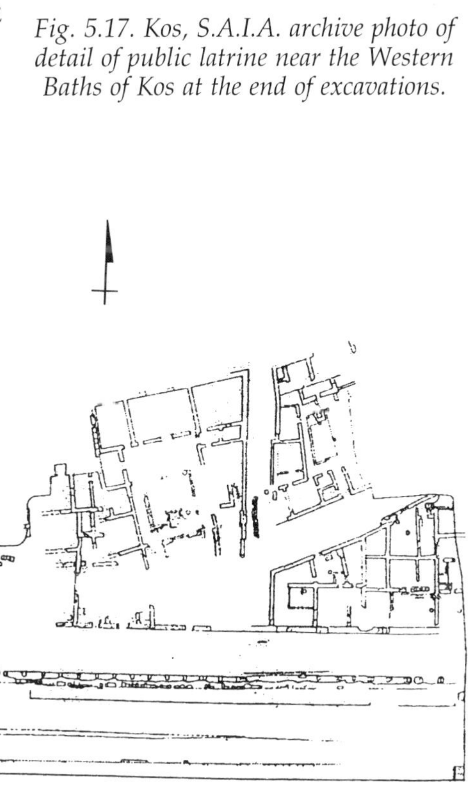

Fig. 5.16. Kos, plan of the area of the Western Baths of Kos (drawing M. Livadiotti, G. Rocco).

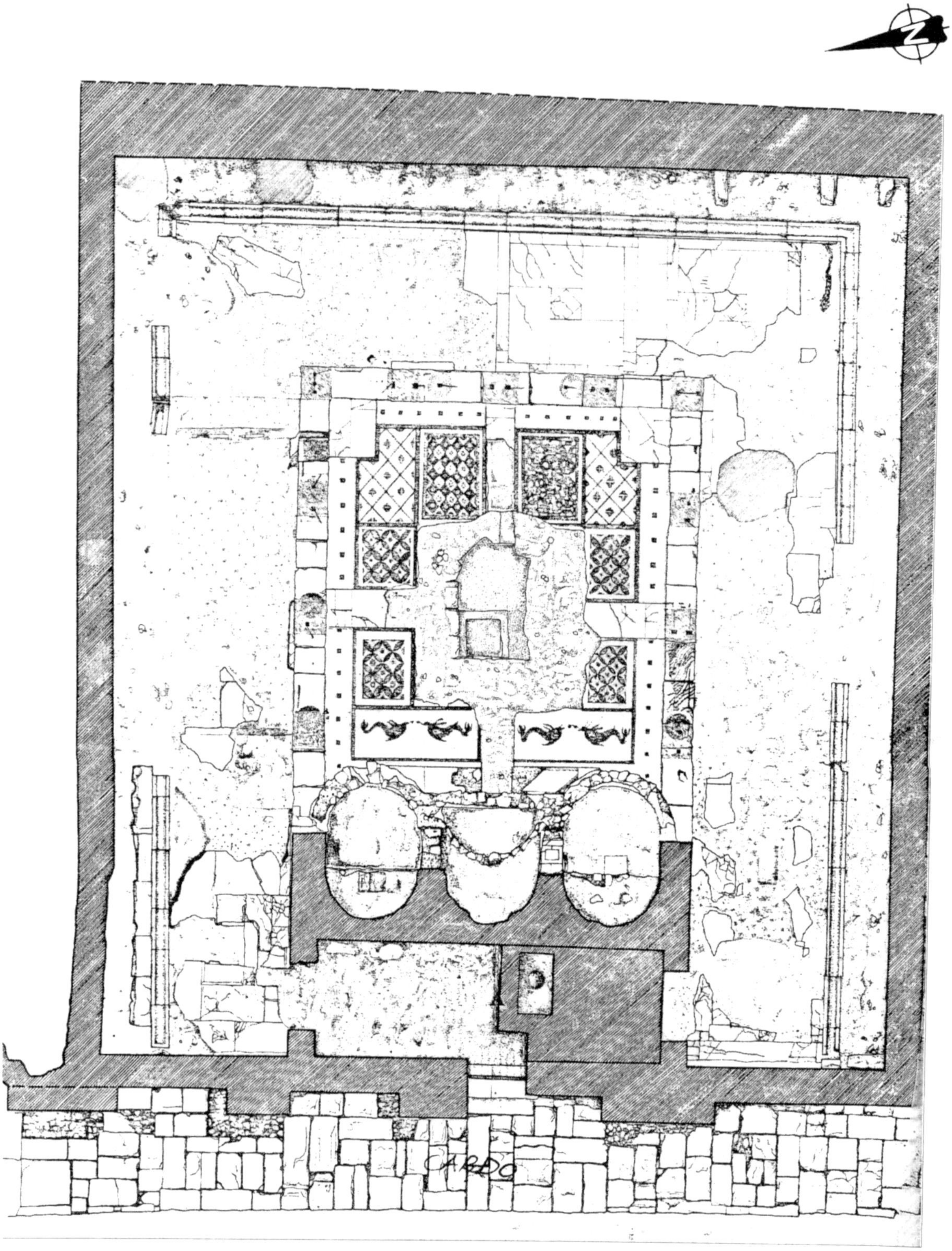

Fig. 5.18. Kos, plan of the public latrine near the Western Baths of Kos, at the end of excavations (drawing A. Merletto).

Case Study: Rottenburg Latrine *(Stefanie Hoss)*

The latrine of Rottenburg am Neckar (50 km SW of Stuttgart) is the only Roman latrine on the right side of the Rhine and one of the largest and most luxurious installations of its kind in Germany.[62] Roman Rottenburg, *Sumelocenna*, was founded around 85/90 (probably in connection with a military fort) and destroyed in 259-260 by the Alemanni. At first, the vicus and the surrounding region were administrated as an imperial estate by an equestrian procurator, whose official residence was *Sumelocenna* itself. Later it became the central place of the *civitas Sumelocennensis*.

The latrine is a long and narrow building, not associated with a bathhouse and dating in its present state to the late 2nd/beginning of the 3rd centuries AD (*fig. 5.19*). It sits on top of the main sewer of the city (w. 80 cm, d. 1 m), which ran under the street but curved in a wide bend to run under the centre of the latrine. The entrance from the street lay on the narrow NW side. From here, an angled staircase of eleven well-worn steps led the visitor ca 1 m downwards into the latrine proper, a room 5.3 m wide that has been excavated to a length of 32 m without reaching the SE rear wall of the building. The room was divided in the longitudinal axis by at least seven 3 m high columns of plastered sandstone, standing 4 m apart and slightly to one side of the central axis, so that they were placed above the southern sewer wall rather than directly above the sewer. The whole room was laid with flagstones of local sandstone. On the northern wall ran a channel (w. 50 cm, d. 90 cm) with a brick floor, which was filled with water from a branch of the main city sewer. Above this channel, the 60 cm deep wooden seats ran in a height of 40 cm. The worn places in the flagstones attest that the holes must have been placed ca 90 cm apart, making it possible for at least 35 persons to use the latrine at the same time. A small and shallow channel in the flagstones ran in front of the seats. Another channel ran next to the southern wall. It is interpreted as carrying fresh water to the round sandstone-basin with a scooped-out bowl (d. 30 cm) found in the room. As the basin has one straight outer side, it is assumed that it stood against the southern wall of the latrine, ca 20 m from the entrance and was used for hand washing. Two foundations running across the flagstones from one long wall to the other were observed in the eastern part of the building. This could point to a later partitioning of the latrine into a male and a female section.

Both the northern and southern walls of the latrine were decorated with wall-paintings. The remains of the northern wall show a roughly plastered base in red, which lay behind the wooden seats. Directly above the seats, a white zone of 60 cm was decorated with yellow and black garlands, bound with thin red string, with a series of horizontal stripes of varying width in red, white, sand and brown above it. Above that, a zone of at least 1.8 m height was painted with floral patterns in yellow, purple and green on a white background. The windows must have been placed in or above the latter zone. On the southern wall, the visitors had left many graffiti on the paintings. The latrine has not been published in a final report yet. It has been preserved under a parking garage and the complex has been turned into the Roman museum of *Sumelocenna*.[63]

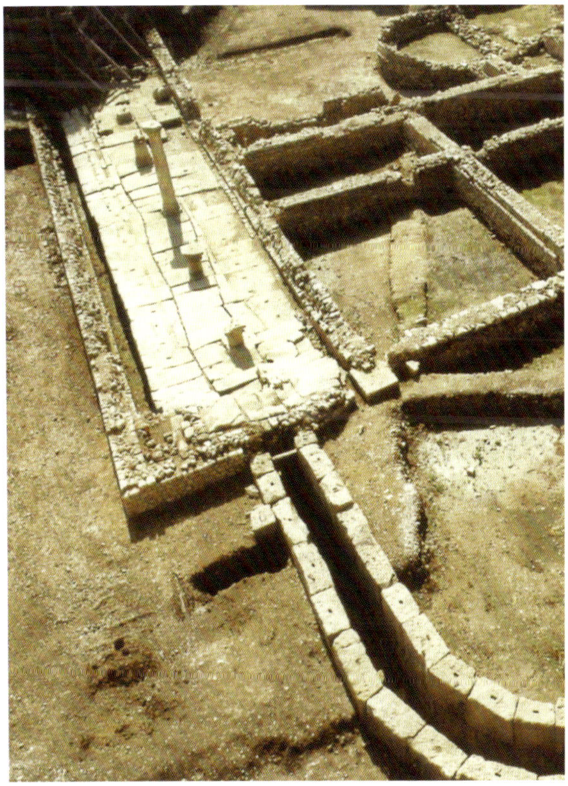

Fig 5.19. Rottenburg, overview of the latrine during excavation (photo Landesdenkmalamt Baden-Württemberg, in Heiligmann 2003, 48).

Notes

1 Waslander 1994, 14. I am extremely grateful to the late Marianne Boissevain and to Thomas and Pieter Burgess for help in the translation of this Dutch article.

2 Waslander 1994, 14, reports (fig. 6) on a squat toilet from Çavustepe in east Turkey, which dates to the 1st millennium BC.

3 Waslander 1994, 14, believes that one major intermediary between East and West was the Hellenistic/Parthian city of Dura Europos on the Euphrates.

4 Chamonard 1922, 181. For other more detailed references, cf. Neudecker 1994, 16, nos 37 and 39. See also chapter 3.4, pp. 33-39 on Hellenistic latrines by Monika Trümper.

5 Cf. Coarelli/Musti/Solin 1982; Castrén 1975, 38-39; Zanker 1988, 32, with n. 5, discusses inscriptions found throughout the eastern Mediterranean region, particularly common on Delos, which was a free port from 166 BC, with the names of traders from Campanian towns.

6 Neudecker 1994, 16.

7 Neudecker 1994, 16.

8 Macrobius, *Satyrae* 3.16.14-16, cited by Neudecker 1994, 16, n. 40. This work (late 4th century AD) is certainly expressing the nostalgia of a Christianized elite in a diminished Rome for the city's great and pagan past, and hence must be used with caution in this context.

9 Koloski-Ostrow, forthcoming.

10 Waslander 1994, 13-23.

11 *OCD*[3], 1996: 1041. Cf. Plautus, *Curculio* 4.4.24: Therapontigonus says to Cappadox: *...ego tua magnufica verba neque istas tuas magnas minas non pluris facio quam ancillam meam quae latrinam lavat* ('I bother no more with your bragging words and big threats than I do with my slave girl who cleans my toilet.') and Varro, *De Lingua Latina* 5.118: *Trua qu<a> e culina in lavatrinam aquam fundunt; trua, quod travolat ea aqua*. R.G. Kent, trans. *Varro On the Latin Language*, Vol. I., Loeb Classical Library (Cambridge, Mass., 1951) 114-115: 'A *trua* "gutter" is that by which they pour the water from the kitchen into the privy; *trua*, because by it the water *travolat* "flies across".' Also *Varro, De Ling. Lat.* 9.68: *Primum balneum (nomen e<s>t Graecum), <cum> introiit in urbem, publice ibi consedit, ubi bina essent coniuncta aedificia lavandi causa, unum ubi viri, alterum ubi mulieres lavarentur; ab eadem ratione domi suae quisque ubi lavatur balneum dixerunt et, quod non erant duo, balnea dicere non consuerunt, cum noc antiqui non balneum, sed lavatrinam appellare consuessent*. Kent, trans. Loeb Vol. II., 492-493: 'The first *balneum* "bath-room" (the name is Greek), when it was brought into the city of Rome, was as a public establishment set in a place where two connected buildings might be used for the bathing, in one of which the men should bathe and in the other the women. From the same logical reasoning each person called the place in his own house where baths were taken, a *balneum*; and they were not accustomed to speak of *balnea* in the plural, because they did not have two in one house - though our forbears were accustomed to call this not a *balneum*, but a *lavatrina*, "wash-room".' Kent, *ibidem*, 492, n. 7, points out that *lavatrina* is more commonly contracted into *latrina*, which by Varro's time (116-27 BC) certainly meant 'privy' or 'water closet'. See also Thédenat 1904.

12 Cf. Juvenal, *Satyra* 3.36-40:
munera nunc edunt et, verso pollice vulgus
quem iubet, occidunt populariter; inde reversi
conducunt foricas, et cur non omnia, cum sint
quales ex humili magna ad fastigia rerum
extollit quotiens voluit Forunta iocari?
G.G. Ramsey, trans. *Juvenal and Persius*, Loeb Classical Library (Cambridge, Mass. 1950), 35: 'Today they give shows on their own and win applause by killing whomever the mob commands with a turn of a thumb, and from that they go back to contract for public toilets (foricae), and nothing they won't take on, since they are the type that Fortuna raised from the gutter just to enjoy a laugh.' In another translation by R. Humphries, trans. *The Satires of Juvenal* (Bloomington, 1958) 35, the word *foricae* becomes 'private privies,' which shows, at the very least, that modern translators do get confused and are not always consistent.

13 The term seems to have been out of use by the 4th or 5th century AD. The writer of the *Scholia ad Iuvenalem in Vetustiora* (*Schol. Vet. ad Juv.*), P. Wessner (ed.) Berlin 1941, comments at some length on the word, as if he is trying to pinpoint a correct meaning, which has long been lost. He states the following: *'Foricas' cloacas. 'Forire' enim (inquit Probus) veteres dicebant deicere ac de (h)onerare ventrem. hinc 'forire' foras eicere. aut 'foricas' foro vicinas tabernas et confines...alii domos publico sumptu aedificatas ad locandum, quarum conductores lucra capiebant Valla;...hinc 'foricas' dicimus cloacas, in quibus publica civitatis stercora defluunt...'Foricas' id est stercus, purgandas latrinas vel cloacas*. My translation: '*Foricae* are sewers. Probus tells us that old men used to say *forire* when they described discharging the stomach (i.e. defecating). *Forire* derives from *foras iecere* "to throw outside". Moreover, *foricae* are shops bordering upon or near the forum...others think that they are structures built at public expense that *conductores* lease for profit...From this we say that *foricae* are sewers in which the excreta of the general public flows...or the excreta is the *forica* itself, which must be cleared away in latrines and sewers.'

14 Private conversation and correspondence with Antonella Merletto. She concurs that while the first documented public latrines were constructed in the 2nd century BC in Greece (Thera and Paros in addition to Delos), Roman expansion of the 1st century BC brought latrine design to the Northern Provinces as it was added to the construction of forts and *castella* in these regions.

15 Neudecker 1994, figs 9-14.

16 Neudecker 1994, 26, with n. 99.

17 Neudecker 1994, 17: 'Domini nämlich bevorzugten die Lasana oder Colocyntha, tragbares Toilettengeschirr, dessen Bereitstellung als besonders erniedrigender Sklavendienst galt.'

18 For research, especially on private toilets in Roman houses, see Jansen 1991, 151-173; 1997, 121-134; 2000, 275-279; 2002c; 2007, 165-181.

19 Koloski-Ostrow 1996, 79-86; 2000, 289-295.

20 A. and M. De Vos 1982, 90-96.

21 A. and M. De Vos 1982, 250-253, on Villa of Oplontis, modern Torre Annunziata. The ample latrine is no 48 on their plan, 251.

22 Jansen 2002, 257, an abstract of the paper she gave at the AIA convention, but see further Jansen 2007, 165-181. Jansen and her team, in fact, studied more than forty toilets at Hadrian's Villa with two questions in mind: (1) Which people used which toilets? and (2) How much privacy did the toilets offer?

23 Cf. Boethius/Ward Perkins 1970; Sear 1982; MacDonald 1982. Robinson 1992, 119-122: a short section on latrines.

24 Tiles: e.g. Houses of Silver Wedding and Golden Cupids at Pompeii (Ehrhardt 2004, 159, fig. 648; Seiler 1992, 52 and 69, figs 335, 338 and 496). Marble threshold: e.g.

House of the Golden Cupids (Seiler 1992, 52, fig. 339).

25 Jansen 1993, 30 speaks of 'lines' on a white background, but these clearly belong to (partially lost) panel systems.

26 See two simultaneously published studies on this pattern: Goulet 2001-2002 (possibly *bardiglio*); Laken 2003 (not necessarily *bardiglio*).

27 Jansen 1993, 30. In the same vein Laken 2003, 173; the zebra dados in other rooms can be explained in the same way.

28 White marbles are cheaper than coloured ones; so it might even be a question of finances.

29 On terminology see Hallier/Humbert/Pomey 1982, 60-61 n. 23 and here Koloski-Ostrow, p. 52.

30 Apparently there is a previous layer with a figure, but the description in Chini 1997 is not very clear at that point. As to the floors, see Chini 1995.

31 Scheibelreiter 2005, 73-74. As the author makes clear, the technique is very rare in Asia Minor.

32 Neudecker 1994, 60; Cappel 1994, 97; Scheibelreiter 2005, 73 n. 45 Clarke 2007, 78-80 (vulnerability: nakedness and squatting attitude, p. 80). On Egypt as motif of *truphe* Versluys 2002, 294-296.

33 See Carandini 1981, 115 on the social differences between the three toilet groups.

34 Ovid, *Metamorphoses* 13.765-778, 844-850.

35 A similar text can be read on the outer wall of the not yet excavated *insula* V 6, here pp. 170-171, *fig. 12.11*: *cacator sic valeas ut tu hoc locum trasea(s)* ('shitter, may you fare well if you do not stop at this place'). It stands next to a huge altar flanked by *agathodaimones*, a clear example of a public *lararium*. See Fröhlich 1991, 319 cat. F35, pl. 56.2. Txt: *CIL* IV 664. Not in *PPM*. It must have been applied briefly before Vesuvius' eruption.

36 Fröhlich 1991, 40. On her iconography Fröhlich 1991, 132-134. See here G.C.M. Jansen, chapter 12, pp. 167-170.

37 The complex was obliterated by the construction of Domitian's Domus Flavia.

38 The whole decoration formed a 'Nobilitierung' of these users (Neudecker 1994, 99).

39 Leblanc 1995, 250.

40 Neudecker 1994, 58-59.

41 Zimmermann 2002, 113, plate 100 ('orange group').

42 On the philosphers' mosaic in the Rheinisches Landesmuseum at Trier (inv. Mos. I 1240: Schefold 1997, 382-383) Anaximander carries a sundial, a device apparently invented by him (cf. W. Rehm, *RE* VIII (1913) 2416-2433, esp. 2417). A sundial also appears on the well-known mosaic of the Seven Sages or the Academy of Plato (or another gathering of philosophers or sages) from Torre Annunziata in Naples (Museo Nazionale, inv. 124545; Schefold 1997, 294-296) and on a mosaic from Antioch, saying that the ninth hour has finished (Levi 1947, 220-221, pl. XLIX).

43 I am grateful to Professor Leonard C. Muellner of the Department of Classical Studies at Brandeis University, for translating the Ephesus latrine inscriptions.

44 Weisshäuptl, and in his vein, Strocka refers to epigrams pertaining to toilets in the *Anthologia Palatina*, ascribed to Agathias Scholastikos (9.642-644, 662).

45 Strocka 1977, 89, n. 300: has ἁπλάς as an abbreviated form of ἁπαλός or ἁπλόος.

46 Neudecker 1994, 5. 32, 58, 114, 128; Scheibelreiter 2005, 72, with n. 42.

47 See on this topic Neudecker 1994, esp. 44-46. Pozzuoli: Neudecker 1994, 53, figs 1, 23-25; 163 (bibliography). Here pp. 187-189.

48 PR: private. P: public. SP: semi-public. This is not an easy distinction.

49 The room has been seen as a *nymphaeum* by K. Dunbabin. See Cappel 1994.

50 Combined with a brothel, according to an inscription (text in Börker/Merkelbach 1979, no 455, who do not accept this interpretation). See esp. Neudecker 1994, 129 n. 401. The latrine was re-decorated in the time of Scholastikia in the 4th century.

51 Versluys doubts Becatti's interpretation. He believes that the latrine is a complete reconstruction by Becatti. 100-150 AD.

52 S.C. Nappo calls it an 'ambiente di servizio'.

53 The Italian School of Archaeology of Athens has the most complete documentation on the excavation of Kos. The specific archives are Fondo Paolini (F/P), Fondo Morricone (F/M) and Archivio della Scuola (ASAIA). The surveys of the building are by me, and are also in the archives of the school. Before my comprehensive study, the main source was Morricone 1955.

54 The plan of the area is in Livadiotti/Rocco 1996, fig. 309.

55 Archivio ASAIA inv. 933.

56 For the plan, see Merletto 2001, fig. 2.

57 The reconstruction of the *nymphaeum* at the end of the excavation and at the end of the restoration can be seen among the drawings in Merletto 2001, figs 5-6.

58 Study of the mosaic decoration in De Matteis 2004, 57-60, table XVII.

59 Merletto 2004, 251-262. Some terracotta pipes can be seen in the western wall and in the back of the *nymphaeum*. See Neuerburg 1965, 73-80, who places the building in the façade-type group due to the presence and size of the cistern. Walker (1979, 223) accepts and develops this theory. As the top of the structure is totally rebuilt and nothing more is said in the notes of Morricone, there is absolutely no evidence to support or strengthen this theory.

60 Kalopissi-Verti 1991, 233-251, dates these invasions to the 7th century, precisely to 654-655 AD.

61 For the earthquakes that hit Kos see Guidoboni 1989, 671-677. Only the central courtyard was used in the fourth phase, and a passage was opened from the exterior through the central lower niche.

62 The following after Heiligmann 2003, 47-51; Gaubatz-Sattler 2005, 287.

63 For more information on the museum see article 'Sumelocenna - Römisches Stadtmuseum' in the German Wikipedia.

Toilets in the Urban and Domestic Water Infrastructure

6.1 Introduction *(Gemma C.M. Jansen & Jeroen Van Vaerenbergh)*

After visiting a toilet, a Roman user would have wanted water both for cleaning and for flushing. Roman toilets required a drain to dispose of faeces and urine. To get this water in and to get urine and faeces out, several methods were possible, depending on the local infrastructure for water and drainage. To remark on these systems, however, we need a city whose toilets ánd urban water infrastructure have been studied. Only a few Roman cities provide this information, for example, Pompeii, Herculaneum, Ostia and Ephesus. Another good dataset of toilets is available at Hadrian's villa near Tivoli. Gemma Jansen has studied the provisions of water supply and the toilets of these cities and this villa, and therefore they serve as the basis for in this chapter.[1]

Baths have a special position within the urban water infrastructure, since they needed much more water coming in and going out than any other building. The water systems of bath toilets, with emphasis on their flushing systems, are given a special treatment in this chapter. Jeroen Van Vaerenbergh has investigated the toilets in or near baths in Roman Italy. He draws his conclusions from this dataset.

6.2. Water Supply into the City and to the Toilets in the Town and Houses *(Gemma C.M. Jansen)*

Every Roman town government ensured its people of enough drinking water. The method with which the water was provided was not the same in all places of the Roman world; it even could change in one place over the years. In pre-imperial times most towns depended on public and private wells and rainwater cisterns. Later, when the need for water increased, because more inhabitants lived in the cities, and when it was safe enough to build outside the cities walls because Augustus brought peace, only then were long water lines built to bring in running water from springs farther away from the city. Not all of these systems delivered an equal amount of water. For example, piped water at Pompeii seemed to meet the town's needs, but apparently not at Ostia, as a lot of reservoirs and basins for storage have been excavated, which themselves indicate that water was not running day and night in this crowded city.[2] In this section we treat the different water supply systems and their effects on the toilets.

Many cities could draw water from a shallow groundwater table with the help of wells. When the water table was very deep, people had to dig additional underground tanks to store rainwater. This water was gathered on the roofs and brought with channels and pipes to underground cisterns that kept the water cool. How both these methods of gathering water were combined differed from city to city. For example, Ostia had a very shallow water table (2-3 m under street level) and therefore relied in the early years only on wells. Herculaneum with a water table at a depth of eight meters, combined wells with small rainwater cisterns. In Pompeii, where the groundwater table could be reached at only thirty meters deep, many, large rainwater cisterns where the common form of water supply. For daily use, groundwater was preferable as this was a constantly flowing water supply that normally did not dry up, whereas the system for gathering rainwater required a lot of maintenance: all the functioning elements such as water spouts, terracotta downpipes, *impluvia*, peristyle gutters, and the cistern itself, of course, had to be kept clean and free from debris. Another inconvenience inherent in this system was stretching the supply over the summer and autumn months. It would have been most inconvenient to experience a water shortage or no more water available at all. Therefore, even in Pompeii with such a deep groundwater table, groundwater was preferred to rainwater for economic facilities, such as fulleries and baths, that needed a lot of water. How did this water arrive in the toilet room? Water from the cistern or well had to be transported in a container all the way to the toilet and stored there. We can surmise that the Romans did not waste much fresh water to flush the toilet, but they used waste water from cooking and cleaning (from the kitchen or from elsewhere in the house) and in this way the toilet also served as a waste water disposal.

In imperial times many cities got water delivered from an aqueduct. The distribution system of this water within cities is different from town to town, due to geologic conditions and local

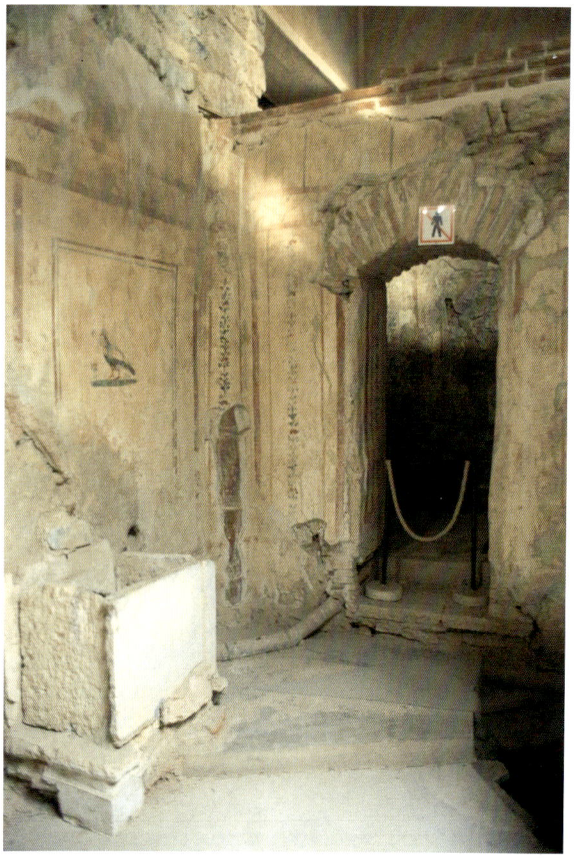

Fig. 6.1. Ephesus, Terrace House 2, 2: courtyard with water basin. Overflow is channelled to the toilet (photo G.C.M. Jansen).

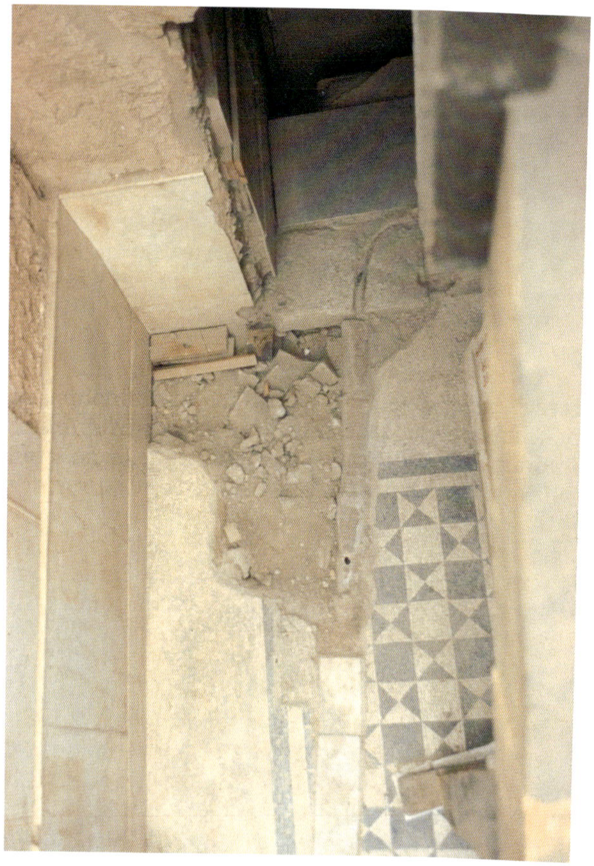

Fig. 6.2. Ephesus, Terrace House 2, 4: water pipe leading to a toilet room (top of photo) terracotta pipes and then lead pipes (photo G.C.M. Jansen).

habits. For example, at Pompeii water towers reduced the height of the flow chamber and the water pressure. At Ostia, on the other hand, water tanks were placed on upper stories to maintain the height of the flow chamber and thus maintain the pressure. In the Italian part of the Roman Empire lead pipes distributed the water, whereas in the eastern empire (modern Turkey), we find mainly terracotta pipes. The details of these distribution systems go beyond the scope of this book,[3] but the effect of the distribution was the same in every town: water was brought to important buildings, such as baths, and to street fountains or *nymphaea*. Many independent group toilets (not belonging to a specific building) were connected directly to the water mains. A few were connected in an indirect way: they received the overflow water from a public fountain or *nymphaeum* for flushing.[4]

Of course, water pipes also delivered water to the houses. Piped water provided quite a revolutionary change, as now water came to houses in large quantities, delivered right at the place where it was needed, with significant pressure so that it could be used to serve house fountains. In theory, every toilet in the house could be connected to this water supply. Surprisingly enough, however, in Pompeii and Herculaneum hardly any toilet received running water. Instead, the surplus water from the fountains was stored in the rainwater cisterns, and we can imagine that from there, water was taken to the toilet as needed. People who had no connection had to fetch water at public fountains (or still had to use water from their cisterns or wells) and had to store it in jars, basins or *dolia* in the toilet room. In Ostia, many more houses were connected to the mains, and lead water pipes filled small basins at various places in the house. From these basins water could be carried to the toilets. In a few cases, the surplus water from the fountains in the courtyards of the houses was directed to these toilets.[5] This can also be seen in Ephesus where the overflow of a water basin in

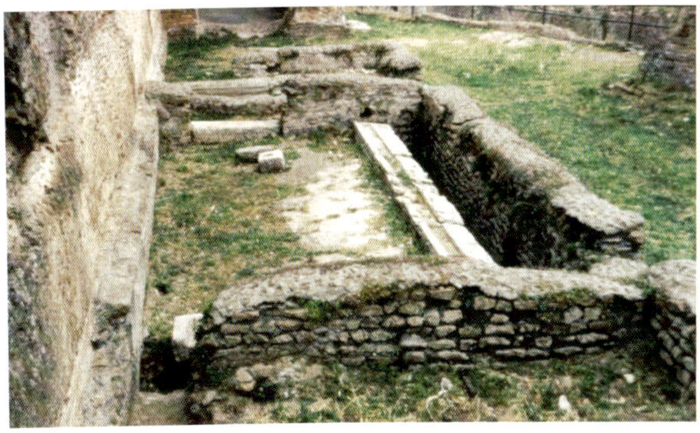

Fig. 6.3. Hadrian's Villa, the Firemen's Barracks, toilet, overview with water reservoir in front (photo G.C.M. Jansen).

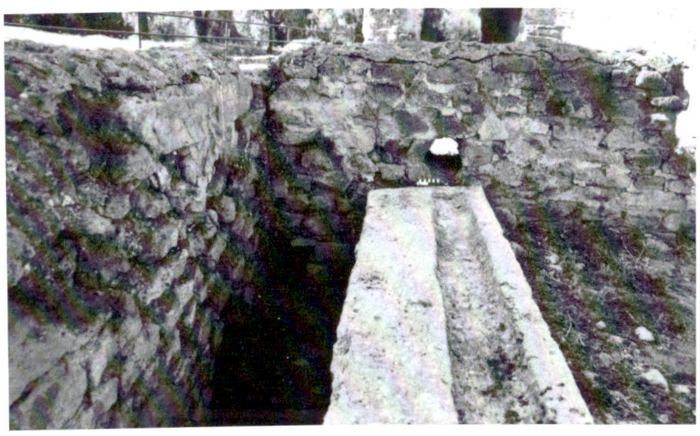

Fig. 6.4. Hadrian's Villa, the Firemen's Barracks, hole for lead pipe and sponge gutter (photo G.C.M. Jansen).

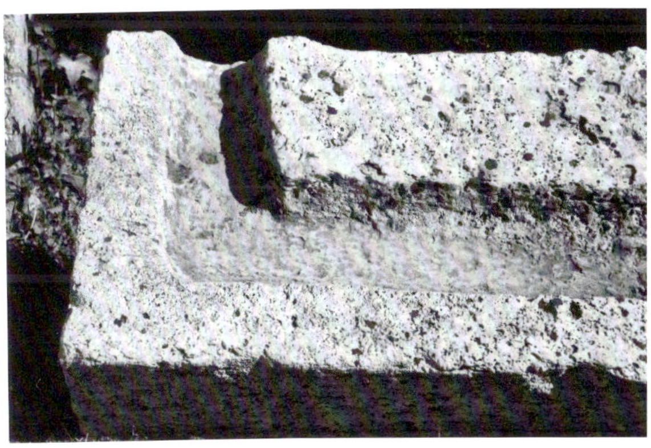

Fig. 6.5. Hadrian's Villa, the Firemen's Barracks, toilet, overflow from sponge gutter into the canal underneath the seats (photo G.C.M. Jansen).

a courtyard of a house leads to the sponge gutter of the toilet, providing a constant flow of fresh water (*fig. 6.1*). At Ephesus water delivery in toilets was organized differently from sites in Italy: terracotta pipes ran to the toilet and the last part of the system (about 50 cm) was laid with a small lead pipe. Lead piping is more flexible and easy to adjust and its small size also added pressure, hence its use in this last complex part of the system. This is the Ephesian way of laying out a water pipe system in a house, and not only for toilets (*fig. 6.2*).

We see in all Roman towns that rainwater not stored was directed to the sewer through the already existing wastepipe of the toilet. The water, however, was not to flush the toilet, as the rain falls only in winter and spring (especially in the Mediterranean). Toilets would have been flushed on a very irregular basis, and, in summer, not at all.

6.3. Water Use and Flushing Activities *(Gemma C.M. Jansen & Antonella Merletto)*

The water use at a toilet can best be illustrated with an example: the servants' toilet in the firemen's barracks at Hadrian's villa (*fig. 6.3*). The entrance is staggered with a small *nymphaeum* in the porch. The toilet room with seats along two sides provided places for thirteen people. Water was brought in with a lead pipe and the hole for it (ø 5 cm) is still visible (*fig. 6.4*). It filled the shallow gutter made of travertine in front of the seats. At the far end, the overflow (*fig. 6.5*) was led into a deep channel (150 cm) underneath the seats. This channel, partly hewn out of the underlying tuff bedrock and partly built in masonry, was made waterproof with layers of *opus signinum*. The channel is connected with a drain *a cappuccina* (pyramidal in form, made by two tiles) to the villa's main sewer network farther down. In addition to wastewater from other unknown sources, which was directed into this channel, spillages and dirty water previously used for cleaning also fed into it, aided by the slightly sloping toilet floor. Figure 6.6 presents all the different elements working together to establish a good water supply and drainage system.

From this example several things can be deduced. As this system requires large amounts of running water, we can assume a connection to the water mains. Clean water was needed for certain visible elements of the toilet, such as the *nymphaeum* and the sponge gutter, and for cleaning the floor. The water to flush the channel underneath the seats did not have to be so clean and indeed, in many cases, water from the overflow from fountains, *nymphaea*, baths, and swimming pools was utilized for this purpose (see Van Vaerenbergh below).

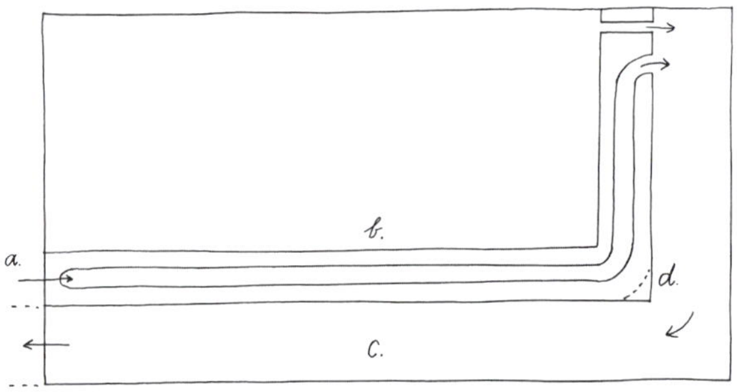

Fig. 6.6. Hadrian's Villa, the Firemen's Barracks, toilet, schematic presentation of the water supply and disposal systems (drawing G.C.M. Jansen).

Let us now look at the different elements needing water. In the example above, a small *nymphaeum* stood in the porch of the toilet. This is a rare phenomenon. Sometimes we find a fountain in the toilet room itself, for example at Kos. But these installations needed water with pressure, which was only possible with a connection to the water pipe system, or when a water tank was placed high enough to create some pressure. More commonly, but also not present in every toilet, was a water basin. Some researchers regard these as hand washing basins, others as places to store or wash the sponges.[6] In eight of the twenty-seven group toilets of Ostia such a basin is present, one in the form of a *labrum*. The overflow of these basins was channeled into the sponge gutter. The drain at the bottom, only to be used when the small basins needed cleaning, opens directly to the toilet floor (*fig. 6.7*). These floors would have had to be frequently washed so that no impurities would form between the tiles or *tesserae* that could decompose and chemically invade the concrete. To facilitate regular cleaning many floors have a slight slope towards a drain or to the gutter underneath the seats.[7] Sponge gutters are always present in toilets. In fact, this is the element that most frequently indicates that a room is a toilet. In whatever material they were executed (marble, travertine or masonry with *opus signinum*) their function was the same: to provide water for the toilet users. The water mains fed these gutters directly or they were fed by the overflow of the water basin in the same room.

Water was also needed to flush the toilet. To get rid of waste materials rounded drains (i.e. drains without corners) served best. From this point of view round and semicircular toilets and corresponding drainage channels were very functional. It is surprising that the Romans - practical as they were - did not prefer this type of toilet.

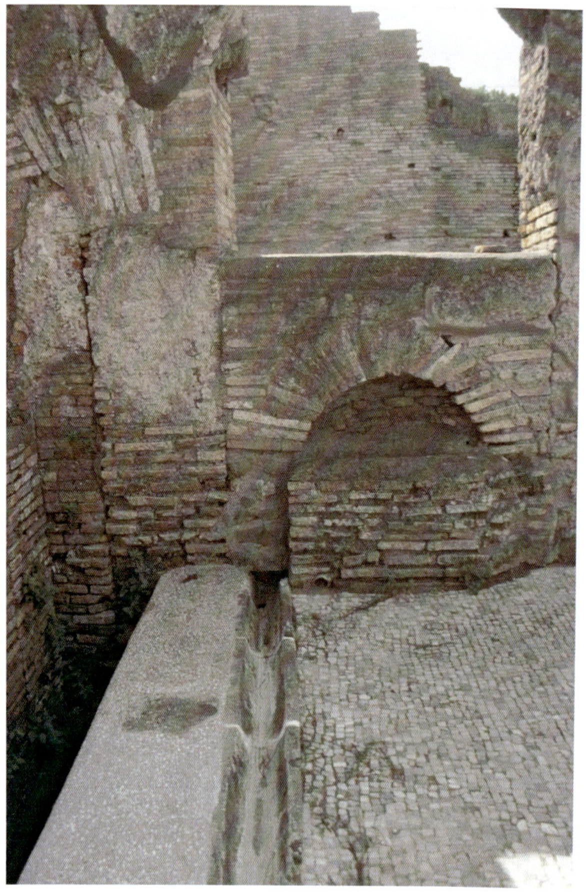

Fig. 6.7. Ostia, Baths of the Six Colums (IV v, 11), toilet room with water basin in toilet (cleaning hole at floor level) (photo G.C.M. Jansen).

The reason is not clear, but it is clear that a rounded drainage channel was not their main priority when constructing a toilet. By far, most toilets are rectangular, and so too are their drainage channels. Here some precautionary measures were taken to smooth the flow of water, urine and faeces. The channels of many toilets show rounded edges to streamline the drain. Tiles were placed at the bottom, and the channel was then completed with a waterproof layer of *opus signinum*. The inclination of the channel is of fundamental importance and most toilet drainage channels have a slight slope.[8] Some channels are frighteningly deep (up to 3 m). This seems not to be related to the flush system, but to the connection of a nearby sewer at a remarkably lower level.[9]

In sum, lots of preparations were made to get the flushing system to work. One question remains and that is: 'Was there enough water available to prevent stagnation?' Water from the sponge gutter

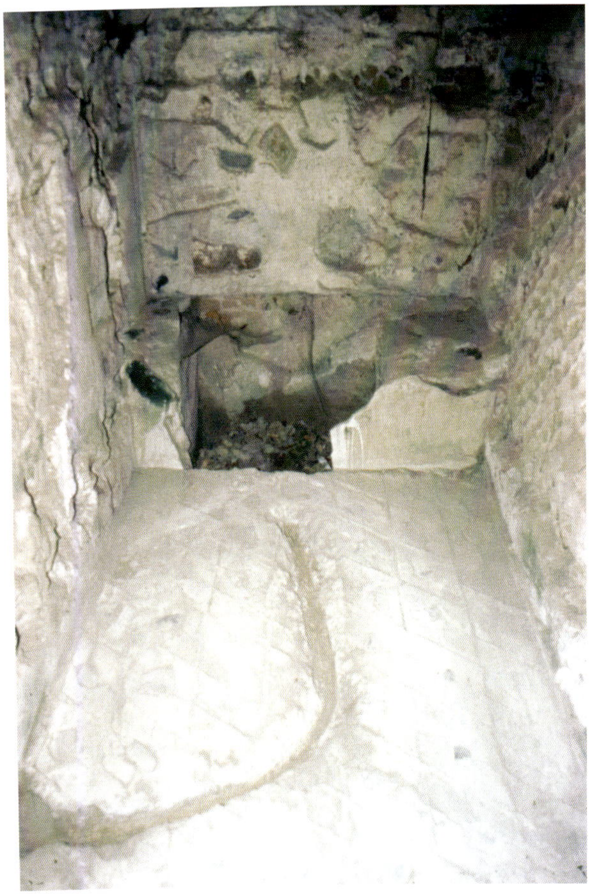

Fig. 6.8. Hadrian's Villa, Canopus, toilet subfloor with imprint of lead water pipe leading to a (now missing) basin in front of the toilet seat (photo G.C.M. Jansen).

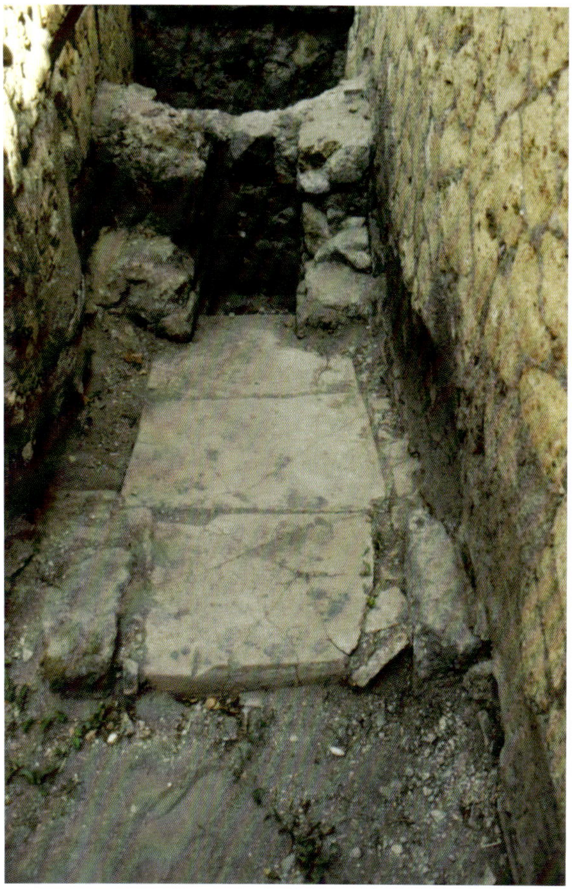

Fig. 6.9. Herculaneum, House of the Painted Papyrus (IV 8-9), flush toilet with sloping floor (photo G.C.M. Jansen).

was led at the far end into the drainage channel underneath the seats. At this point the drainage channel is at its highest elevation and has a decline to the place where it empties into a drain or a main sewer line. We can conclude from this that overflow water was intended to flush the channel underneath the seats. In this way the surplus could be used efficiently. The sponge gutters are rather shallow, for example, those at Hadrian's villa show an average depth 9 cm and an average width of 12 cm, while those at Ephesus are even more shallow with average depth of 5 cm and a width of 13 cm.[10] This does not suggest a large stream of water flushing the drainage channel underneath the seats. It seems that additional flushing was needed to keep the excreta flowing and at some toilets extra flush water was provided. This was mostly done in baths (see Van Vaerenbergh below), though some toilets had large water tanks at hand, for instance the example cited above from Hadrian's villa and several toilets at Ostia.[11] These tanks are too small to provide continuous flushing, but they might give an extra boost once or twice a day.

So far we have looked at public group toilets, and they show some remarkable uniformity. This is due to the fact that they almost always had a connection to the water mains and that they were almost always linked to the city sewer network. This was not necessarily the case with private toilets, and these show much more diversity. In toilet rooms that provided less seating capacity than three or four persons, there was no sponge gutter, but a water basin, apparently with the same function as the gutter. Some of these basins were connected to the city mains and had an overflow; others must have been filled by hand, taking water from a nearby cistern, well, or street fountain.

Continual flush toilets do not occur much in private contexts, the ones in Hadrian's villa, the estate of the emperor, form the major exception.[12] Although most lead pipes have been removed by robbers in later times, the imprints of the pipes under the floors tell us where the water mains were heading (*fig. 6.8*). In toilets they led to a small basin in front of the seats, while the overflow produced a constant flush. In other, more common households, toilets could be flushed with buckets of water (*fig. 6.9*). These hand-flushed toilets occur mostly in kitchen areas.[13] To flush the toilet a small plateau of tiles was built in front of the toilet seat that slanted slightly towards the drain underneath. To facilitate flushing, toilets had no front cover. Households that were not connected to the water pipe system or apartments on upper floors had toilets built into niches in the wall. Thus one could sit right above the drainpipe that was built into the wall. For these drop toilets not much water was required for efficient flushing (*fig. 6.10*). Whether these toilets were connected to a sewer or a cesspit did not determine their form. Only at Herculaneum do we see drop toilets in households with enough water available. They were installed here for a different reason: they were connected to badly functioning cesspits. These pits were dug into the hard lava banks underneath the city, and as the fluids were blocked from seeping away, the pits would have filled up very quickly. Extensive flushing was, therefore, prevented here, and not because of a shortage of water, but because of the demands of the local geology. Drop toilets simply served the town's needs more efficiently.

Just as public toilets and multi-seaters had facilities that made flushing more effective, so did private toilets and single-seaters. In Hadrian's villa under every toilet there is a kind of receptacle smoothed out with several layers of very fine *opus signinum* and plaster (*fig. 6.11*). Everything was so designed to get the faeces washed away without sticking to any surfaces or without getting obstructed by anything. Hand-flushed toilets of Pompeii often had a small slide in form of a roof tile underneath the seat, to direct the faeces into the middle of the cesspit without dirtying the cesspit walls.

6.4. Waste Disposal from Toilets (*Gemma C.M. Jansen*)

What happened with the urine and faeces? Once it was dropped, it remained invisible to the toilet user. The toilet seat and the front plate blocked the view to the drainage channel or cesspit underneath. As the Romans had no odor traps in their toilets, toilet rooms must have held powerful smells even when the faeces and urine of the user were washed away immediately. Because of the open connection, the stench of the cesspit or sewer pervaded the toilet and adjoining house or building. Here we explore cesspits and sewers to which toilets evacuated the faeces and urine. The topography of the city and the choices of the city board determined what methods of disposal were available for individual households. From earlier investigations it appeared - contrary to what a modern person might think - that the Romans preferred all other options of waste disposal over a sewer line: only when there was no other choice left did they lay out an expensive sewer network that required a lot of maintenance.[14] For example, at Pompeii where the sloping streets provide a very good framework to get rid of surplus water, and where the underground of porous lava was very suitable for cesspits, a sewer network was not needed. In this town a sewer line was laid only at places where large amounts of water had to be

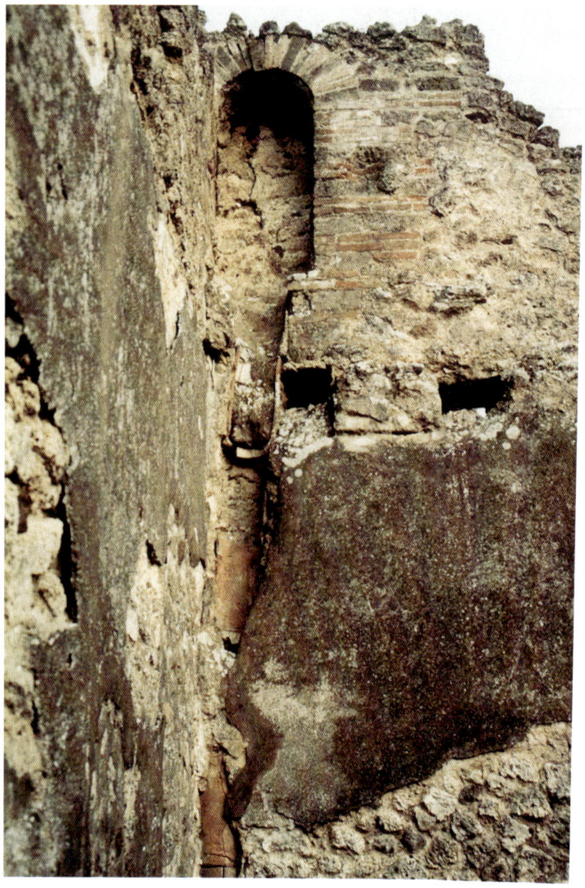

Fig. 6.10. Pompeii, House V 1, 30, drop toilet on upper floor and connecting drain in wall (photo G.C.M. Jansen).

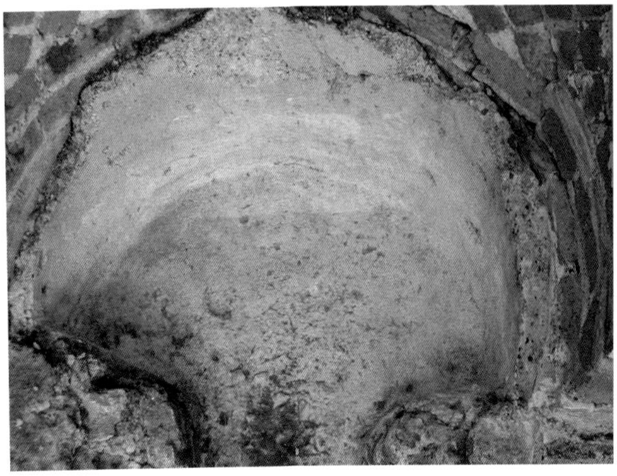

Fig. 6.11. Hadrian's Villa, Rocca Bruna, receptacle underneath toilet (photo A. Vela).

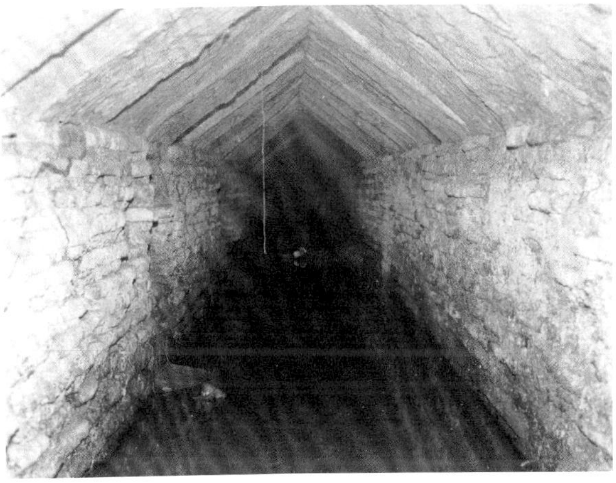

Fig. 6.12. Ostia, sewer underneath the Street of the Tempio Rotondo (toilet connections are visible at places where earth has accumulated) (photo G.C.M. Jansen).

disposed of, such as baths, or where rainwater started to flood a particular area. The geologic conditions of Ostia were not so fortunate: the city was situated on rather flat sand dunes in the middle of a swampy lagoon next to the ever flooding Tiber. The high groundwater table caused problems with the proper function of cesspits, and since streets did not slope enough to guide liquid waste out of inhabited areas, the town was forced - from the very beginning - to install a systematic sewer network.

Thinking of Roman sewers, we have to let go the vision of our modern well functioning sewer networks. Our V-shaped sewers - given enough declination and flush water - are almost self-cleaning. Roman sewers were absolutely not. Their right angles, shallow slope, and irregular flushing must have caused clogging many times over. That people had to go down into the sewers to clean them is also indicated by the many sewer entrances at Ostia. This might be for inspection, but more likely the reason is cleaning. There is some written testimony on sending slaves into sewers to clean them.[15] Sewers were not only very expensive to lay out and to build, but they were constantly on the minds of the city council. Cesspits, on the other hand, were in private hands and did not burden the city government in any way.

Cesspits could be dug by individual house owners and city government would have nothing to do with that. A cesspit was a hole in the ground underneath a toilet seat. It was easy to build, and in most cases, when operating well, it could provide some profit, too (see chapter 10, pp. 147-148). In a cesspit the liquid material seeped through seams between the bricks into the subsoil, and solid material remained in the pit. The Pompeian pits were either round or square and they could be up to 11 m deep. The opening through which the cesspit had to be emptied was often situated in the pavement of a nearby street or in an adjoining garden. In this way, the pit could be emptied without causing a mess in the house. When, by any chance, an underground sewer line passed such a house, the toilet was connected to it.

The sewer system of Ostia is one of the best-preserved Roman sewers thanks to the stable underground temperature and humidity (*fig. 6.12*). The typical Ostian sewer is about 80 cm wide, built in masonry and is covered by two large tiles leaning against each other at the top. The sewers, which are high enough to walk through, could be entered through the manholes; fifty of them can still be seen in the streets of Ostia. They have been laid out in a rather uniform way, but do not date from just one period. All the toilets in Ostia were connected to the sewer system.

The connection between toilet and sewer or cesspit was very direct. We must realize that, as there was no odor trap (as we have seen above), one sat directly above the drain leading to the sewer or the cesspit. Some toilets were built right above the sewer line, as one toilet in Ephesus, another was connected to the sewer in the street by simply breaching the sewer wall.[16] In most cases things were done more neatly, and in these cases, lined channels transported toilet contents to the sewers. The drains emptied into the upper half of the sewer, which can be seen well at Ostia; at

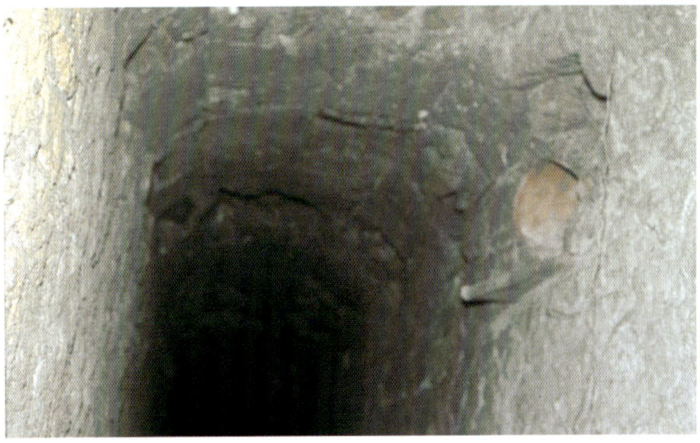

Fig. 6.13. Herculaneum, sewer along Cardo V, connection to house IV 12-13, 15-16 (photo G.C.M. Jansen).

Herculaneum we also see that a chute was used to prevent faeces from sticking on the sewer wall (*fig. 6.13*).

A lot of precautions were taken to have a good flow in the toilet, and some water was added to flush it. The big question of whether the toilets were flushed adequately remains open for debate. The next sections of this chapter will ask this question for toilets in the neighborhood of baths.

6.5 Flush Water for Toilets in and near the Baths *(Jeroen Van Vaerenbergh)*

The supply of flush water was essential for latrines that could receive large numbers of visitors. Because of this, flushing by hand was insufficient and a supply of running water was necessary. A repeated manual emptying of the latrines, as often happened in individual cesspit toilets, was obviously no option. In the following section we see to what extent freely flowing water was attainable for bath-connected latrines.

The study of the toilets near Roman baths must be seen as part of the research on Roman toilets that has been neglected for many years. Because of a lack of comprehensive studies on bath-connected latrines,[17] we have chosen to start with a detailed study of the latrines in and near baths in Italy, the Roman motherland.[18] We have found about forty researchable examples.[19] Certainly, we must be conscious of the fact that these examples are still only a glimpse of the big picture. Nevertheless, we compiled a diverse sample; from the late-Republic and the early empire, from the sites destroyed by Vesuvius, and from sites like Ostia and others that date to the late Roman period.

The earliest Roman examples of flushed multi-seater latrines can be found in the public baths of Pompeii. It is characteristic that the multi-seater latrines of the Stabian (VII 1, 8)[20] and the Forum Baths (VII 5)[21] only came into being when the baths were connected to the city's water supply. Before that, an efficient flushing of a large latrine would have been impossible. It seems that, in contrast to individual latrines, the rise of this kind of toilet is inextricably bound up with a sufficient water supply and the existence of discharge possibilities. The fact that baths contained large amounts of water that repeatedly had to be drained off, made them a logical place to build latrines in this system. Creating large toilets was not the objective of bath builders, and they were of secondary importance within the water systems of these baths. From the perspective of water technology, builders simply made logical use of the existing conditions within the baths in terms of flushing and other water needs.

Within the set of latrines in and near the baths within Italy we can distinguish eight different sources of water supply. Besides the supply of bathwater, it is remarkable that most of the latrines made use of several other flushing facilities to achieve the most feasible flush solution. Ultimately, there is also an internal flush supply that has its origin in the latrine room itself.

Flush Water Supply from the Baths

Although a constant flow of flush water could not always be guaranteed for latrines in baths, we must not forget that at the moment when the bathtubs were emptied, an enormous amount of pressurized water was conducted through the latrine channel under the seats. Possibly this big gush of water was more important for the Romans than a steady flow of a smaller amount of water. Roman designers could often partially compensate for the lack of such a large gush of water for flushing by connecting a toilet to other external and internal water sources that also had to be drained off. Why waste this water if it still could be used for flushing the latrine, or, at least, keeping its drainage channel moist?

Within the context of the bath complexes most of the latrines were connected to one or more bath basins (*piscinae*), generally the cold-water pools of the *natatio* or the *frigidarium*. Only three toilets, namely those of the Grand Palaestra (II 7),[22] the Central Baths (IX 4, 5.10.18)[23] and the Baths of the *Praedia* of Iulia Felix (II 4)[24] in Pompeii, were flushed by water that came from a large open-air swimming pool, *natatio* (*fig. 6.14*). All others were connected to the smaller bath basins of the *frigi-*

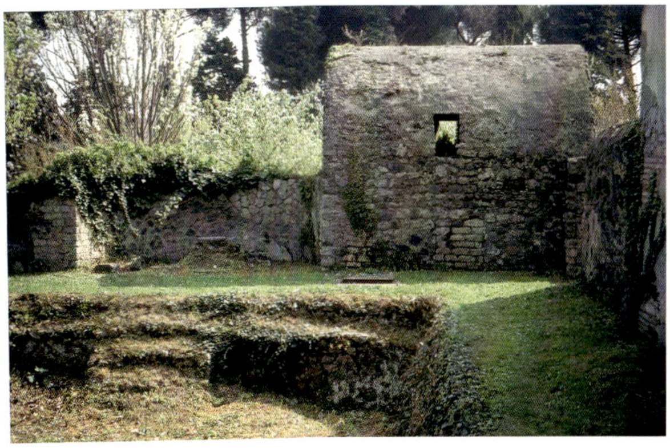

Fig. 6.14. Pompeii, Praedia *of Iulia Felix (II 4),* Natatio *in front of the barrel-vaulted latrine (photo J. Van Vaerenbergh).*

darium. In some cases the *frigidarium* water was supplemented by the discharge water of hot-water tubs and/or other (unknown) water features within the baths.

Surprisingly, all these latrines drew their flush water from a discharge opening at the bottom of the bath basin. Not one bathtub of the researched examples shows an overflow at the top that was connected to a latrine. This is a crucial observation, assuming that a connection to an overflow was the best way of guaranteeing a constant discharge of (superfluous) bath water towards the latrine. We can expect that many drainpipes at the bottom of bathtubs were closed by bath plugs or other stopping mechanisms. These were only opened when the baths were emptied, alhough there also seems to be some evidence to suggest a regulated supply of running water, with or without regular intervals of use.

Without going to deep into the question of a constant water flow into cold baths, we nevertheless can make some remarks to put the issue into a larger perspective. Besides the mention of coldwater pools with flowing water in written sources, there are also archaeological arguments that at the least indicate a sporadic supply of running water.[25] In fact, many of the *natationes* and *frigidaria* were equipped with fountains and waterspouts. Therefore, we can assume that flowing water formed an asthetic and acoustic component within the overall picture of the cold baths.[26] A fine example of such a water feature can be found in the *frigidarium* of the Suburban Baths (VII 16 a) in Pompeii.[27] The lack of an overflow at the top of many of the bathtubs simply shows that the bath was periodically filled and emptied.[28] When the water in the bathtubs became too high, the bath attendants probably had to open the bottom drainpipes for a little while. This resulted in an irregular flushing of the connected latrines. Such a closing mechanism of a drainpipe was found in the big *natatio* of the Grand Palaestra near the amphitheater in Pompeii.[29] It consisted of a simple valve system with a vertically sliding panel that closed off the drainpipe. Only when the valve was pulled up could the water flow towards the latrine.[30]

We also have to keep in mind that some bath basins just had no stoppage system at the bottom drainpipe.[31] Logically inverted, water flowed out as fast as the fresh water to the bath basin. Obviously, this was only possible when the baths were connected to a lavish water supply system.

Whether there was a constant water flow throughout the opening hours or not differs from city to city and from bath to bath. Only a detailed study of the overall hydraulic system can answer this question. As we saw earlier in this chapter (Gemma C.M. Jansen) every Roman city had its own specific water infrastructure with individualized adaptations, specially put together in favor of its local possibilities and needs. In contrast to Pompeii, Ostia probably had no constant supply of running water day and night.

More specifically, for example, a study in the Baths of the *Praedia* of Iulia Felix in Pompeii has shown that a constant water flow was not feasible in those baths.[32] It is clear that the *natatio* only could be emptied to a certain limit. As a result, the multi-seater latrine could only properly be flushed from time to time. In the meantime, the overflow water from the little water basin and the sponge gutter just prevented the faeces from accumulating too much in the drainage channel. This again stands in stark contrast to the conventional picture of large amounts of freely flowing water in the Roman *thermae*.

The availability of running water depended, of course, on the city's overall water infrastructure, the connection of the baths to an aqueduct, and was inextricably bound up with the opening hours of the bath complex. Still, it cannot be fully ruled out that some latrines remained accessible when the baths were closed. The location of many latrines near the entrance to the bath complex made it possible that they could even be used at moments when a decent flushing could not be guaranteed.

Furthermore, there are many baths without a connection to an aqueduct. Freely flowing water was therefore impossible. For example, the Mutatio baths in Valesio were fully supplied by a well that could not guarantee a constant water flow to the *frigidarium*-tub.[33] Since a drainpipe connected the latrine to this bath basin, it could only be flushed when the tub was emptied. Undoubtedly, this four to five-seater was used without a constant water supply.

In some rare cases, a connection with the hot-water basins (*caldaria*) can be established, although always in combination with flush water coming from the cold baths. This is logical, since the hot tubs were filled with water that first had to be heated in a water heater (*miliarium*). A constant water flow was therefore out of question. As a result, these bathtubs were less reliable water providers. In addition, these tubs contained less water than the cold-water pools, and the hot water would have caused a much bigger stench problem. Even in the thermal baths of Terme Taurine in Civitavecchia,[34] where we find a sufficient natural supply of hot water,[35] the Roman hydraulic engineers preferred to connect the toilets to the cold water supply.

Other External Flush Supplies

Flush Water Supply from Public Fountains

The most efficient way of compensating for the lack of freely flowing flush water in numerous baths was a connection to a public fountain. Many toilets that are located in or near baths are, therefore, linked to fountains. We can make a distinction between big ornamental fountains (*nymphaea*) and smaller drinking fountains.[36]

A fine example of a latrine that is fully flushed by a big ornamental fountain is the one behind the *nymphaeum* at the corner of *Cardo Maximus* and the Street of the Round Temple in Ostia.[37] Although this multi-seat toilet was situated next to the Forum Baths (I xii, 6), its builders preferred it to be flushed by the fountain. Since ornamental fountains had no purpose without freely flowing water, they can be considered the most reliable water providers for the latrines.[38] They often contained a large amount of water and continued to be supplied day and night. Whether these latrines also were used at night is difficult to say.

Smaller, more functional public fountains had the same effect. But because of their modest size they could only provide a smaller amount of flush water. In city contexts these fountains were often the only sources of water for most of the citizens. An assured water supply was therefore of vital importance. In turn, the latrines could make use of a part of the fountain's overflow water. In the case of the latrine in the *palaestra* of the Baths of Neptune (II iv, 2) in Ostia, the flush water was partially supplied by a public fountain in the adjacent street (*fig. 6.15*).[39] It is noteworthy that a toilet that was situated within the walls of the baths still made use of an extramural water provider.

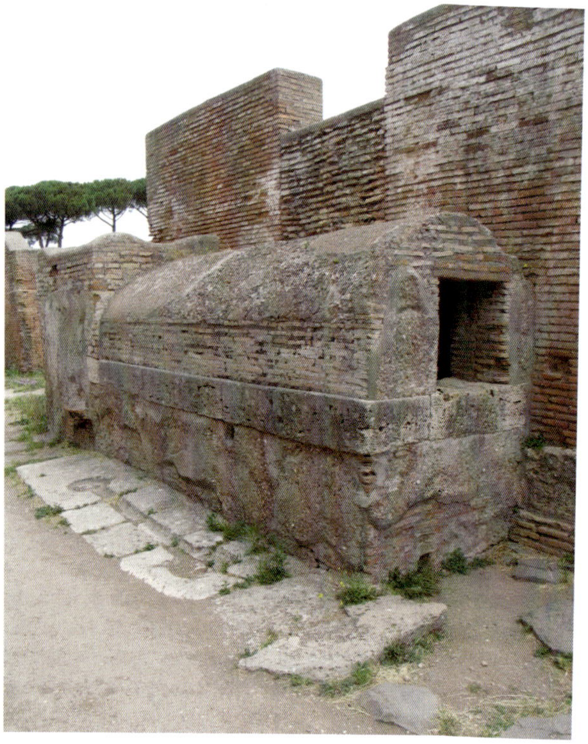

Fig. 6.15. Ostia, public fountain adjacent to the latrine in the palaestra *of the Neptune Baths (II iv, 2) (photo J. Van Vaerenbergh).*

It becomes clear that the toilets in bath complexes were not necessarily dependent on an internal water supply. Although baths offered a good chance of getting a sufficient amount of flush water, the Romans still searched for other water sources, even if this source was located outside of the bathing complex. Using a combination of water suppliers was common, and, in fact, stimulated an easy discharge of the faeces from the latrine canal. In the long run, a direct connection to the bathtubs still assured the greatest amount of additionally pressurized flush water, although its flow was intermittent.

Flush Water Supply from Private Water Basins

A connection to a private water basin (a sink, for example) from a neighboring room could be an additional flush water supply for latrines. Such latrines were less dependent on the water supply of the baths, even after opening hours. Because of the small size of the sinks and the often limited water flow from the water taps, such a flush water supply can, in most cases, only be considered a secondary source of water.

Flush Water Supply from an Adjacent Toilet

The latrine in the Baths of the Philosopher (V ii, 7) at Ostia was also connected to the latrine channel of a neighboring property, in this case the House with the Porch (V ii, 5).[40] It is clear that the Romans tried to make use of this water until it was too filthy to use it further. Such a system stands in strong contrast to conventional depictions of Roman systems squandering water. The Romans apparently knew well that they had to be sparing with their water use.

Flush Water Supply from Vertical Chutes

Too often vertical terracotta drains that discharged into latrine channels are without any question wrongly identified as rain pipes. On the basis of material evidence, it is very difficult to prove that a direct supply of rainwater actually existed for these latrines. In Ostia, it is even doubtful that rainwater was systematically captured, in contrast to towns like Pompeii and Herculaneum, where numerous underground rainwater tanks were found.[41] Tanks on upper floors were mostly not collecting points for rainwater (see water reservoirs, section below). If rainwater was collected, this almost always happened at ground level.

Since the upper structures of latrines with vertical chutes are seldom preserved, we can only guess about the starting point of their water source. Recent analysis of the residue in some vertical terracotta pipes in Pompeii has shown that it contained faecal remains (see chapter 2.4, Andrew Jones). These pipes were possibly connected to individual latrines on upper floors that also could be used to discharge domestic water (see above). Therefore, it is possible that a part of the vertical pipe system in some bath-connected latrines had the same function, certainly when the pipes were situated underneath living quarters.

In all these cases, the often small amount of water moving from time to time through these chutes would not have improved the flush system of the receiving latrine. In fact, the likely possibility that the water carried filth in it could have hampered a swift discharge of the faeces from the latrine channel. These chutes only used the latrine channel as a means for conducting its own contents towards the sewer.

Flush Water Supply from Water Reservoirs

Latrines connected to water cisterns that are on a higher level seem to be arranged in the same manner as those with vertical terracotta drainpipes, supposedly supplied with rain water. Ground level and underground reservoirs also existed. They were filled with water by water lifting devices or by aqueducts.

Within the context of bath-related latrines in Italy, we could only find two examples with a clear connection to a water tank.[42] The latrine of the Stabian Baths (VII 1, 8) in Pompeii was partially flushed by a tank on the upper floor. Also, the latrine on the Street of the Latrine (I xii, 1) in Ostia was linked to an adjacent underground water reservoir.[43] Both tanks were built primarily to contain a water reserve for the baths and other water consumers. Flushing the latrines was only a secondary function.

The flush supply of the toilet in the Stabian Baths was connected to the overflow of the reservoir, and, therefore, only functioned when it was full. Although this flush water had not been used for other purposes, it cannot be considered as a wasteful use of precious fresh water. In certain respects, the water that came through the overflow was redundant water that needed to be discharged in order to prevent flooding. Given the Roman attitude towards unnecessary waste of water, it is logical that they tried to use the overflow for the benefit of the latrine's flushing system. Parsimony was clearly the rule. The connection of a latrine to such an overflow was one of the possibilities for preventing the waste of precious water.

Examples in Italy outside our research domain of the bath-connected latrines show that, besides the overflow connection, a direct connection to a water tank also existed. Among other places, such toilets can be found near the so-called firemen's barracks at Hadrian's villa (see above in this chapter Gemma Jansen) and at Poitiers (see case study at the end of this chapter). The closing mechanism at Poitiers combines the two necessities of a well-flushed Roman latrine: namely, a continuous modest flow of water; and a pressurized water boost from time to time (perhaps, once a day?).

Fresh Water: a Direct Connection of the Latrine Canal to the Water Mains

In bath contexts, only in very rare cases the Romans used 'fresh water' to flush their toilets. By fresh water we mean water that was led directly into the latrine's drainage channel underneath the seats without first being used for other purposes (e.g. the sponge gutter). Only in two latrines, in the Stabian Baths (VII 1, 8) in Pompeii and in the Small Baths at Hadrian's villa, can a direct supply of fresh water to the latrine channel be determined. In both cases, we find imprints of lead pipes that discharged directly into the latrine drainage chan nel (fig. 6.8).

Evidently, the Romans only resorted to the use of fresh water, when they had no other option. By its location at the highest point of the site, the latrine of the Stabian Baths could not benefit from the discharge water that came from the lower baths. Flushing this latrine, which could receive as many as twenty users, was fully dependent on the water tank above.[44] Since the reservoir was not always filled to the top, because of bath supply and possible pressure problems,[45] the overflow functioned only on occasion. As a result, the latrine could be flushed only sporadically. Moreover, because of the unfortunate position of the intake of the overflow, both ends of the latrine channel could not be flushed adequately. Consequently, the toilet needed an additional, more reliable water supply. Eventually the flushing problem was solved by connecting both ends of the latrine channel to fresh water piping. Nevertheless, we cannot fully rule out that this fresh water flow could be regulated by water taps or other closing mechanisms.

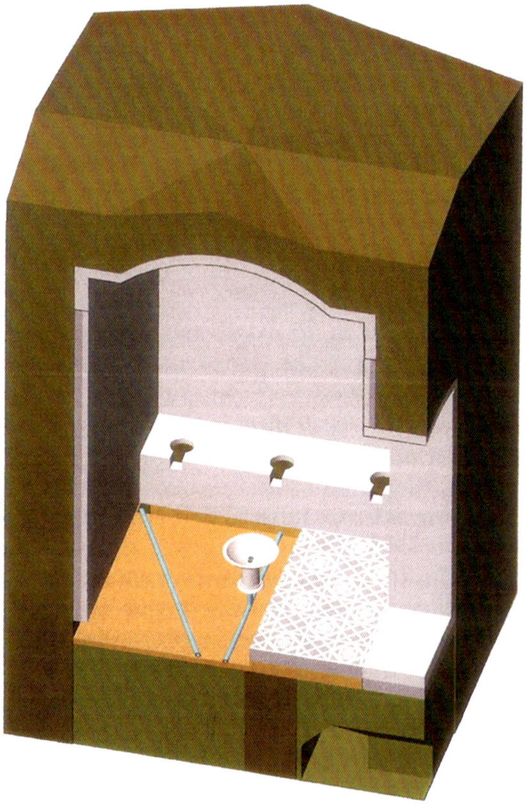

Fig. 6.16. Hadrian's Villa, Small Baths, hypothetical reconstruction of the latrine (from A. Blanco, 2007, Fig. 3, printed with permission).

The three-person latrine of the Small Baths in Hadrian's villa[46] also could only be flushed sporadically by a considerable amount of water. This water entered the toilet gutter by a diversion of the main sewer drains of the baths. Because the intake of this diversion was at a higher level, only if the water level in the main sewer drain was higher than some 30 cm, could the toilet be flushed; perhaps once a day, when all pools were emptied. Therefore, an additional supply of fresh water was conducted to the latrine by two lead pipes, maybe first passing through a water basin (*fig. 6.16*). Since this latrine was located in the most luxurious imperial residence of its day, sparse use of fresh water was not really an issue. Again, this is a fine example of a continuous moderate water flow combined with a sporadic bigger water surge.

In both cases, it is very doubtful that the additional supply of fresh water was sufficient enough to remove all the excrement. The same can be said about most of the previous additional flush water supplies. Only a small part of the waste must have been flushed away. In the first place, this only prevented the faeces from sticking and drying out. In my opinion, a periodic, bigger flush supply was crucial. As we see later, a frequent manual cleansing of the latrine gutter must have been common and even necessary.

Flush Water Supply from a Small Water Basin with Sponge Gutter in the Latrine itself

Latrines were also flushed by a connection between a small water basin and the sponge gutter in the toilet room itself. Most of the time these basins were linked to the latrine channel by the sponge gutter.

Without going too deeply into the issue of the function of these facilities (see chapter 7) the water of the basin and the sponge gutter were supposedly used for cleansing after a visit to the toilet. Whether this was always related to the use of a sponge stick is not clear. The sponge gutter must have had a function in cleaning the latrine room as well. Because many sponge gutters were equipped with discharge holes that opened directly into the latrine channel, we may assume that these gutters had a constant supply of water. This, how-

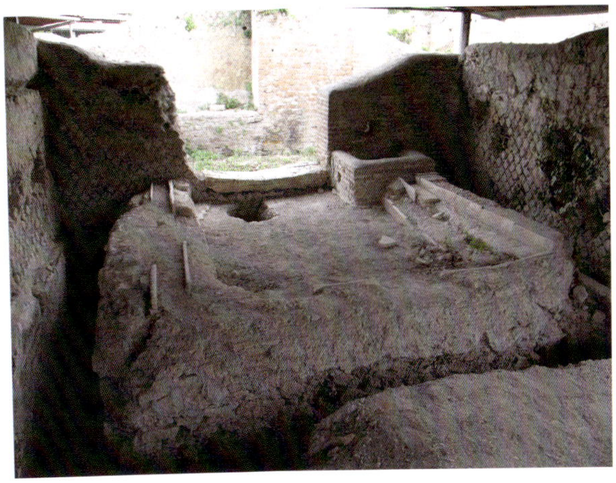

Fig. 6.17. Ostia, Baths of the Swimmer (II iv, 2), second phase of use for the latrine with lowered floor (photo J. Van Vaerenbergh).

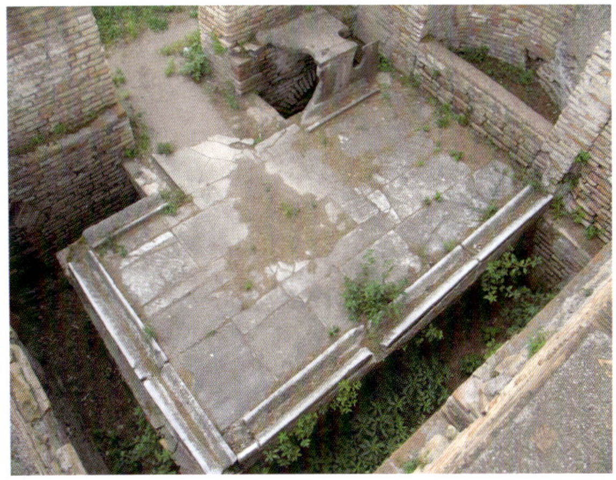

Fig. 6.18. Ostia, Baths of the Philosopher (V ii, 7), latrine channel, sponge gutter and water basin (photo J. Van Vaerenbergh).

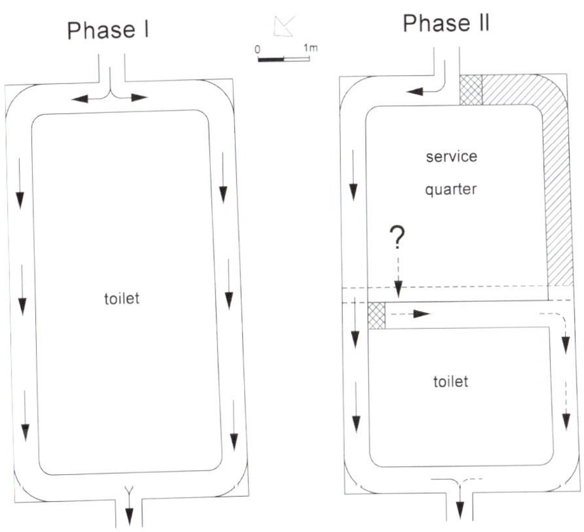

Fig. 6.19. Ostia, Baths of the Swimmer (II iv, 2), two phases (drawing B. Maris).

ever, was not the case in all toilets. In some very rare examples, these discharge openings towards the latrine channel are completely lacking. The water of the sponge gutter had to overflow its rim and flooded the floor in which a drain hole was present. In situations like this, we can suggest a sporadic water supply to the gutter (perhaps once a day).

This certainly was the case during the second phase of the multi seat latrine in the Baths of the Swimmer (V x, 3; *fig. 6.17*). The only way of renewing the water in the sponge gutter was by letting it overflow onto the central white mosaic floor. Near the door there was a drain hole in the floor that led directly into the sewer. In addition, the water basin could also be emptied directly onto the floor. This was probably the reason why the floor level was situated some 40 cm lower than the rim of the sponge gutter. The water could then be used to keep the floor clean after closing time. A similar situation, although with a small overflow slit, can be determined at the much earlier latrine of the Stabian Baths in Pompeii.

I think it is clear that gutters without direct discharge holes towards the latrine channel were only filled once a day. Only when the toilet room needed to be cleaned, was the water renewed and 'flooded' onto the floor. This clearly shows that the internal water system (water basin/sponge gutter) of all the toilets in general must have had an additional function for cleaning the latrine room itself.

The water basin in the toilet of the Baths of the Philosopher (V ii, 7) in Ostia could only be emptied by discharging its contents over the marble floor (*fig. 6.18*). Again, this was probably a way of keeping the floor clean. We can assume that this flooding only happened when it was needed. As a result, the water basin had no continuous water supply.

That toilet floors got filthy, certainly near and around the seats, is obvious. We might explore the latrine in the substructures of the Baths of the Domus Tiberiana along the Clivus Victoriae in Rome in order to verify this point.[47] The broad sponge gutter of this toilet was originally covered by metal grating. The grate probably prevented the users from stepping into it and still left enough space to rinse the sponges. Besides this grating, a wooden foot-rest in front of the latrine seats prevented the users from getting wet/dirty feet while sitting down.[48] Stone protrusions in the sponge gutter of the latrine in the Stabian Baths perhaps indicate a similar solution.

Conclusion: Efficiency and Conservation of the Water Supply in the Latrines of Roman Baths

We can conclude that toilets always were located near a source of water that offered the greatest chance of an assured and reliable water supply. Although most baths could not always guarantee a constant water flow towards the latrines, in the long run, they offered the biggest potential for getting a large amount of flush water. The connection to the overflow of a public fountain might imply a more constant water flow, but, in most cases, the overall amount of flush water could not be compared to that of emptying the baths. Other suppliers of flush water, like the overflow of water basins, cisterns, etc., can only be seen as a less important, additional source of water in this respect. This combination of a more or less constant water trickle, which prevented large accumulations of filth, and a periodic pressurized water surge from the baths, ensured that in Roman times bath complexes were the best places to locate big, multi-seat latrines. As we shall see, however, this does not mean that flushing problems did not persist.

It is remarkable that in order to flush these toilets the Romans almost always recycled water that already had been used for other purposes. Only in very rare cases was the latrine additionally flushed by fresh water. This implies that in order to get flushed the latrines were always dependent on other water-using facilities. As a result, the reliability of water supply between different water sources could vary a great deal. Instead of pursuing the utopian image of a perfectly flushed latrine, the Romans looked for the most feasible water supply in relation to minimal waste of that water. With this perspective, baths can be regarded as the perfect compromise. Moreover, as we shall later see (chapter 8, pp. 114-119), the large number of bath users could take advantage of the latrines, as they were already engaged in body care.

6.6 Disposal from Baths and Malfunctioning of the System

Despite the fact that baths were a fairly reliable source of large amounts of flush water (as discussed above), this was not sufficient to maintain a well functioning toilet system.

Disposal of the Soiled Flush Water

An easy water circulation within the latrine channel was a second important factor engineers had to take into account when constructing latrines. The bottom line was, the fewer corners in the drainage channel, the better. When there was just one straight latrine channel along one of the walls, good water circulation was guaranteed. But in smaller rooms, placing the toilet seats only along one wall would drastically limit the total number of seats. A better design was a circular or semi-circular layout, like the latrine of the so-called Large Baths of Hadrian's villa,[49] which ruled out the accumulation of faecal sediments in corners and could receive more toilet users. The layout of surrounding rooms, however, often prevented a circular design. Rounding off the corners with water resistant mortar (*opus signinum*) was often the only solution, and also protected the channel walls from urinal and faecal corrosion. Furthermore, the gradient of the toilet gutter had to be large enough to ease the flow towards the outlet.

Ultimately, the Romans also had to look for the quickest way to evacuate the soiled flush water, mostly through a nearby sewer. Again, the latrine could take advantage of its location near the baths, since sewers were inextricably bound up with baths. This is certainly true in the early periods, such as we find in Pompeii and Herculaneum, when the sewers were to a great extent designed to drain the large amounts of water from the baths to outside the city walls.[50]

The only bath-related toilet without a connection to the sewer[51] was the latrine of the *Praedia* of Iulia Felix (II 4) in Pompeii, which was connected to a pit dug into the porous tuff, a so-called soakaway, that made it possible to use the residue as manure in the big, surrounding gardens.[52] This solution combined a flushed multi-seat latrine with an 'economical use' for its contents (see also chapter 10). This latrine shows that the arrival of large toilets did not necessarily mean that agriculturally important faeces were wasted. Nevertheless, it is evident that in most cases faeces were not used from large public latrines.

The closer the toilet was located to the place were the baths discharged its used water, the quicker the foul-smelling flush water would have left the complex, and the fewer nuisances it would have caused. It is not surprising that most of the latrines were the last facility connected to the internal discharge system of bath complexes, the place just before water went into the sewers. Toilets could benefit by emptying their smelly contents directly into an underground canal that often contained a greater flood of water than the latrine channel itself. As a result, human waste could be removed pretty efficiently from living spaces by a quick discharge.

Several latrines have a special adaptation that assured an even quicker discharge into the sewer. Just before the soiled water left these latrine channels, there was a final inlet of water, either from underground canals or from the overflow of the so-called sponge gutters/water basins. Sometimes, as in the latrine of the Suburban Baths in Pompeii, this final inlet even provided a greater amount of water than the normal flushing system of the toilet. It is almost as if the Romans gave more priority to an easy underground flow than to a decent flushing of the latrine itself. It is just a fact that a latrine channel was easier to clean than a clogged sewer. This remark puts the malfunctioning of many latrines more into perspective.

In brief, the latrines near baths in Italy seem to have been more or less well accommodated to remove urine and faeces quickly out of daily living spaces. Nevertheless, in some cases, there is reason to believe that there were still some difficulties and inconveniencies that the engineers could not fully correct. Compromises were, therefore, inevitable.

Malfunctioning of the System

We have already seen that the Romans tried to compensate for an irregular water supply of the baths with additional water sources. The toilet of the Baths of the Swimmer (II iv, 2) in Ostia, however, proves that in most cases these extra sources were not sufficient, even in apparently well equipped latrines. The latrine of these baths shows that faecal accumulation could not always be avoided. Such an accumulation problem as a result of a malfunctioning of the flushing system is probably one of the reasons why the latrine was made smaller, from 21 (?) to eleven seats, after a period of time,[53] and finally even went out of use, about 100 years after its first use.[54]

Thanks to the outstanding excavation of this latrine, we get a unique chance to study its actual function throughout its existence. At first glance, during its first phase of use, the toilet with 21 (?) seats seems to be excellently accommodated with water to accomplish a swift flow towards the sewer. The flush water was provided by several bath basins, a water tank and other water features. Together with the indirect overflow of a sponge gutter and maybe a water basin, this seemed to be sufficient to flush the entire toilet. In addition, the sides of the latrine channel were covered with *opus signinum*, the inner corners were rounded off, and the bottom gradually sloped towards the outlet. Nevertheless, great quantities of faecal accumulation were discovered in a part of the latrine canal, which later on was cut off. Although almost all the best conditions were present, they did not seem to be adequate to flush away all the faeces.

Most certainly, as said, this was one of the reasons why the number of seats was almost halved to some eleven seats (*figs 6.17 and 19*). During the second phase of use, there did not seem to be any improvement, and, on the contrary, the situation even worsened. By reducing the toilet's capacity, part of the latrine channnel could not be reached by the flush water supply that came from the baths.[55] Evidently, the part with a malfunctioning flush water supply had to cope with greater amounts of faecal accumulation than the better flushed part of the toilet. Still, the latter was not at all free of dirt. The numerous artifacts that were found in these deposits were clearly affected by their faecal surroundings.[56]

Even in apparently well flushed latrines, an accumulation of faeces could not be totally eliminated. The same problem must have been common in countless other latrines. This is no surprise at all, because in most latrines, there was a constant fluctuation in the amount of flush water. In calm flush periods, the faeces would have stuck more to the bottom. A gentle flow of water just would have prevented it from sticking too much and drying out. Depending on the size of the latrine, and the possibilities it had for a regular, large, and pressurized flush supply from the baths, frequent manual cleaning of the latrine channel must have been common and even necessary.

Another example of a well-excavated latrine, which shows the complexity of the flushing system and the problems the Roman builders had to face, is the latrine in the Small Baths in Hadrian's villa.[57] Besides water from two lead pipes (*fig. 6.16*), which clearly was not sufficient, this three-person latrine was sporadically flushed by a diversion of the main sewer of the baths, maybe once a day. In spite of its rich decoration, even the latrines of the emperor and his guests left much to be desired in terms of modern attitudes towards cleanliness and smell. In the last phase of use, a faecal deposit was found at the bottom of the channel.

In the future more meticulous and methodologically correct excavations, like the one in the

Baths of the Swimmer, will give us better insights into the actual (mal)functioning of Roman flushed toilets. A multidisciplinary approach is a necessity. Analyses (archaeobotanical, palynological, etc.) of the deposits can give us insights into the users of the toilet and its surroundings.[58] In addition, we can hope that this chapter will motivate future water engineers to make more detailed studies of the resulting pressure on the flush water in Roman latrines. Such studies seems to be crucial for understanding the function of these toilets, after it clearly has been shown that at least a sporadic pressurized water surge was necessary for an adequate flush of multi-seat toilets.

Again, it becomes evident that the Romans always looked for the most efficient hydro-technical solutions possible, even if not necessarily perfect. The result was 'a nice compromise with a bad smell'. From this perspective, the Romans were not as extravagant as they are often depicted. Obviously, by modern Western standards, the hygienic conditions of Roman latrines would have been inferior. The question is to what extent the Romans were bothered by this. This issue will be considered in detail in chapter 11.

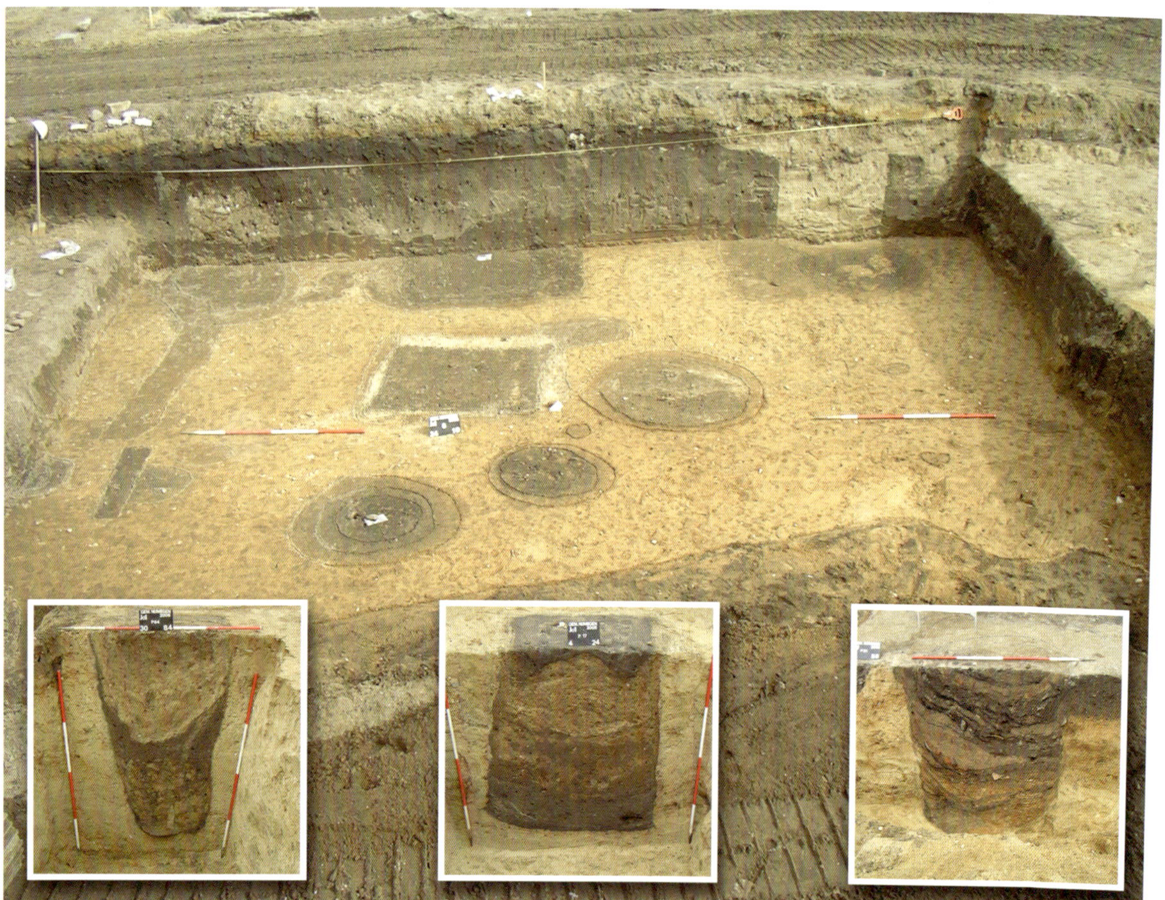

Fig. 6.20. Nijmegen, square, rectangular, round and oval cesspits: some of them still contained remains of the original filling (photos Bureau Archeologie en Monumenten van de gemeente Nijmegen).

Case Study: 1st-Century Roman Cesspits in *Oppidum Batavorum* (Nijmegen, NL)
(Elly Heirbaut)

Oppidum Batavorum was originally a ribbon village, established around 5 BC to house the first veterans of the legions encamped in *Germania Inferior*. In the following decades, the village developed into the chief settlement of the *civitas Batavorum*. Besides veterans, Gallo-Roman civil servants, artisans, traders, and shopkeepers also lived in *Oppidum Batavorum*. According to Tacitus, the entire settlement was destroyed during the Batavian Rebellion in AD 69/70, in a fire started by the Batavians. Recent research in the center of this settlement has led to fresh insights into the layout of the private dwellings that predate this fire, and the property located behind. A total of eleven lots have been identified, of which five (nos 3-7) have for the most part been excavated. The strip houses (*tabernae*), which all have the same floor plan, are located on the northern side of the lot and connect directly to the settlement's principal road running from east to west. Numerous rubbish pits, ditches, and cesspits have been located on the parcels that stretch at least 100 m behind the dwellings.

A total of 84 cesspits have been excavated, with the number of pits ranging from nine to fourteen on lots 3-7. One remarkable aspect of the cesspits is their location. A small group is located indoors. Stratigraphic analysis shows that these are the oldest cesspits and can be attributed to the first phases of Roman settlement. The majority of the pits is found in the areas behind the dwellings. Remarkably, with the exception of two pits, all these pits are situated at the same distance from the houses. The pits' contents allow them to be dated to the Claudian-Neronic period.

The majority of pits are barrel pits and square-shaped cesspits. A smaller number are rectangular or oval in form (*fig. 6.20*). The barrel pits are lined with multiple barrels that are positioned on top of each other. Placing these barrels involved either digging a hole or undermining the barrel from below, which allowed the barrel to subside ever further into the ground. The diameter of the barrels varies from 0.9 m to 2.4 m. The square and rectangular cesspits (with minimum dimensions of 1.25 x 1.25 m/1.8 x 1.4 m and a maximum size of 2.1 x 2.1 m/ 2.3 x 1.3 m) are lined with wooden boards, and in some cases the corners of this casing have been reinforced using beams placed on the inside. In the case of the rectangular casings, one occasionally finds additional beams placed in the center of the longest sides. The boards are sometimes nailed one to another and/or to the posts, but occasionally also placed against the posts without any further means of fixation that can be determined through archaeological research. In the latter case, the boards stay in place thanks to the pressure of the earth that has been thrown back into the pit after the casing was placed. Finally, the oval cesspits were constructed by placing the boards of the casing directly against the side of the pit or a braided basket was used. On occasion, it appears as if the bottom of the pit had a wooden floor. Holes in the floor would have allowed for the drainage of fluids, while more solid matter remained in the pit. The wood of the casing or floors has not been preserved in any of the pits.

It was only possible to make out wooden outhouses at 14 locations. In most cases, the ditch lining the wall on the eastern, southern and western sides is situated in close proximity to the cesspit construction. On the northern side, room is left for a 1.5-m to 2-m wide entrance. Although no evidence has been found to support this, it can be assumed that these outhouses were similar in appearance to the private toilets in the Mediterranean area, except for the fact that they were made from wood rather than stone.

Most cesspits are separate from one another. A few are linked via ditches that were used to carry water to and from the facilities. Considering the many excavations that have since taken place on the site, it is not inconceivable that several pits were connected by ditches that have now disappeared. In addition, several cesspits are connected to cesspools via small, wooden overflow ducts. These cesspools are located at a short distance from the cesspits and have a similar construction to the barrel pits or the square/rectangular pits.

All cesspits were emptied on a more or less regular basis and after falling into disuse, the empty cesspits were filled in. In a small number of pits, remnants of the primary contents - night soil - were found in the bottom-most level. In other words, faeces were saved and used for other purposes, such as the fertilization of the gardens behind the houses or the fields located outside the settlement.

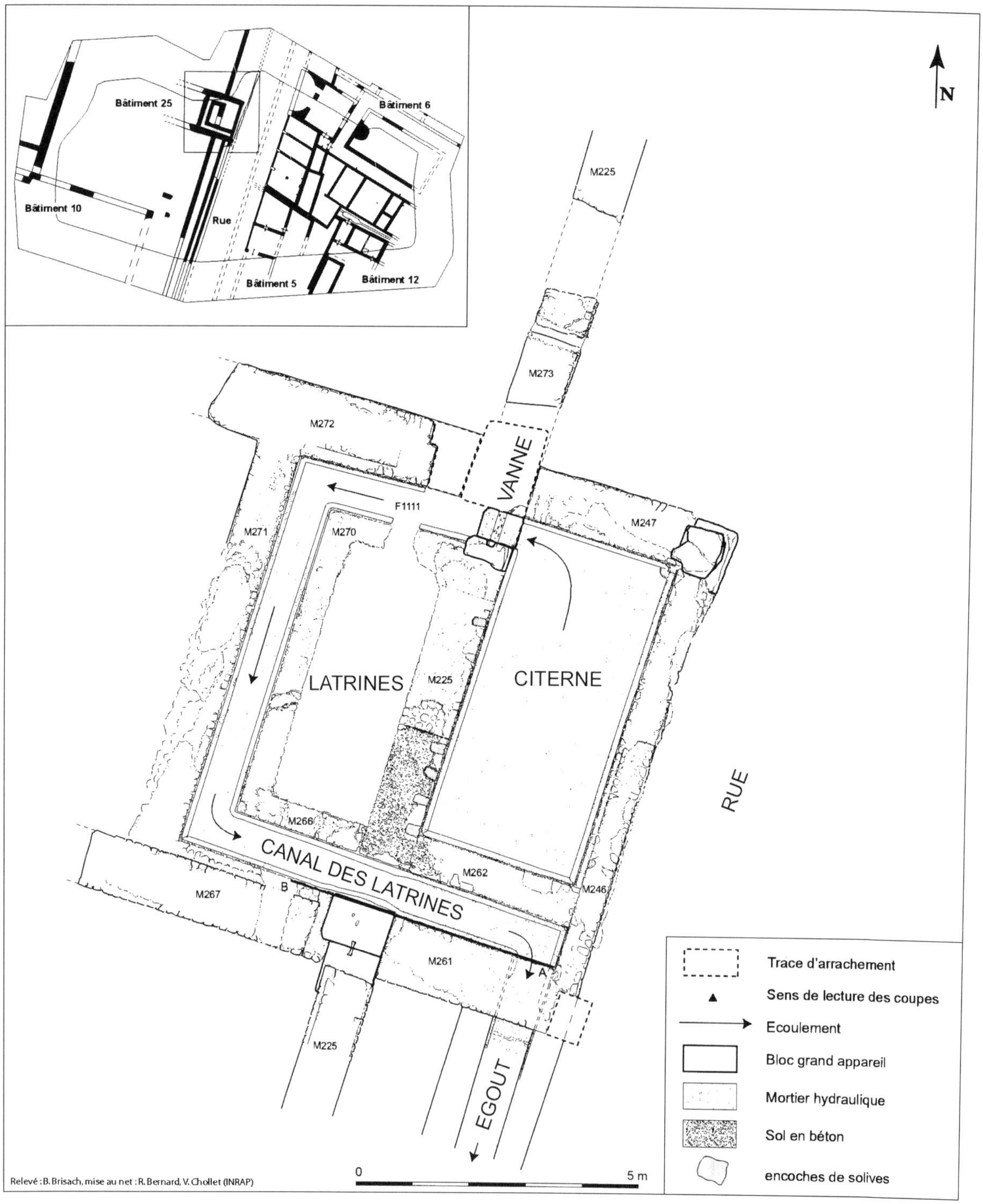

Fig. 6.21. Poitiers antique, latrines publiques (dessin B. Brisach et R. Bernard, Inrap).

Case Study: Poitiers antique: latrines publiques et chasse d'eau
(Anne-Marie Jouquand-Thomas & Jacques Seigne)

En 1998, les vestiges bien conservés de latrines publiques datables du IIIème siècle de notre ère furent mis au jour à Poitiers (France) (*figs 6.21-22*). De plan rectangulaire (9,50 m sur 8,50 m), elles étaient aménagées à l'extrémité d'un bâtiment très mal conservé situé en bordure de rue et correspondant peut-être à l'une des entrées, vraisemblablement condamnée à cette occasion, d'un grand monument public établi sur une terrasse. Le puissant pilier de maçonnerie, restituable au centre du bâtiment, apparemment clos de murs sur au moins trois cotés, servait peut-être à supporter la toiture. Le sol de la pièce, en grave compactée liée au mortier de chaux sur remblais de terre, n'était conservé qu'à l'état de traces. Par contre, les structures en «sous-sol» étaient totalement et remarquablement préservées.

Au nord, à l'ouest et au sud, un étroit (0,75 m) et profond (1,10 m) canal maçonné et enduit longeait intérieurement les murs de la structure, suivant un dispositif bien attesté dans les latrines publiques en exèdre.

Au sud, ce canal se retournait, traversait le mur méridional et se prolongeait par un égout en forte pente (4%), implanté le long de la rue. Il a été reconnu en bordure de chaussée sur 95 m de long.

La moitié orientale du bâtiment, construite sur le trottoir de la rue, abritait une vaste citerne (5,80 m sur 2,80 m, profonde de 1 m) entièrement enduite de mortier hydraulique. D'une capacité assurée de 11 m^3, elle était couverte d'un plancher sur poutraison simple, établi au même niveau que le sol de la salle. Le canal d'égout des latrines prenait naissance dans son angle nord-ouest. Des blocs de calcaire de grand appareil marquaient la jonction citerne/canal. Munis de feuillures verticales, ils appartenaient à un dispositif de fermeture/ouverture de la citerne (vanne en bois). En position fermée, cette vanne, haute de 0,70 m, permettait au trop plein du réservoir de se déverser dans l'égout des latrines, assurant un nettoyage minimum, permanent, du canal. Le système d'alimentation en eau du dispositif n'est pas connu, mais une canalisation d'adduction d'eau en boisseaux de bois frettés a été reconnue au pied du portique de la rue, sur toute sa longueur. Elle longeait la façade orientale des latrines. Une alimentation de la citerne via un tuyau de dérivation, probablement en bois lui aussi, branché sur cet aqueduc sous pression, est donc très vraisemblable.

De nombreux fragments d'enduits peints ont été découverts dans le canal. Ils appartenaient à un panneau figurant probablement une scène de combat de gladiateurs et révèlent qu'au moins l'un des murs de la salle avait reçu un décor peint.[59]

Tel que mis au jour, le bâtiment est complet et il est possible de restituer des latrines publiques en exèdre, vraisemblablement richement décorées, pouvant accueillir une vingtaine de personnes. La particularité remarquable de l'édifice réside dans la présence, en tête du dispositif, d'une citerne dont les 11 000 litres d'eau pouvaient être brutalement libérés dans le canal de l'égout, grâce au relèvement d'une vanne, permettant ainsi le nettoyage rapide et complet des matières accumulées. Ce dispositif de «chasse d'eau» intégré à des latrines publiques semble être le seul actuellement connu pour l'Antiquité.

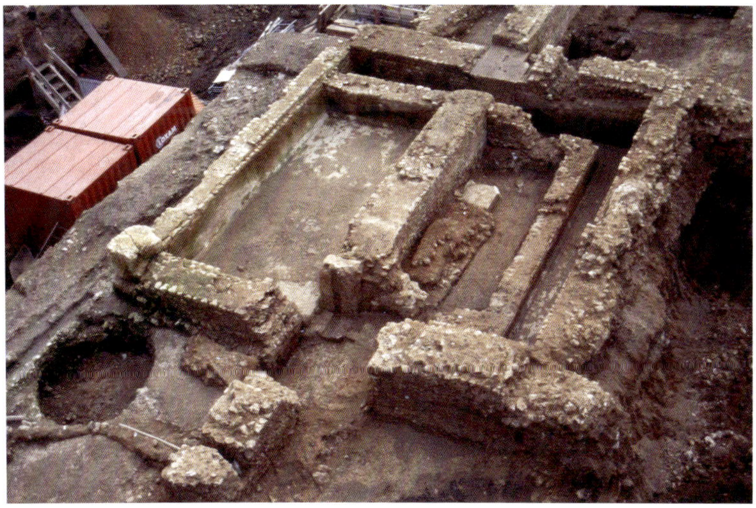

Fig. 6.22.
Poitiers antique, latrines publiques (photo F. Champagne, Inrap).

Case Study: Ercolano: la ricostruzione dei sistemi fognari *(Domenico Camardo)*

La città romana di Ercolano, distrutta dall'eruzione del Vesuvio del 79 d.C., disponeva di un organico sistema di smaltimento delle acque che è da suddividersi in pubblico e privato.[60] All'interno di diverse domus sono stati infatti individuati pozzi utilizzati per scaricare le acque piovane e le acque reflue delle latrine.[61] In altri casi le acque piovane erano incanalate in condutture che le scaricavano direttamente sulla pubblica via. Tuttavia accanto a questi sistemi privati la città di Ercolano era anche dotata di un sistema pubblico di smaltimento delle acque, rappresentato da fognature costruite sotto la pavimentazione stradale.

Il III *Cardo* presenta, per tutta la sua lunghezza, una fognatura larga 60 cm ed alta 1,05 m, pavimentata con tegole (*fig. 6.23*). La fognatura corre rettilinea fino all'estremità meridionale della strada, dove le acque erano convogliate in un pozzo che, tramite un cunicolo, le scaricava sull'antica spiaggia. Dalle *domus* le acque erano convogliate, tramite condutture, direttamente nella fognatura pubblica.[62] Anche le Terme di Foro erano collegate a questo ramo fognario. Recenti indagini hanno infatti permesso di svuotare questo condotto, alto circa 1 metro e largo 60 cm, e che conserva una pavimentazione in tegole. Questo si sviluppa al di sotto del corridoio di servizio delle Terme. Circa a metà della lunghezza del corridoio, dopo un pozzetto di ispezione, la fogna cambia radicalmente sezione trasformandosi in una canaletta di circa 25 cm di larghezza per 25 di altezza, che serviva per scaricare le acque della vasca del *calidarium* delle terme.

A differenza di quanto accade per il *Cardo* III, la presenza di numerose bocche di scarico lungo il marciapiede del IV *Cardo* aveva fatto ipotizzare che questa strada non fosse servita da una fognatura pubblica.[63] Tuttavia una chiara indicazione dell'esistenza di una fogna sotto questa strada è venuta dalle prospezioni geognostiche realizzate lungo il IV Cardo fino all'incrocio con il Decumano Inferiore (*fig. 6.23*).[64] Sono state eseguite sia indagini geoelettriche sia di tipo georadar. Entrambi le analisi hanno mostrato l'esistenza, al centro della strada, immediatamente al di sotto del basolato, di un condotto fognario largo circa 60 cm ed alto circa 90 cm, ancora pieno del flusso piroclastico dell'eruzione del 79 d.C.

Anche il Decumano Inferiore era servito da una fognatura presente sotto il marciapiede del lato meridionale che serviva per raccogliere le acque della strada e quelle degli edifici circostanti (*fig. 6.23*). Questa fogna, alta circa un metro e larga circa 60 cm, pavimentata con tegole, era stata già parzialmente individuata durante i lavori del Maiuri, che nei diari di scavo parla di feritoie esistenti lungo il marciapiede del Decumano Inferiore che servivano a portare le acque nella fogna.[65]

Diversa appare la situazione del V *Cardo* dove è stato individuato un complesso sistema fognario che permetteva lo scarico delle acque della palestra e di tutte le abitazioni dell'*Insula Orientalis* II. Questa fognatura corre lungo il lato orientale del V *Cardo*, sotto tutto il fronte dell'*Insula* (*fig. 6.23*). Fu costruita in fase con la realizzazione della palestra e delle botteghe che si aprono sul V *Cardo*. Tutta l'*Insula Orientalis* II fu edificata compensando il doppio dislivello del terreno che da Nord andava verso Sud e dal V *Cardo* andava verso Est.

Il dislivello a ridosso del V *Cardo* fu superato con la costruzione, circa 3 m più in basso della sede stradale, dei muri perimetrali dell'isolato. Questi furono fondati nel livello compatto dell'eruzione vesuviana delle 'Pomici di Avellino'. Infatti il muro di facciata dell'*Insula* sul V *Cardo* non è altro che il muro occidentale del lungo braccio N-S della fogna che parte circa 3 m al di sotto della strada. Questo braccio presenta una copertura a volta, ed è composto da un cunicolo rettilineo lungo, in senso N-S, ben 86,30 m (*fig. 6.24*). Mostra una larghezza costante di 80 cm ed un'altezza che aumenta gradualmente verso Sud, seguendo il pendio della terrazza su cui sorge la città, fino a raggiungere i 3,60 m.

Lo scavo completo della fognatura ha rivelato l'assenza di scarichi verso il mare e quindi ci ha dimostrato che più che ad una fogna il sistema è assimilabile ad una gigantesca fossa settica nella quale si accumulavano gli scarichi delle latrine ed i resti di pasto provenienti dalle cucine, dalle quali erano gettati nel condotto anche ceramiche ed oggetti che si rompevano quotidianamente durante l'uso. Le pendenze dei piani portavano il sedimento ad accumularsi in un largo braccio E-O che si immetteva nel braccio principale N-S in corrispondenza della fauce n. 2 della palestra. Questo braccio ha una larghezza di ben 1,75 m ed un'altezza circa 3 m. Al momento dello scavo fu scoperto al suo interno un accumulo di sedimento organico di oltre 1,35 m di spessore. Questo deposito era poi periodicamente svuotato ed il sedimento era probabilmente utilizzato per fertilizzare i campi.[66]

Lo scavo stratigrafico completo di questo deposito ci ha permesso di recuperare ben 770 sacchi di deposito organico ed oltre 170 cassette di reperti ceramici interi o in buona parte ricomponibili. La straordinaria ricchezza del deposito organico ci ha spinto a coinvolgere il Prof. Mark Robinson dell'Università di Oxford che si sta occupando dello studio del materiale organico. Una prima campagna di indagini con un'equipe di esperti e studenti dell'Università di Oxford ha portato a setacciare e studiare circa il 10% del deposito organico, permettendo il recupero di moltissimi frammenti di gusci d'uova, semi di papavero, di fico, noccioli di olive, scaglie e lische di pesce, ossa di piccoli animali ed uccelli, larve di grano, di aculei di riccio di mare, e gusci di molluschi. A questo punto la prosecuzione delle analisi permetterà anche di aprire inediti scenari di quantificazione statistica dei diversi alimenti e perfino delle diverse specie di pesci recuperati nel deposito. Di pari passo si sta portando avanti il delicato lavoro di ricomposizione e studio dei reperti ceramici che, allo stesso modo, provengono da un contesto chiuso di grande ricchezza, destinato ad aggiungere altri elementi alle nostre conoscenze sulla circolazione delle ceramiche nell'area vesuviana nel 79 d.C.

La fossa settica dell'*Insula Orientalis* II probabilmente non era il solo sistema fognario esistente lungo il V *Cardo*. Le altre *domus* che si aprivano su questa strada dovevano servirsi di un diverso condotto fognario. Infatti la presenza di un canale di scarico individuabile sotto il primo fornice della terrazza di Nonio Balbo,[67] ed un piccolo tratto di fognatura individuato sotto il marciapiedi E del V *Cardo*, sembrano confermare l'esistenza di un altro percorso fognario, che portava sull'antica spiaggia gli scarichi delle case e delle botteghe delle altre *insulae* che si aprono su questa strada.

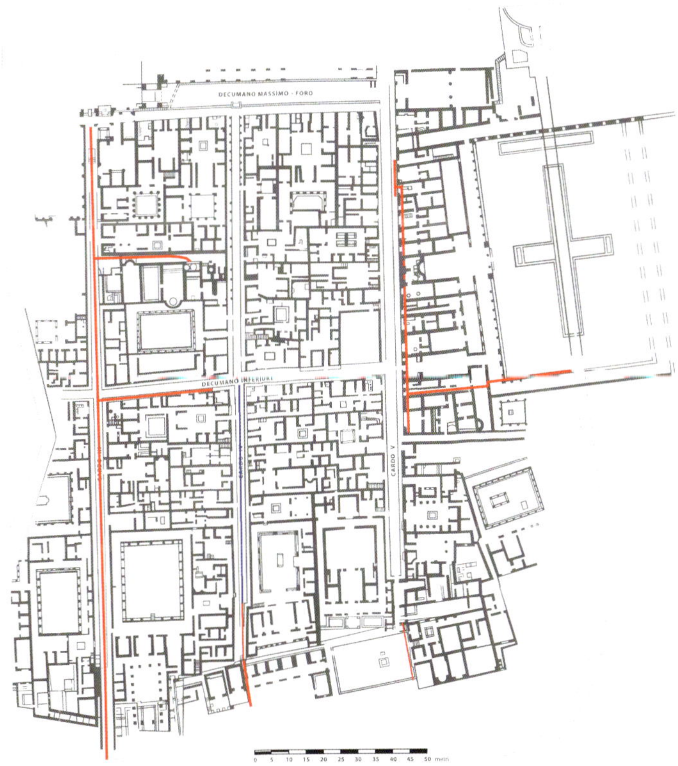

Fig. 6.23.
Planimetria dell'antica Ercolano con evidenziata in rosso la rete fognaria indagata dal Progetto HCP. In blu il tratto ipotizzato sulla base delle indagini geognostiche (disegno D. Camardo).

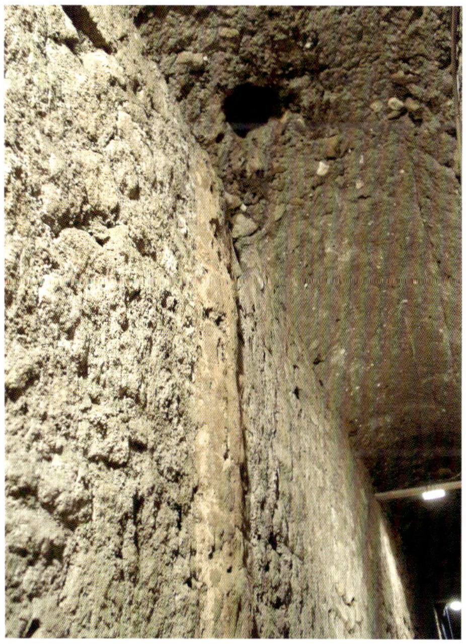

*Fig 6.24. Ercolano, Lo scarico di una latrina all'interno della fossa settica dell'*Insula Orientalis II. *Si riconosce la striscia di materiale organico ancora conservato lungo la parete del condotto (foto D. Camardo).*

Notes

1 For Pompeii see Jansen 1997; for Herculaneum and Ostia, see Jansen 2002a; for Hadrian's villa, see Jansen 2007; for Ephesus see Jansen 2006b.

2 Jansen 2006a.

3 For more information see Jansen 2002a and 2006a.

4 For example, at Ostia the toilet IV iv, 4 behind the *nymphaeum* at the Street of the Round Temple, the toilet behind the large *nymphaeum* at Miletus, and the large toilet next to a street *nymphaeum* at Magnesia. I want to thank Wolfram Letzner for providing two more examples: the agora toilet at Side and the toilet in the Bains des Lutteurs at Saint-Romain-en-Gal.

5 For example, in the House of Amor and Psyche (I xiv, 5) and the House of Fortuna Annonaria (V ii, 8).

6 There is only one indication in classical texts about washing hands in relation to toilet use. In Petronius' *Satyricon* (2.27) there is a reference to washing hands after urinating. We have to be cautious, as this might be a modern projection.

7 Boon 1972, 155 refers to this been found in many British sites. Another good example is the *Nymphaeum* Latrine at Kos - see case study in chapter 5, pp. 64-65.

8 Comprehensive studies on the subject have still to be published. Hallier/Humbert/Pomay (1982, 61) give for the public toilet of Bolsena an inclination of 4%. The average slope of the drainage channels in the toilets of Hadrian's villa is approximately 30 cm per toilet (Jansen 2007, 171). The average slope at the toilets of Ephesus is 50 cm per toilet drain (under study by Jansen).

9 The floor of the drainage channel of the toilet of the Scholastikia baths at Ephesus is more than 3 m below floor level. The same goes for the latrine channel of Hadrian's Baths of Lepcis Magna (see Bartoccini, 1929, table IV). This is rather deep for a Roman toilet, the average depth of these channels at Ephesus is 1.2 m. The drainage channel underneath the seats of the Roman agora toilet at Athens is 1.8 m deep and much more normal, see Travlos 1971, 342-343.

10 We do not know to what level this gutter was filled with water. For Hadrian's villa see Jansen 2007, 171. The measurements from Ephesus are still under study by Jansen.

11 Although waste water from elsewhere was discharged in some drainage channels, this was not done to flush the toilet, but rather to find an easy way to dispose of that water in an already existing drain. This disposal can be deduced from the fact that waste water drained randomly into the channel and not at the far end where it could be helping to flush the toilet gutter.

12 Jansen 2007, 171-174. Ephesus has also continuous flush toilets in private context.

13 For household toilets at Pompeii see Jansen 1997 and Hobson in chapter 5, pp. 53-54.

14 Jansen 2000c.

15 See Scobie 1986, 412 n. 104 and 105.

16 First example is the late antique toilet in a house west of the Bouleuterion, the other is in toilet 2a in Hanghaus 2, 1.

17 Latrines are only briefly mentioned in studies on baths. Neudecker (1994, 83-91) is one of the first to dedicate a whole chapter to this special type, although mainly focusing on non-technical topics. For a more exhaustive study on the hydro-techniques of Roman baths, see Garbrecht/Manderscheid 1994 and Manderscheid 2000, 467-535.

18 For a summary of the comprehensive study 'The latrines in and near the Roman baths of Italy' see Van Vaerenbergh 2006, 453-459.

19 Pompeii: Stabian Baths (VII 1, 8): 1 (2?) latrine(s); Forum Baths (VII 5): 2 latrines; Central Baths (IX 4,5.10.18): 1 latrine; Palestra Baths (VIII 2, 23): 1 latrine; Baths of the *Praedia* of Iulia Felix (II 4): 1 latrine; Suburban Baths (VII 16, a): 1 latrine. Ostia: Baths of Neptune (II iv, 2): 3 latrines; Forum Baths (I xii, 6): 3 latrines; Baths of the Swimmer (V x, 3): 2 latrines; Baths of the Seven Sages (III x, 2): 3 latrine; Baths of Mithra (I, xvii, 2): 1 urinal; Baths of the Philosopher (V ii, 7): 1 latrine. Rome: Baptisterium baths: 1 latrine; Palace baths of Maxentius: 1 latrine; Substructures, Baths of Domus Tiberiana: 1 latrine; Baths of Trajan: 2? latrines; Baths of Caracalla: 2? latrines; Baths of Diocletian: 2 latrines; Baths of the Arvales: 1 (2?) latrine(s). Tivoli: Small Baths: 1 latrine; Large Baths: 1 latrine. Canosa di Puglia: Lomuscius Baths: 1 latrine; Fiesole: Baths: 1 latrine. Valesio: Mutatio Baths: 1 latrine. Fuorigrotta: Baths of the Via Terracina: 1 latrine. Massaciucolli: Baths of Nero: 1 latrine. Civitavecchia: Taurine Baths: 8 latrines. Agnano: Thermal baths: 4? latrines.

20 Eschebach 1979, 24, 36, 38, 64-73, pl. 26, 67.

21 Eschebach 1991, 261.

22 Maiuri 1939, 188-193.

23 De Haan/Wallat 2006, 418.

24 Parslow 1998, 206.

25 Manderscheid 2000, 467-538.

26 Cf. Schönbeck 1962, 19-27, for the optical and acoustical effects of flowing water within the ideal landscapes of ancient poetry.

27 With thanks to H. Manderscheid for information on his new study on hydro-techniques of the Suburban Baths in Pompeii (Manderscheid 2009).

28 It cannot fully be ruled out that the water flowed over the rim of the bathtub and was drained off by a drain hole into the floor of the room. Nevertheless, none of these drain holes were connected to a latrine.

29 Maiuri 1939, 188-193.

30 This specific system made it possible to open the valve only partially. This would suggest a more regular water flow towards the latrine. Yet the resulting vortex would make it fairly hazardous to use the bath.

31 Manderscheid 2000, 503, 508.

32 Parslow 2000, 208.

33 Boersma et al. 1995, 102-105 (latrine), 222-223, 230 (water provision).

34 Köhler 2000, 190, n. 55; here pp. 121-122. Cf. also Timgad, case study in chapter 7, pp. 106-108.

35 Manderscheid 2000, 509-514, for more information about the hydro-techniques of the thermal baths. Here pp. 121-122.

36 Information on street fountains in Ostia (following examples): Jansen 2002a, 142-145.

37 Ricciardi/Scrinari 1996 II, 227.

38 Since the Forum Baths were built in the second century, it must have been difficult to connect the new toilet to the water disposal of the still functioning baths. The fountain was, therefore, a better water supplier.

39 Ricciardi/Scrinari 1996 II, 65-68.

40 Boersma 1985, 392-393.

41 Jansen 2002a, 135-136.

42 Many times there was a supposed connection, but no proof. This is a result of the often dreadful conservation of many of these tanks. More detailed research is necessary.

43 Ricciardi/Scrinari 1996 I, 106.
44 Eschebach 1979, 32; Oleson 1996, 67-70.
45 The big cistern was built on an earlier construction.
46 Jansen 2003, 142; 2007; Blanco 2007,183-190; Van Vaerenbergh, forthcoming.
47 Krausse 1994, 144, 158-159, 168.
48 As often can be seen in individual kitchen toilets.
49 Jansen 2003, 142, 149; 2007, 171.
50 Jansen 2002a, 68-70.
51 Within the studied dataset mentioned in the introduction of this chapter.
52 This hypothesis has been put forward by Parslow 2000, 208. Since we know that in Roman times faeces were collected to use as manure, the theory of fertilizing the *hortus* in the *Praedia* of Iulia Felix with human sewage seems very plausible. In Belgium people still use human faeces from their cesspits as manure in their vegetable gardens and on fields.
53 Possibly in combination with the need for more service quarters (Carandini et al. 1973, 30.).
54 Carandini et al. 1973, 26-31, 91-93.
55 It is not clear from where this additional flush water came. Probably it arrived through a partition wall, which was demolished in a later phase. Anyhow the amount of water must have been very limited.
56 The archaeological objects found in the deposits are mostly in fragments: ceramics (fine and common ware and oil lamps), glass vessels, metal objects and coins (Carandini et al. 1973, 30, 78-82 (Strato IIIA), 87-89 (Strato IVA)). Possibly, a considerable number of the artifacts originated from other places in the bath complex and were transported here by the water flow. Another part may have sunk down from the final deposit of fill, after the latrine was closed down. For the situation I personally discovered at the excavation of the latrine of the Small Baths in Hadrian's Villa at Tivoli, see Van Vaerenbergh, forthcoming.
57 Jansen 2003, 142; 2007; Blanco 2007, 183-190; Van Vaerenbergh, forthcoming.
58 Such an approach has been carried out in the recent excavation of the latrine channel in the latrine of the Small Baths in Hadrian's villa. See Van Vaerenbergh, forthcoming. As a result, the specific way this exceptional latrine functioned can be reconstructed. Unfortunately, bad preservation conditions have made it impossible to obtain results from the archaeobotanical analyses.
59 Décor mentionné in Barbet 2008, 296. Les peintures sont en cours d'étude par Claudine Allag (CEPMR de Soissons CNRS-ENS E). Sur les peintures dans les latrines v. la contribution d'E.M. Moormann, Ch. 5.2.
60 Questa ricerca si è sviluppata nell'ambito dei lavori dell'*Herculaneum Conservation Project* in corso di realizzazione da parte del Packard Humanities Institute e della Soprintendenza Archeologica di Pompei, della British School at Rome. Il Progetto è diretto dal Prof. Andrew Wallace Hadrill e si avvale della direzione scientifica della Dott.ssa Maria Paola Guidobaldi, Direttrice degli Scavi di Ercolano.
61 Un buon esempio in tal senso è una latrina recentemente scavata che si trova nell'ambiente 4 della casa IV, 18. Questa, situata in un sottoscala, si presenta come una tipica latrina ad acqua con pavimentazione in tegole e con bordo in cocciopesto. Gli scarichi erano incanalati tramite un tubo in un pozzo di forma circolare sottostante. La copertura del pozzo era stata realizzata ponendo in posizione orizzontale sull'imboccatura del pozzo un'anfora del tipo Dressel 2/4, sulla quale era stato poi posto un piano di tegole rivestito di malta. Tale apprestamento rendeva semplice la riapertura del pozzo per la manutenzione o per lo svuotamento. Infatti per la natura compatta e poco permeabile del sottosuolo di Ercolano non si aveva un buon funzionamento dei pozzi neri o d'assorbimento collegati alle latrine, che dovevano essere periodicamente svuotati. Una prova in tal senso è nell'iscrizione *Exemta ste(r)cora a(ssibus) XI* ('il pozzo nero è stato svuotato per 11 assi'), trovata presso una delle colonne del peristilio della Casa del salone nero (*CIL* IV suppl. 3.4.10606; Jansen 2000b, 43).
62 La fogna del III *Cardo* è stata recentemente completamente ripulita nel corso dei lavori dell'*Herculaneum Conservation Project* che hanno realizzato una completa mappatura degli scarichi presenti nella stessa aprendo notevoli prospettive di ricerca per lo studio dello smaltimento delle acque di questo settore della città.
63 Maiuri 1958, 50.
64 Guidobaldi et al. 2006, 10-11.
65 Ercolano - Diari di scavo, 20 ottobre 1932. Questo ramo fognario è stato negli ultimi mesi parzialmente ripulito e si è potuto verificare il collegamento diretto alla fogna esistente sotto il III *Cardo*.
66 Arthur 1993, 195.
67 Pagano 1993, 596 n. 12.

7

Urination and Defecation Roman-Style

7.1 Introduction *(Andrew Wilson)*

This chapter is concerned with people's behavior and experience of bodily evacuation between entering and leaving the toilet, across the full spectrum of private to public toilets in the Roman world.[1] Our written sources for this aspect of latrine use, while of some help, are relatively meagre (see Thüry, chapter 4.1, pp. 43-47), and much of the reconstruction has to rely on a close reading of the archaeological evidence. Inevitably, this is weighted towards the multi-seater public latrines (*foricae*), since being larger and more monumentally built they are more likely to preserve incidental details that can provide clues to behavior, but many of the insights thus gained can be transferred to less public settings also.

7.2 Children

Once children were of an age when they were toilet trained they could use the same toilets as adults, though at first small children (two to three years) might have to be held in place by an adult. Before this age we have little evidence, and what we have is more abundant for the ancient Greek world than the Roman world. We do not know when children were toilet trained (probably earlier than many modern children in the Western world whose highly absorbent nappies shield them from much of the discomfort of a wet nappy) - perhaps around two years in the case of girls and a little later for boys. Toddlers, at least in the warmer parts of the Roman empire, could be left to run around much of the time without any nappy on, and it would be easier to clean up after them than to clean any kind of cloth nappy. Ancient texts refer more to swaddling clothes for newborns than to cloth diapers for babies;[2] nappies may have been used, but must have been difficult and unpleasant to wash by hand in a world with limited detergents.[3] Several Greek vases of the 5th century BC depict a small child in a kind of potty-cum-high chair, and one complete and several fragmentary examples, some dating back to the 7th century BC, have been found in the Athenian Agora excavations (see chapter 3.3, pp. 25-28),[4] but no counterpart is known from the Roman world; the known portable toilets and chamberpots are all designed for adults.

7.3 Chamberpots

The simplest forms of toilet provision were pisspots and chamberpots (Greek ἀμίς or λάσανον; Latin *matella, matellio, matula, scaphium, lasanum*), which had the advantage that they did not need a dedicated, built space and could (in theory) be used anywhere.[5] Latin terminology distinguishes between a pisspot for a man (*matella*), a pisspot for a woman (*scaphium*), and a chamberpot used by both sexes for defecation (*lasanum*); presumably they had different shapes, the *scaphium* being a shallower bowl than the *lasanum*, and the *matella* probably a narrower-necked vessel, perhaps having a handle so it could be held while standing (as in the *Satyricon* passage discussed below).[6] One imagines that the bedroom was the commonest place for chamberpot use. In Pompeii a graffito in VIII 7, 6 purports to record the unhappy consequences of equipment shortage in an inn (*CIL* IV.4957):

> *Miximus in lecto. Fateor, peccavimus, hospes.*
> *Si dices: Quare? Nulla matella fuit.*
> 'We've peed in the bed. Host, I admit - we've done wrong.
> If you ask: Why? There was no pisspot.'

Since this is clearly an elegiac couplet, however, the graffito might simply be an epigram current at the time.[7]

The chamberpot is revealing of the extent to which slave-owning Romans might expect to be waited on hand and foot - there are numerous references in literature to slaves being summoned to bring a pisspot and hold it for people as it was used. Martial's epigram (14.119) on a clay *matella* gives the idea:[8]

> *matella fictilis*
> *Dum poscor crepitu digitorum et verna moratur,*
> *O quotiens paelex culcita facta mea est!*
> While I am summoned with a snap of the fingers and the slave delays, oh, how often has a mattress become my rival!

If the lack of private latrines or cesspits in elite houses at Volubilis (Mauretania Tingitana) is real rather than apparent (the site was poorly excavated and some evidence may have been missed), it is possible that the houseowners simply relied on slaves bringing them chamberpots as and when necessary.[9] But while the use of chamberpots was clearly necessary in houses or premises without built latrines, Petronius' *Satyricon* (27.3-6) contains a remarkable scene in which the vulgar freedman Trimalchio, playing ball in the *palaestra* of the public baths, urinates into a silver chamberpot held for him by a eunuch slave:

> *nam duo spadones in diversa parte circuli stabant, quorum alter matellam tenebat argenteam, alter numerabat pilas ... etiamnum loquebatur Menelaus, cum Trimalchio digitos concrepuit, ad quod signum matellam spado ludenti subiecit. exonerata ille vesica aquam poposcit ad manus, digitosque paululum adspersos in capite pueri tersit.*
> For two eunuchs were standing on the opposite side of the group, of whom one held a silver chamberpot and the other was counting the balls ... Menelaus was still speaking, when Trimalchio clicked his fingers, at which signal the eunuch held the chamberpot out for him as he played. When he had relieved his bladder he called for water for his hands, sprinkled a little on his fingers and wiped them on the head of the boy.

The scene occurs in a set of public baths - a type of establishment regularly equipped with latrines, but Trimalchio simply cannot be bothered to break off his game and go to them. His use of a silver vessel is as grossly ostentatious as his public micturition; most chamberpots were bronze (Juvenal 10.64) or ceramic, and the use of precious metal for them becomes something of a trope in discourses on luxury (e.g. Pliny; *NH* 33.14.152 on silver chamberpots). Golden chamberpots are the ultimate extravagance:

> *Messalla orator prodidit Antonium triumvirum aureis usum vasis in omnibus obscenis desideriis, pudendo crimine etiam Cleopatrae ... Antonius solus contumelia natura vilitatem auro fecit*
> The orator Messalla has told us that the triumvir Antony used vessels of gold in satisfying all the indecent necessities – an enormity that even Cleopatra would have been ashamed of. ... Antony alone cheapened gold by this contumely of nature (Pliny *NH* 33.14.50, Loeb translation).

Golden chamberpots are ridiculed also by Martial (*Ep.* 1.37):

> *ventris onus misero, nec te pudet, excipis auro,*
> *Basse, bibis vitro: carius ergo cacas.*
> You receive your belly's load, Bassa, in unlucky gold, and are not ashamed of it, but you drink out of glass. So you shit more expensively.[10]

The theme recurs in *SHA Elagabalus* 32.2:

> *onus ventris auro excepit, in murrinis et onychis minxit.*
> he received the load of his belly in gold, and urinated into fluorspar and onyx vessels.[11]

It is picked up by early Christian writers as part of their general discourse against consumer luxury and a concern with material goods.[12] Clement of Alexandria derides men who carry around silver urinals and alabaster chamberpots with them 'like personal advisors', and the use of gold chamberpots by 'rich but stupid women' (*Paedagogus* 2.3. 39.2-3). An anecdote in the *Life of St Theodore of Sykeon* (ch. 42), who lived in the late 6th century AD, tells how a chalice and paten made of silver turned black when used for communion in Theodore's monastery because the silver had been recycled from a prostitute's chamber pot. Notwithstanding the element of rhetorical exaggeration in such passages from pagan and Christian moralists, the *Digest* shows that silver chamberpots were actually in use to the extent that it was worth ruling on whether they were to be considered part of a legacy of silver:

> *argento legato non puto ventris causa habita scafia contineri, quia argenti numero non habentur.*
> I do not believe that chamberpots are included in a legacy of silver, because they are not considered part of the silver collection (34.2.27.5, Ulpian; trans. Watson).

The poet Juvenal makes it clear that in densely populated cities like Rome, empyting chamberpots from the upper storeys of apartment buildings into the street was a common practice, resulting in nuisance and sometimes injuries for passers-by (Juvenal, *Sat.* 3.276-277). *Digest* 9.3 and 44.7.5.5 deal with the general hazards of things being thrown out of apartments and buildings into streets or public places.[13] A rescript of Augustus (6 BC) to the town of Knidos passes judgement in a case where a house was besieged for three nights by angry neighbors, until the owner instructed a slave to throw excrement on the besiegers to drive them off. The slave, either inadvertently or by design, threw the pot as well as its contents and killed one of them; Augustus' judgement exonerates the defendants on the grounds they were acting in self-defence, and one detects in the closing sentences of the letter a note of annoyance that the town council has bothered him with such a case.[14]

Despite the numerous references to chamberpots in the written sources, archaeologists have been slow to identify them in the material record. Ceramic examples, however, are known from an early 3rd-century AD domestic latrine fill at Ordona, and also from Luni, Ostia, Agrigento, Pollentia (Spain), sites on Cyprus,[15] and now *Carnuntum* (see here below). They are tall tapering vessels with an ovoid mouth and a wide rim to sit on; the homogeneity of their form suggests mass production, and they may well have been widely traded, though apart from the demonstration that the *Carnuntum* chamberpots were lovelly produced, I am not aware that any petrological provenancing studies have yet been undertaken that might address this question. If the distinctions that seem apparent in Latin terminology are to be applied to these artefacts, they would seem to be *lasana* rather than *matellae* or *scaphiae*.

Case Study: Chamberpots from the Civil Town of *Carnuntum*. Excavations at the '*Weststrasse*' (*Silvia Radbauer & Beatrix Petznek*)

Several chamberpots were found during excavations in the civil settlement of *Carnuntum* (preserved in the Archaeological Park Carnuntum, Austria; *figs 7.1-2*). The finds were made in the urban center on the '*Weststraße*' in the infrastructure under the street.[16] A number of fragmented, but complete chamberpots came from two sewers with different construction dates and different times of going out of use: one sewer was filled up during the third quarter of the 2nd century AD; the other was built later and clogged up with settlement deposits during the last quarter of the 3rd century AD. The settlement refuse in the sewers was plentiful, well preserved, and contained both private and commercial objects from the surrounding dwellings and neighboring bathhouse. Fragments of chamberpots were also found in the massive levelling layers of the street. These small sherds belonged to settlement refuse that had been redeposited several times within the fill.

Because of the well-dated, closed contexts of the finds, a typological development of the form of the chamberpots can be determined, which runs from the late 2nd to the late 3rd century AD. We can note a clear development in both the form of the body and the rim as well as changes in material.

The chamberpots - λάσανα - manufactured in the second half of the 2nd century AD usually are very large, high and conically oval vessels with a round base and wide, flat, oval rims. The rim is frequently thicker on the outside. Two shallow grooves usually decorate the upper side of the rim. Because of the oval form, the diameter of the rim varies between 26-40 cm, while the height is ca 31 cm. Some chamberpots have a support on the inner side of the rim to widen and reduce the seat. The steep vessel walls taper from the oval rims to the bases giving these vessels their conical form. The uniform thickness of the vessel walls is ca 1 cm. The bases are round and were turned on potters' wheels. They have a diameter of ca 20 cm and are slightly concave. The capacity of one whole pot is around 11 liters, while the height of the incrustations on the inside shows that it was usually filled with ca 1-2 liters.

The chamberpots from the sewer filled up in the late 3rd century resemble common vessels and are usually characterized by a large, bellied vessel form with a round base and a flat rim. Rims are raised like a funnel and sometimes decorated with two shallow grooves. The mouths are slightly oval, and the diameter of the rims are 27-28 cm with vessel heights of 25 cm. The upper vessel walls are bellied and taper somewhat to the base. The thickness of the vessel walls is between 0.8-1.0 cm, with the base being a bit thicker. The round bases have a diameter of ca 11 cm and are slightly concave. The capacity of the pots is ca 7 liters.

Some characteristic features indicate the use of these vessels as chamberpots. Analyses of incrustations on the inside of the chamberpots, especially on the base and the lower vessel wall which reach up to ca 4 cm, also give some indication of their usage (see contribution below). The production took place in the potteries of *Carnuntum* with clay also used for coarse wares on a fast rotating wheel. The upper part of the chamberpots was pressed into an oval form after turning, providing a comfortable seat. There are no handles on the pots. The vessels were fired in an oxidizing atmosphere, resulting in a fine, homogenous and thoroughly oxidized fabric. The paste is very homogenous, showing few pores, and containing only badly sorted natural temper particles. The temper grains are characterized by a small amount of transparent (or mostly white) fine quartz grains, fine mica flakes, a few carbonate grains and dark red and dark grey iron oxide aggregates. Typologically dissimilar vessels also show slightly different fabrics.

The size and capacity of the chamberpots suggests the use of one pot for several people, perhaps including the members of one family or household. Smaller pots are also common; some of these have a lateral round open attachment on the vessel wall, resembling a spout, but not connected with the vessel interior. This could be used to thrust a wooden stick into it and thus handle the pot. There are no finds of ceramic lids to cover the pots (against the smell). It is possible that wooden lids or textile material were used; but perhaps the pots were left uncovered.

The form of the chamberpots is completely functional and can be found in Italy and the provinces of the Roman Empire as a common Roman vessel form with local typological variants.[17] Direct typological comparisons for the chamberpots of *Carnuntum*[18] can be found in the north eastern provinces, especially in the area of the Danube, in Vransko (*Celeia*, Slovenia), Vienna (*Vindobona*) and Bruckneudorf (both Austria), Budapest (*Aquincum*), Belgrade (*Singidunum*) and Sremska Mitrovica (*Sirmium*, both Serbia), Vinkovce (*Cibalae*, Croatia), Stara Zagora (*Augusta Trajana*) and Dewnja (*Marcianopolis*, both Bulgaria) and Gála Mare (*Drobeta*, Roumania). Chamberpots were also found in Italy at Rimini (*Ariminum*), Ordona (*Herdonia*), Luni (*Ortonovo*), Milan (*Mediolanum*) and Pompeii. The pottery of Carlino in northern Italy produced glazed chamberpots during late Antiquity. In the Mediterranean area chamberpots are known from Carthage, Pollentia (*Pollentia*, Spain), Hyères (*Olbia*, France) and Knossos. Completely different forms of chamberpots, low basins, were found in the Gallic provinces. In all of the listed find places, the chamberpots are concentrated in the residential part of the Roman settlements.

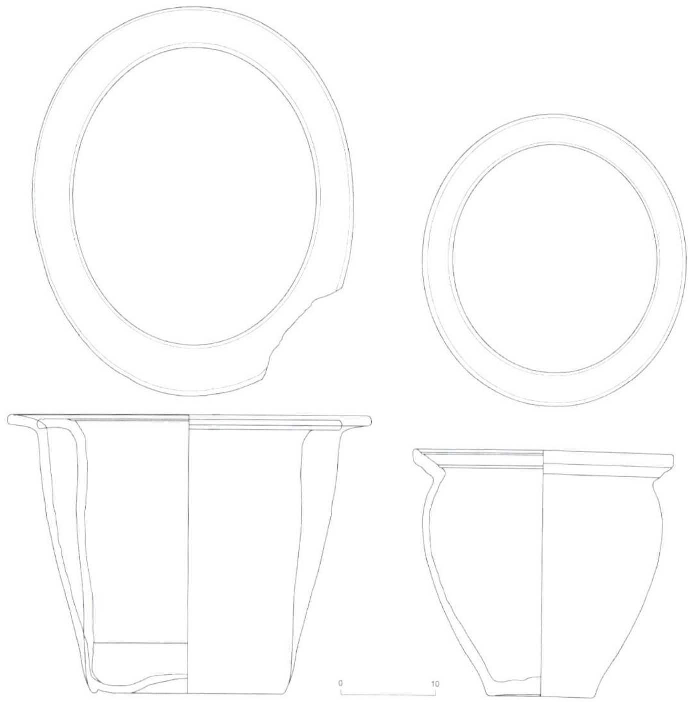

Fig. 7.1. Carnuntum, Weststraße, *chamberpots from the late 2nd (left) and the late 3rd (right) century AD (drawing B. Petznek and S. Radbauer).*

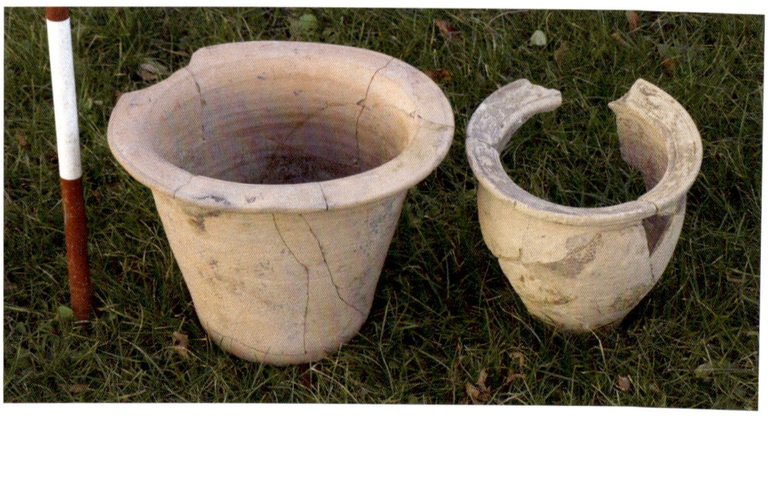

Fig. 7.2. Carnuntum, Weststraße, *chamberpots from the late 2nd (left) and the late 3rd (right) century AD (photo S. Radbauer).*

Case study: Mineralogical Analyses of Incrustations Found on the Interior Part of Some Chamberpots from *Carnuntum* *(Roman Sauer)*

The incrustations were analyzed by microscopic thin sections, X-ray diffraction analysis, and also tested by chemical analyses (*figs 7.3-4*). The incrustations are only patchily preserved. The analysed samples show a layer thickness of approximately 0.5 mm-1.5 mm and show variable, whitish to yellowish to dark brownish colors. An irregular color lamination can be observed in parts of the cross sections. The incrustations also show partly elongated pores of variable pore sizes. The incrustation surfaces and the pores are frequently contaminated by sedimentary material.

The microscopic analysis showed that the incrustations consisted of an intense intergrowth of very fine calcite and practically isotropic phosphate minerals. The phosphate-rich areas frequently show shadows of former, rhombohedral-shaped crystals (size from 86x80 µm up to 270x30 µm). Occasionally the incrustations show inclusions of very fine organic material.

The XRD-analyses showed the presence of poorly crystallised apatite and calcite in all analysed samples. A chemical test also confirmed the presence of abundant phosphorus in all samples.

The outer rims and partially also the pores of the analyzed samples are contaminated with clayish, silt to fine sand sized sedimentary material, composed of clayish material, quartz, feldspar, dolomite and calcite grains, iron oxides, traces of heavy minerals (hornblende). The mineralogical and chemical compositions of the analyzed incrustations seem to be similar to urine stone scalings, frequently occurring in recent sewer systems.

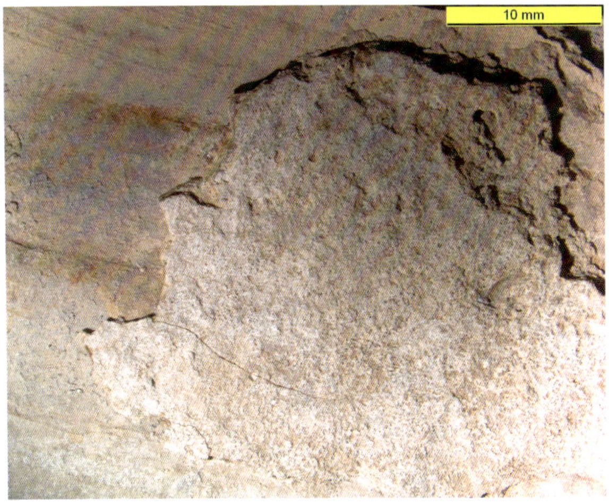

Fig. 7.3.
Carnuntum, Weststraße, *Macro-photograph of an incrustation inside of a chamberpot (photo R. Sauer).*

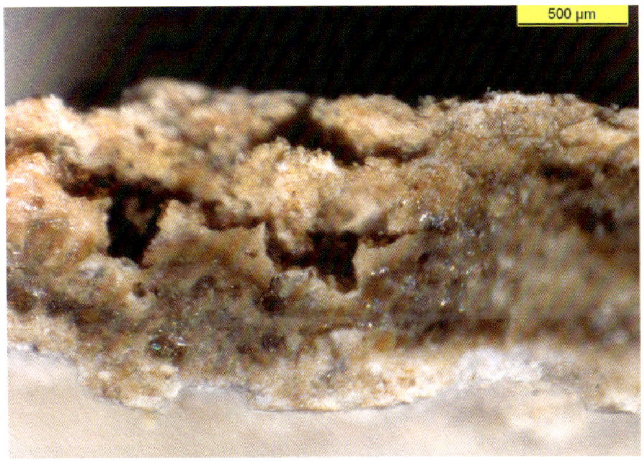

Fig. 7.4. Carnuntum, Weststraße, *chamberpot. Cross section: incrustation consisting of irregular, porous carbonate and phosphate layers (photo R. Sauer).*

7.4 Toilets *(Andrew Wilson)*

As regards constructed toilets, a first question is: how did one find the toilet? There were no signs or visual clues that might have helped a stranger in an unfamiliar town to locate the public latrines, or that might have guided the customer in an inn or the visitor to another person's house to the toilet within the building (carved phalli on buildings sometimes pointed out to tourists at Roman sites as signs to the latrines are simply apotropaic symbols on usually unrelated buildings). The relatively predictable locations of certain toilets must have helped here - public bathhouses, often recognizable by their domed or vaulted roofs would have been obvious places to look; public toilets were also likely to be found near the forum. Ancient cities were physically much smaller than their modern counterparts, so that a stranger from out of town probably faced a less perplexing and complicated search than a visitor trying to locate public conveniences in a modern city; but it must often have been necessary to ask the way. In bars and houses, the common location under a staircase, or down a service corridor must also have provided an obvious place to start looking.

The physical layout of the toilet usually afforded some privacy from external gaze. Despite the fact that public latrines were multi-seater affairs in which people urinated and defecated communally, there was evidently a recognition that people engaged in the act of voiding themselves should be shielded from the view of those who were not, and vice versa. Approach passages and doorways to private latrines therefore often turned a corner to avoid a direct line of sight to the toilet. Talmudic texts indicate the importance, for Jews at least, of establishing whether there was anyone in a single-seater latrine before entering (see Hoss, chapter 4.2, pp. 47-48). Public latrines had doors - the two doors to the possibly 4th-century latrines in the Street of the Latrine at Ostia revolved on pivots in the center of the threshold, minimizing the amount of the interior that could be glimpsed from the street when a person entered or left. Writing in the late 6th century AD, but referring to events in the time of Sidonius Apollinaris (late 5th century), Gregory of Tours relates the story of a wicked priest who died on the toilet and was eventually discovered when the servant who had been waiting outside with a candle became worried when his master failed to reappear, and pulled aside the curtain.[19] The anecdote may be fictitious but suggests that, at the time, a private toilet screened by a curtain was not unusual.

Graffiti on the wall of a room in a toilet complex in Ordona (southern Italy) may have been written by people waiting to use the toilet.[20] Even with public latrines with many seats, (ten to twenty seats are common, and some have up to 80),[21] crowding may sometimes have been a problem - a Jewish text, illustrating both cultural oppression by the Roman authorities and the power of God, purports to relate an incident in which a Roman soldier entered a toilet where all the seats were occupied and forced a rabbi to stand up for him, and was then bitten in the anus by a snake lurking in the toilet (see p. 48).[22]

Some evidence suggests that users may have paid to use public latrines. Besides the fact that the operation, daily cleaning and maintenance of public latrines incurred costs that it would have been desirable to defray, the *Digest* (22.1.17.5) refers to the rental of public latrines by contractors - this would only have been desirable or viable if such contractors received a revenue, which can only have come from the users since such latrines discharged into running sewers rather than cesspits whose contents could be sold (see chapter 10, pp. 147-156). Beyond this, however, our evidence does not go (Vespasian's famous tax on urine cannot refer to the regular operation of public *foricae*, for reasons explored in chapter 10). If payment was made, probably on entering, but perhaps on leaving, there must have been an

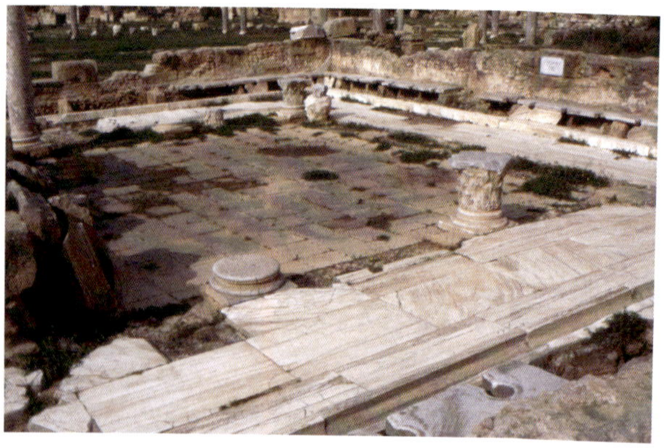

Fig. 7.5. Lepcis Magna, Hadrianic Baths, latrines. Note the distinctly keyhole-shaped plan of the seat apertures (e.g. right foreground) (photo A. Wilson).

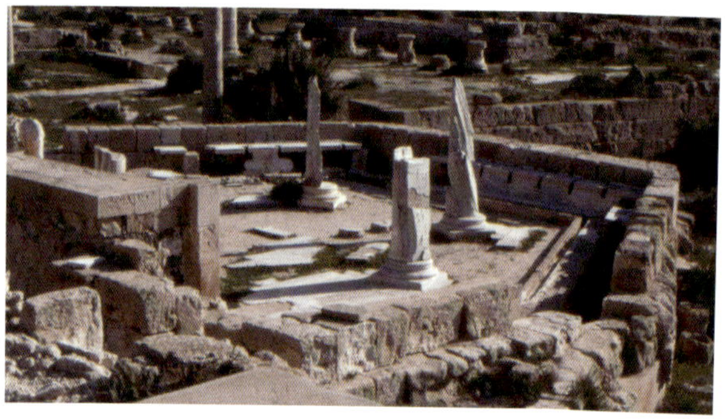

Fig. 7.6. Sabratha, Seaward Baths, latrines (photo A. Wilson).

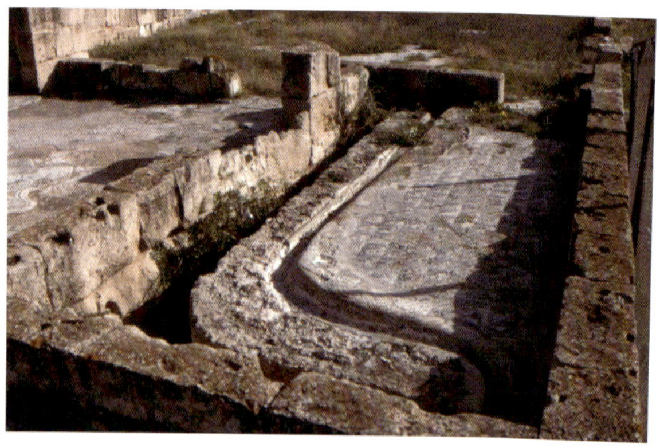

Fig. 7.7. Sabratha, Baths by the Rest House, latrines (photo A. Wilson).

attendant to receive it; he may also have been charged with cleaning the facilities. A parallel of a sort is provided by an inscription from Cirta (modern Constantine) in Numidia, listing valuable items in a monumental public *nymphaeum* - these included chained goblets for people to drink from, and six hand towels, which must have required an attendant to hand out and take back to prevent their being stolen.[23] The forum latrines at Timgad were entered through a vestibule that would have provided space for such an attendant to sit (see below Case Study on Timgad pp. 106-107, see also Kos Case Study pp. 64-66).

Seat Design

It is a cultural choice, not a biological necessity, to sit rather than squat when defecating, and to sit rather than squat or stand when urinating. The traditional custom in the Middle East, Far East and North Africa, and also parts of Mediterranean Europe, of squatting over a toilet which is essentially a hole in the ground, is physiologically more efficient in aiding evacuation than the current Western European habit (apparently a Roman inheritance) of sitting on a seat. Sitting also carries the disadvantage of entailing physical contact with the seat, and with germs or dirt left behind by previous users. Habits of squatting or sitting, fashions of clothing, and modes of cleaning oneself are all interrelated. The Biblical euphemism for defecation, 'covering one's feet', refers precisely to the habit of squatting while wearing a long garment (Judges 3:24 and I Samuel 24:3). It is, in fact, much more convenient to use an Asian-style toilet if one is wearing a loose-fitting robe that can be hoicked up around one's waist, than if one is wearing a Western-style jacket and trousers; conversely, the voluminous folds of a robe are more difficult to keep clear of dirty porcelain, if one is sitting on a Western-style toilet. The position in which one sits or squats, and how one arranges one's clothing, has implications for the relative ease of cleaning oneself - either with hands and water, or wiping with some object or paper. The Roman choice to sit, then, is connected with clothing fashions and with ways of cleaning oneself; and the design of latrine seats is a function of these relationships.

Public latrines, and the larger multi-seater private latrines had seats arranged around three or even four sides of a room (a space being left for the entrance),[24] or along the curved wall of a semi-circular exedra,[25] set over a drain to carry away the excreta (*figs 7.5-6*). A gutter, of U-shaped cross section, ran around the room in front of the users' feet, and provided water which people used somehow to clean themselves - exactly how will be discussed below. Usually this gutter was carved into stone blocks or in the slabs on the floor; sometimes it was a simple channel in an *opus signinum* or mosaic floor (as, respectively, in the latrine in Room 21 in the villa at Oplontis (*fig. 5.6*), or in the baths at Sabratha, baths behind the Rest House, to the south of the main excavated area (*fig. 7.7*).[26] Importantly, there is no regular provision in public or private latrines for a separate urinal (the evidence for possible urinal jars in the street, separate from *foricae*, is dealt with in chapter 10). The implication is that Roman men, like women today, often sat on the toilet even when just urinating. A tunic would present little problem, but urinating standing up while wearing a toga would be rather difficult. Men and women therefore sat on the toilet seat, hoisting up their tunic, toga or *stola* around their waist at the back, but presumably letting it fall in front. In practice, this would mean that people would reveal very little of their private parts even while sitting in a communal latrine, and makes the idea of men and women sharing the same public latrines less shocking than it at first sight appears (see chapter 8.2, pp. 117-118).

In the Mediterranean and Near East the seats in public or private latrines were usually of stone; in the north-western provinces they were more usually of wood, both for reasons of availability of materials and because in northern Europe it would often have been unpleasantly cold to rest one's bare buttocks on stone seats. In the Mediterranean region marble was often although not invariably used; its fine grain and smooth surface was both more comfortable, and easier to clean. Sometimes seats in public latrines might be provided with grandiose dolphin-shaped armrests; and two late antique toilet thrones in *rosso antico*, used in the middle ages in Papal coronations in the Lateran Palace, may have come from a late Roman imperial property (Case Study below on Timgad; Case Study at chapter 12 on porphyry thrones, pp. 187-189). At Ephesus the space allotted per user varied between 46 and 58 cm.[27] Two seats in the latrines by the forum at Timgad are double-width seats, with only one hole in the same space as occupied by the pairs of seats elsewhere in the room (normally 60 cm per person).

The upper surface of a Roman latrine seat had a circular hole connected by a gap to a vertical slot running part-way down the front wall of the seat (*fig. 7.8*). Since there was not space at the back of the toilet seat to insert one's hand to wipe one's bottom, this gap in the front was presumably designed to enable the user to insert something to clean the anus with - his or her hand, either wetted with water or holding something to wipe

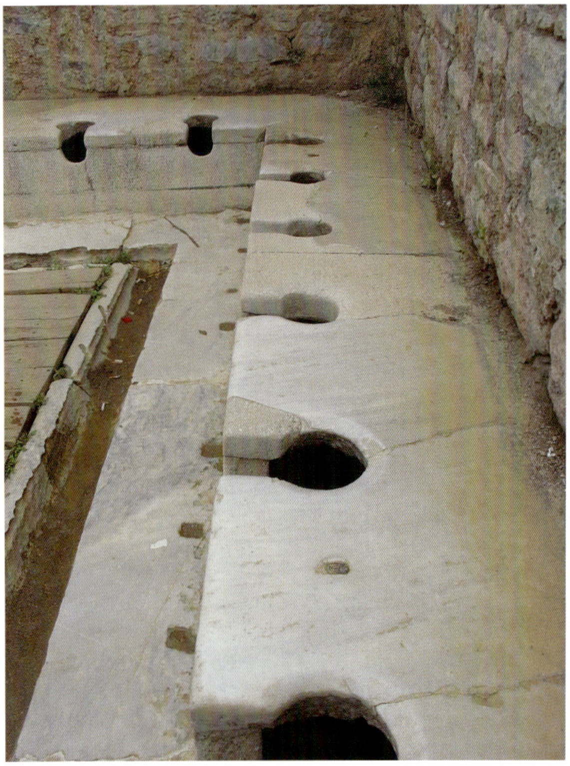

Fig. 7.8. Ephesus, Vedius Baths, latrines with remains of metal stanchions between some of the seats (photo G. Wiplinger).

with, or to insert a sponge on a stick. The front slots in many toilets in North Africa, for example at Dougga or Sabratha, are very narrow (*fig. 7.9*), while at Timgad the slot is reduced to a shallow groove in the top surface of the seat; in all these cases it would have been virtually impossible to insert one's hand, and this design clearly facilitated the use of a sponge on a stick for cleaning oneself (see below). Elsewhere, however, the front slots are often wider - as at Ephesus (*fig. 7.8*) and would have allowed the insertion either of one's hand or a sponge on a stick. At Lepcis Magna the seats in the latrines of the Hadrianic Baths have a slot wider at the front of the seat than towards the circular hole, giving the aperture a keyhole shape (*fig. 7.5*).

Cleaning Oneself

There were a number of different ways of cleaning oneself after going to the toilet, and there may indeed have been regional diversity of practice. The use of parchment or papyrus for wiping is possibly implied by Catullus's disparaging refer-

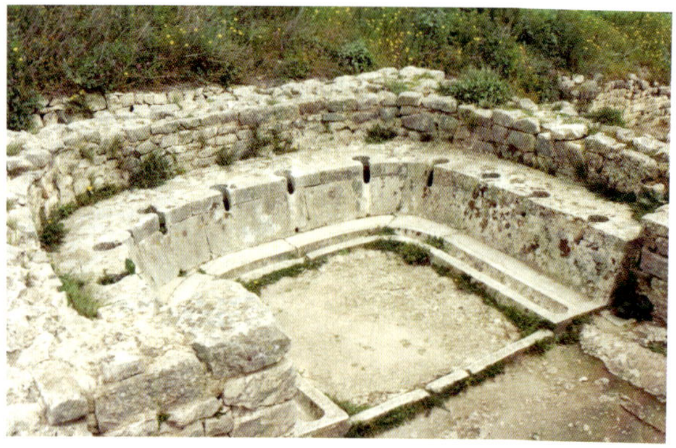

Fig. 7.9. Dougga, Baths of the Cyclops, latrines (photo A. Wilson).

ence (poem 36) to the works of one of his poetic rivals as *cacata carta* - 'beshitted sheets' - but the expense of those materials must have meant that if they were used at all as toilet paper it was rare. Aristophanes (*Frogs* 478-90) has Dionysos wipe himself with a sponge after he has fouled himself in fear. Ancient Greek sources also refer to the use of stones for wiping, and it has been speculated that potsherds may also have been used for this purpose.[28] The Jerusalem Talmud mentions the use of stones, potsherds and grass as wipes, and specifies that the left hand was used for wiping (see Hoss, p. 47).[29] Potsherds found in latrine cesspits do not in themselves provide proof that sherds were used for wiping, since latrines were also used for the disposal of general household waste. It is possible, however, (though not at all certain) that potsherds and shells found in concreted deposits in downspouts from upper-floor toilets at Pompeii may be evidence for this practice, since these toilets are less likely to have been used for the disposal of kitchen scraps.[30]

Papyrus, potsherds or shells are what might be called dry wipes, and particularly suited to use in toilets without running water. But public toilets, and many private toilets, had running water and these toilets usually have a gutter in the floor in front of the seats. There is some debate over the function of this channel, and its connection with the sponge sticks attested as a piece of Roman latrine equipment. The gutter is clearly separate from any arrangement to carry away spilt urine,[31] for reasons discussed below, and as a separate washbasin was generally provided for washing hands, it does not seem to have been for this function either. Where the supply to this channel can be traced, it usually comes from the overflow of the hand-washing basin in the room, and thus supplied water with which one could clean oneself. One way of doing this might have been simply by dipping one's hand into the gutter, and scooping up water with which to wash one's bottom. Small jars or dipper juglets found in some latrines may also have served this purpose.[32] It has been suggested that traces of metal stanchions between each pair of seats in the latrine next to the Vedius Baths at Ephesus may possibly have been for holding inverted juglets when not in use (*fig. 7.8*).[33]

The other possible, and much debated, method of cleaning oneself which would have required water is the famous sponge on a stick, which almost every schoolchild learns was the Roman equivalent of toilet paper. In this case the gutter running in front of the latrine seats would have served to moisten the sponge before use, and for rinsing it off afterwards. Yet despite the fact that the sponge stick is one of the aspects of ancient toilet culture where, at first sight, we appear to have texts that tell us what happened, a number of scholars have doubted the use of this instrument.[34] The primary evidence consists of three texts associating sponges on sticks in some way with toilets or excretion; another text refers to a sponge stick metaphorically, but without making an explicit connection with toilets. Sponges on sticks also appear in ancient veterinary texts as implements for applying ointment to open sores on an animal.[35]

The first, and most explicit, piece of evidence is Seneca *Epistles* 70.20, an anecdote about a German who committed suicide by choking himself with a sponge stick in a latrine rather than face the animals in the arena:

> *nuper in ludo bestiariorum unus e Germanis, cum ad matutina spectacula pararetur, secessit ad exonerandum corpus: nullum aliud illi dabatur sine custode secretum: ibi lignum id, quod ad emundanda obscena adhaerente spongia positum est, totum in gulam farsit et interclusis faucibus spiritum elisit. Hoc fuit morti contumeliam facere.*

A more passing reference is in Martial, *Epig.* 12.48.7-8: where a fine dinner soon will be

> *quod sciat infelix damnatae spongea virgae,*
> *vel quicumque canis iunctaque testa viae*
> what the luckless sponge on a damned stick, or some dog or a pot placed by the roadside will know about.

In the Baths of the Seven Sages at Ostia, in the lower register beneath the figure of Thales, one of the texts representing conversation between people who are apparently seated on a toilet reads *verbose tibi / nemo / dicit dum Priscianus / [u]taris xylosphongio nos / [a?]quas*.[36] The precise meaning is obscure; it has been interpreted (taking Priscianus as nominative for vocative) as 'Nobody gives you a long lecture, Priscianus, as long as you use the sponge-stick' - but the rendering of *verbose dicere* as 'to give a long lecture' is unsatisfactory, and leaves *nos aquas* unaccounted for.[37] Clearly something is elided in the phrase, and J.N. Adams suggests, with ellipsis of *dare* (common in vulgar Latin), some interpretation such as: 'Nobody talks to you much, Priscianus, until you are using the sponge-stick; [let] us [give you some] water' - the implication being that Priscianus stinks until he has cleaned himself up.[38] Whatever the precise meaning, the context again suggests that the use of the sponge stick has something to do with cleansing after defecation.

One other text refers to sponge-sticks, but without illuminating their use. In a papyrus letter of the early 2nd century AD the writer, Claudius Terentianus, reporting a contretemps with one Saturninus, uses the word figuratively to mean something vile or of no value: *non magis quravit me pro xylesphongium sed sum negotium et circa res suas* ('He did not care for me more than for a sponge-stick, but only about his business and his things' - equivalent to saying 'he treated me like shit').[39]

It is possible that the scene in the Gospel accounts of the Crucifixion,[40] when one of the onlookers puts a sponge dipped in vinegar on a reed and offers it to Jesus is intended to recall the *xylosphongium* of Roman latrines. Although in the Victorian and later tradition this has been seen as an act of charity, a bitter liquid is anything but comfort when one is in pain, and if the sponge on a stick was normally seen as a piece of latrine equipment intimately associated with excrement, it is conceivable that it was intended to represent the ultimate humiliation. Against this interpretation, however, is the fact that sour wine was a common drink and that the implement in the Gospel accounts is not a ready-made sponge stick, but a sponge which, naturally, has to be put on a reed in order to get the liquid up to Jesus on the cross.

The direct archaeological evidence - as opposed to the indirect evidence provided by the gutter in front of the latrine seats - is limited to occasional finds of sponge spicules in some sewer, latrine, or refuse contexts. Here the rarity of finds may be largely due to the scarcity of thorough excavations of latrines that have analyzed deposits for organic or biological remains. Both freshwater and marine sponge spicules were found in the fortress main sewer at York; the freshwater sponge spicules are unlikely to have come from toilet sponges, but the marine sponge spicules, found 'in quantity', probably did.[41]

The passage of Seneca implies that sponge sticks were normally kept in the latrines, presumably for communal use, and at the latrines of the Baths of the Cyclops at Thugga a circular depression in the floor by the end of the gutter has been interpreted as the rest for a sponge stick when not in use (Case Study on Thugga below p. 109).[42] Jansen interprets masonry basins at floor level in toilets at Pompeii, Herculaneum and Ostia as for rinsing out sponge sticks rather than as hand-washing basins (see below), since most are at floor level.[43] In the House of the Faun at Pompeii, there is a toilet with a masonry basin supplied originally from the urban water network by a now-robbed lead pipe,[44] while a further three private toilets have masonry basins which were not connected to the water supply network.[45] A couple of examples are known from Herculaneum.[46] Five are known from Ostia, all ultimately connected to the urban supply network, although the one in the House of Fortuna Annonaria received its water indirectly, via the overflow from the elaborate domestic *nymphaeum*.[47] At least one of the Ostian examples, however, is at waist height and might better be seen as a hand-washing basin. Elsewhere sponge sticks might, for example, have stood in a bucket or jar. The hygienic implications, of course, of using a communal sponge stick rinsed only in water need no spelling out; this is the practical downside of the grandiose and visually impressive public latrines. This, perhaps, is one of the reasons why the idea of the Romans using sponges on sticks to wipe themselves with has met with some scholarly resistance.

Spillages

The design of seats, with a slot at the front, will also have had a secondary advantage of avoiding drops of urine being left on the front of the seat as the user - male or female - gets up from the toilet. Specific provision for dealing with urine spillages to the front of the seats was made in several public latrines - in the latrines by the forum at Timgad drain slits in the floor in front of each seat, between the user's legs, seem intended for this purpose (see Case Study on Timgad below pp. 106-108), while in the latrines of the Baths of the Cyclops at Thugga spillages were prevented from entering the gutter in front of the seats by a raised border, and the space between the seat and the gutter sloped backwards towards the seats to allow any spillages to drain into the sewer through small drain holes at the base of the seat wall (see p. 109).[48]

Flushing

In public latrines, and those multi-seater private latrines either connected to a private bathhouse or (as at Timgad) set over a street drain, flushing may have been either continuous or periodic according to whether the latrine sewer was connected to a continuously overflowing public bath (or fountains), or to a bath which was periodically emptied (see Van Vaerenbergh at chapter 6.5, pp. 84-86). In either case, however, from the user's point of view flushing was automatic and did not require intervention on his or her part. Domestic latrines connected to cesspits, however, would need to be flushed by means of a jug or bucket, and these often have a tiled floor that slopes to an opening beneath the latrine seat.[49] A drain with a sloping tiled surface on one side, in a villa at San Giovanni di Ruoti in Basilicata, is probably a small latrine of this type, despite its publication by the excavators as a water-mill.[50] The question of flushing sewers and emptying cesspits is explored more fully in chapter 6, pp. 71-86.

Washbasins

Most public latrines preserve some evidence for arrangements for washing hands after one had finished going to the toilet, arrangements which are separate from the gutter in front of the seats. A washbasin was usually placed either against the wall not occupied by seats, near the entrance, or centrally in the room (Housesteads). At Thugga (see p. 109) the design of the basin, plastered and on a pedestal, looks surprisingly modern. In the Antonine Baths at Carthage a shattered marble basin lies in the exedral latrines on the western side of the complex (*fig. 7.10*). In these cases, where basins were evidently set on a pedestal to be used at waist height, their interpretation as hand-washing basins seems secure. In other latrines the same use may be inferred by analogy; but in some latrines a basin in the same general position in the room may take the form of a stone tank, often set rather lower than the pedestal basins (Housesteads, Timgad, latrines near forum). These basins would require the user to stoop a little, and, as argued above for some private toilets at Pompeii, Herculaneum and Ostia, may instead have been intended for rinsing or keeping the sponge sticks rather than for handwashing. At least one of the examples from private toilets in Ostia, set at waist height, however, may, in fact, have been for washing hands.

The water for washbasins in public toilets usually came directly from the urban supply or via the intermediary of a cistern in the complex in which the latrines were situated, as in the Baths of the Cyclops at Thugga, where the basin is fed directly from the baths' cistern the other side of the wall; but this cistern was itself fed from one of the town's aqueducts. Overflow water from the washbasins usually went into the gutter that ran around the room in front of the seats before emptying into the drainage channel under the seats. One assumes, therefore, that the washbasins overflowed continually into this channel to ensure it was constantly supplied; if so, the inflow to the washbasins would have been continuous too. We may, however, be underestimating the use of taps or stopcocks (which are usually robbed out, since they were made of bronze): at Pompeii there is one private toilet with a stopcock still *in situ* in the House of the Silver Wedding.[51]

The Atmosphere of the Latrine

Latrines in private houses are often cramped and fairly dark places, with a small window (if any) placed high up;[52] they were therefore poorly lit and ventilated. Niches for lamps facilitated their use at night, or helped illuminate the dark space.[53] Despite the emphasis in medical texts on checking patients' stools as an indicator of their health, and the indications that under the empire elites

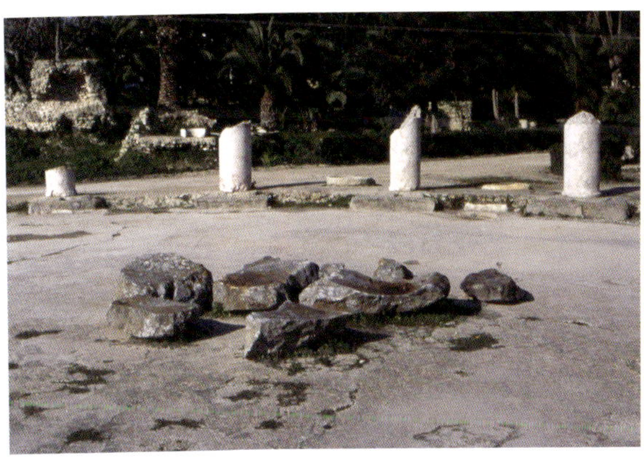

Fig. 7.10. Carthage, Antonine Baths, the broken remains of a marble washbasin in the exedral latrines (photo A. Wilson).

at least became increasingly interested in theories of health and regimen, the Roman latrine was not well designed to facilitate the widespread human behavior of inspecting one's leavings as a basic check on the state of one's bowels - the drain beneath the seats might be quite deep and in continually flushed latrines the faeces would have been quickly carried away by the water. It may not have been felt necessary, therefore, to have had much light to examine what one had done, although enough light must have been provided to see at least in outline what one was doing (and whether one had got sufficiently clean afterwards).

On the other hand, some larger public latrines must have been well lit by natural light, particularly those exedral latrines in North African bath complexes (Thuburbo Maius; Antonine Baths at Carthage) in which the seats were arranged around the curve under a colonnade and the central space was open, or the elongated peristyle design of the public latrine on the main street at Hierapolis in Phrygia. These latrines would also have been much better ventilated, an important consideration in an environment where many people are urinating, defecating and breaking wind.

Other means of managing smells can also be envisaged. Clearly, the frequency or otherwise of flushing will have affected the atmosphere inside public latrines. In latrines that were not flushed regularly or continuously, as for example many domestic latrines, it is conceivable that sand or earth may have been dumped over the waste to absorb and contain the smell. This would have been particularly important in the case of cesspit latrines. There is no hard evidence for antiquity, but earth or sand was sometimes dumped in privies in 18th- and 19th-century Europe and America and the practice of covering faeces with sand is still common in rural Egypt.[54] The frequent siting of Roman domestic latrines next to the kitchen would facilitate the dumping of ash from the oven over the toilet waste, helping to contain and neutralise the smell. Finally, it is possible that incense or scented oils may have been burned in some latrines - it has been speculated that small circular shallow dishes found in the baths and in a sewer at *Carnuntum* might have been used for this purpose.[55]

7.5 Conclusion

The standards of hygiene, or otherwise, achieved by Roman toilets will be considered more fully in chapter 11, but here several points can be noted. There was often quite extensive provision for built toilets in both public and private settings; and this provision increased once running water became common in towns through the provision of aqueducts. People usually sat to use the toilet, whether urinating or defecating; this entailed contact with the seat and therefore some risk of germ contagion, but the seat design at least usually avoided urine droplets at the front. Several methods of cleaning oneself were available, both wet and dry. If one sees the sponge on a stick as the Roman equivalent of toilet paper, there is a major hygienic downside in that this would have been a potential disease transmission route, especially if shared. Although running water was provided for handwashing in public toilets and some private toilets, this was cold and there was no soap.

Case study: The Latrines by the Forum at Timgad *(Andrew Wilson)*

The largest set of latrines at Timgad (ancient Thamugadi, in Numidia) lay along the north side of the forum, on the *Decumanus Maximus* (*figs 7.11-12*).[56] However, they were not entered directly either from the *Decumanus* or the forum, but from a passage running between the *Decumanus* and a side entrance to the forum behind the basilica. Access was through a vestibule (3.15 x 2.85 m) on the eastern side, which may have provided room for an attendant who took fees from users. In the centre of the northern side was a low stone basin set at floor level, with a moulded surround, from which water ran into a gutter with U-shaped cross-section, 0.20 m wide and 0.09 m deep. This gutter ran from the SE corner of the basin around all four sides of the room in front of the seats before entering the latrine drain near the SW corner of the basin. The latrine drain, 1.20 m deep, likewise ran around all four sides of the room under the seats, from one side of the basin back to the other before presumably connecting with the main street drain of the *Decumanus Maximus*. Water for flushing the latrine drain may have come from the basin in the latrines themselves, or from a public fountain on the *Decumanus Maximus* set against the north side of the vestibule, by the NE corner of the latrines; Ballu's plan shows two drain gratings in front of it and the overflow drain from the fountain could easily have fed into the NE corner of the latrine drain.

Ballu, the architect in charge of the early excavations of Timgad, thought that there was an additional blocked doorway at the NW corner of the latrine. He gives no evidence for this but presumably is referring to the patch of different masonry visible in his general photo. There are, however, some difficulties with this interpretation, not least the awkward interruption to the seating it would imply in the putative first phase. An alternative explanation should be considered, in the light of the observations that the latrines actually interrupt the colonnade of the *Decumanus Maximus*; and that their flushing was enabled only by the provision of running water, but that the creation of an aqueduct supply network in AD 146 at Timgad post-dated the foundation of the city while the forum complex is part of the original layout.[57] In other words, there must be a strong suspicion that the latrines by the forum at Timgad, together with the adjacent street fountain, are a subsequent alteration and addition to the original forum plan. In this scenario, the west wall of what became the latrine space existed originally in its southern part as a wall flanking a side entrance to the forum, and perhaps forming part of a row of shops in the *Decumanus* colonnade. When the putative shops were removed to make way for the latrines, and the latrine space had to be extended to the edge of the *Decumanus*, this west wall had to be continued in different masonry in its northern section, to join a pier of the *Decumanus* colonnade. The difference in masonry abutting the original wall at the south end and the colonnade pier at the north end was then misinterpreted by Ballu as a blocked doorway. This is confirmed by the fact that the north wall of the latrines is in similar masonry, differing from that of the south wall, and incorporates the stone piers of the original arcade or colonnade along the *Decumanus Maximus* (*fig. 7.12*).

The seats of the latrine, in local limestone, were socketed with tenons into holes in the inside face of the latrine walls, and supported laterally by socketing into stone slabs that divided the seating area into fourteen stalls with one or two seats in each stall. The upper part of these slabs, visible above the seats, were carved in the shape of dolphins and provided a comfortable armrest (*fig. 7.13*). The seats had circular holes, with a groove to the front for inserting the sponge stick; evidently this was too shallow for inserting one's hand (*figs 7.14-15*). This shallow groove, unlike the normal arrangement of a slot in the front of the seat connecting with a hole in the upper surface, is found also in the latrines of the House of Corfidius at Timgad, and seems to be a local variation.[58]

Ballu suggests a figure of 0.60 m average width per user; most of the seats had a pair of holes in each stall between each pair of armrests, but the reconstructed seats either side of the basin on the north side of the room have only a single, very capacious, seat.

In front of the seats, between the gutter and the latrine drain, are a series of small slits or channels that seem to be designed to enable spillages to enter the latrine drain.[59]

Previous estimates of capacity range from 24-26.[60] Ballu proposes that there was space for a possible 26 users, assuming 0.60 m per seat, but the two especially wide seats next to the basin and the evidence of the urine spillage channels suggests that this figure needs to be lowered. It seems that there was probably one spillage drain slit per seat, and Ballu counts eleven of these on the south side, six on the west, and four on the north (the basin taking up much of this side), for a total of 21. On the east the paving has collapsed and while sockets for seat tenons in the E wall[61] show that there were seats on this side, it is unclear precisely how many; the available space would suggest two, or a maximum of three, seats. The total capacity of the latrines would therefore have been 23 or 24.

As these toilets are the only set associated with the forum at Timgad, there could have been no separate facilities for men and women, and we must either assume that they were only for men (the provision of such facilities for women but not for men being highly unlikely in the Roman world), and that there were no facilities for women; or that these toilets were mixed.

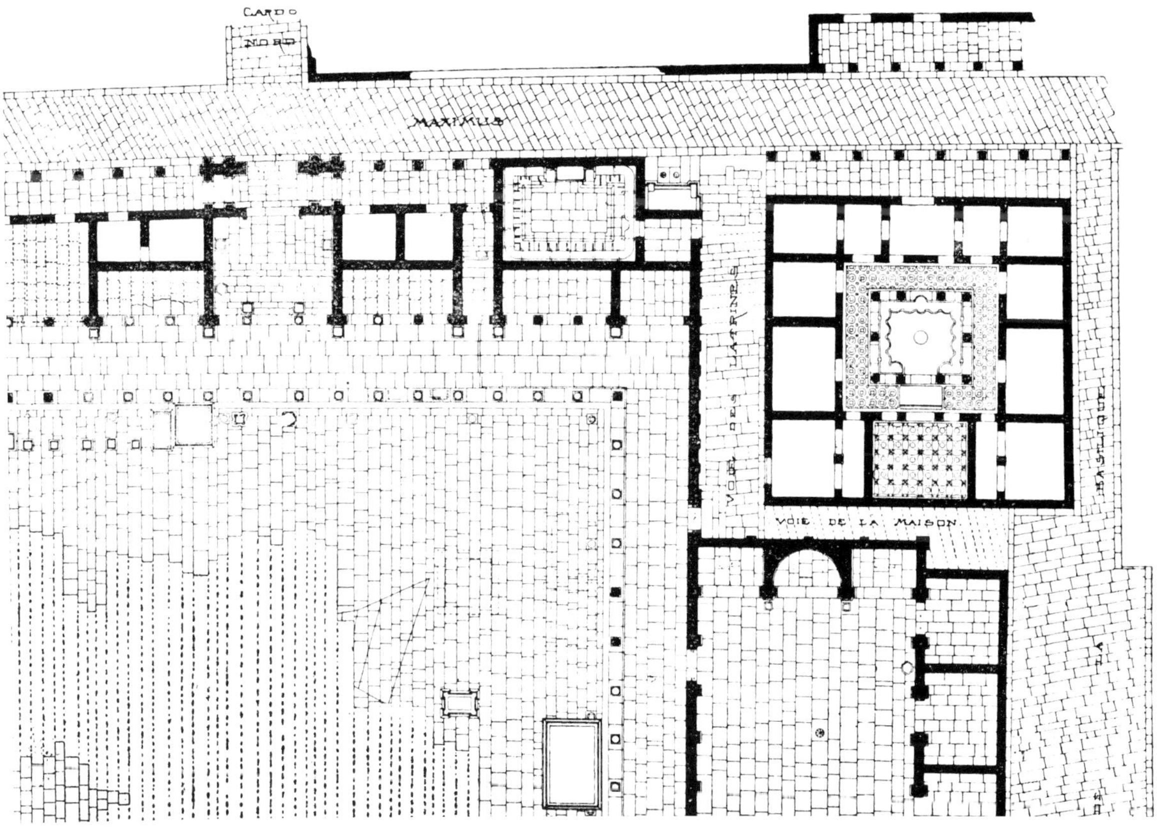

Fig. 7.11. Timgad, Plan of the NE corner of the forum: the latrines are centre-top (from Ballu 1897).

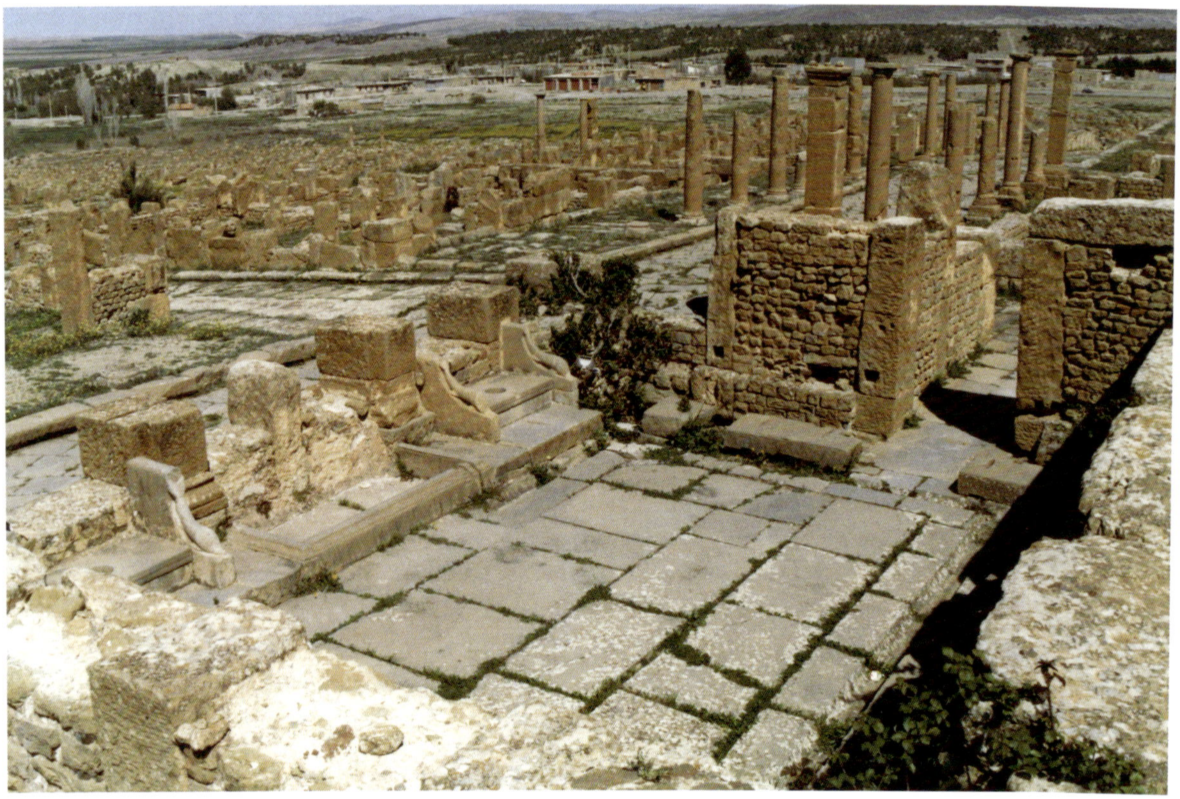

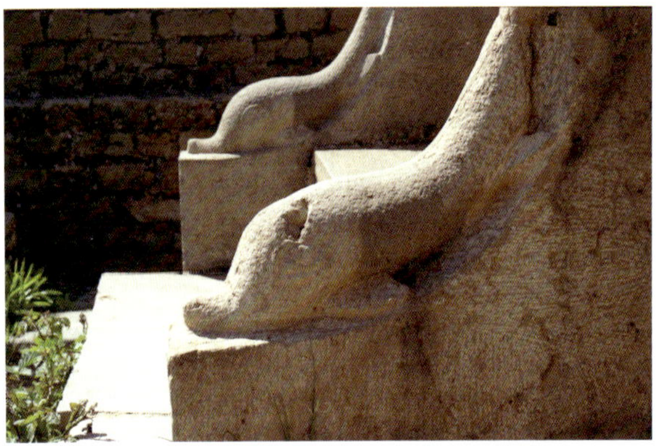

Fig. 7.12. Timgad, latrines, facing NE. The seats either side of the basin in the N wall have been reconstructed (photo A. Wilson).

Fig. 7.13. Timgad, latrines, detail of armrests in the shape of dolphins (photo A. Wilson).

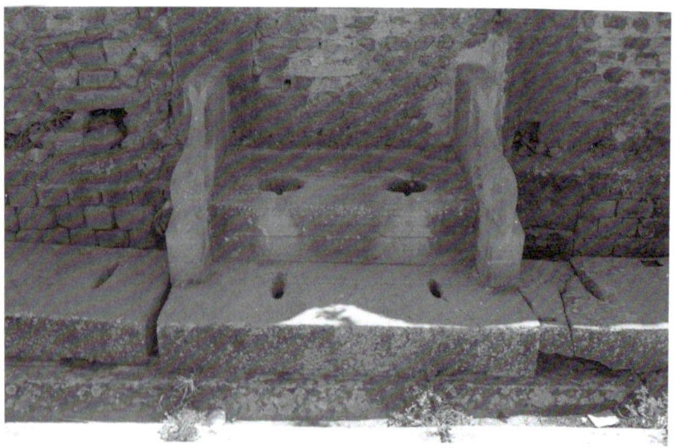

Fig. 7.14. Timgad, a pair of latrine seats, reconstructed (photo A. Wilson).

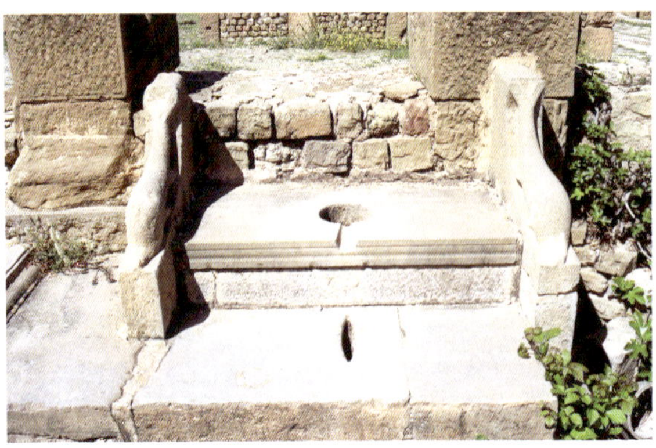

Fig. 7.15. Timgad, wide latrine seat to the east of the basin (photo A. Wilson).

Case study: The Latrines of the Baths of the Cyclops at Thugga *(Andrew Wilson)*

The Baths of the Cyclops are a modest set of neighbourhood public baths in the small town of Dougga (ancient Thugga, in Africa Proconsularis). They have a well-preserved set of latrines, with twelve seats arranged around three sides of a room in U-shaped plan (*fig. 7.9*).[62] The limestone slabs for the top and front of the seats are closely fitted together; the front wall of the seats slopes slightly. The holes in the seats are circular with a narrow slot in the front wall for inserting the sponge stick (too narrow effectively to put one's hand in). In front of the seats runs a water channel carved in blocks of stone; a raised lip separates this gutter from the space immediately in front of the seats where the users would rest their feet (*fig. 7.16*). The surface of this space is inclined slightly towards the seats, and small holes at the base of the front wall of the seats allow spilled urine or water to run into the latrine drain. This arrangement shows that the gutter is separate from any arrangements to deal with spilled urine, and lends support to the idea that it is for wetting the sponge stick. A small circular cavity in a stone block by end of the seats may have served as a place to rest the sponge stick when not in use (*fig. 7.16*).[63]

The fourth side of the room, not occupied by the toilet seats, is of course the side on which the latrines were entered, and was paved in mosaic with a geometric design. Against the wall of this area is a pedestal washbasin (*fig. 7.17*), supplied by a pipe through the wall from a cistern the other side of the wall. Water, either directly from the cistern or more probably as overflow from the washbasin, must have been conveyed to the start of the water channel in front of the seats in a pipe now removed, probably of lead.

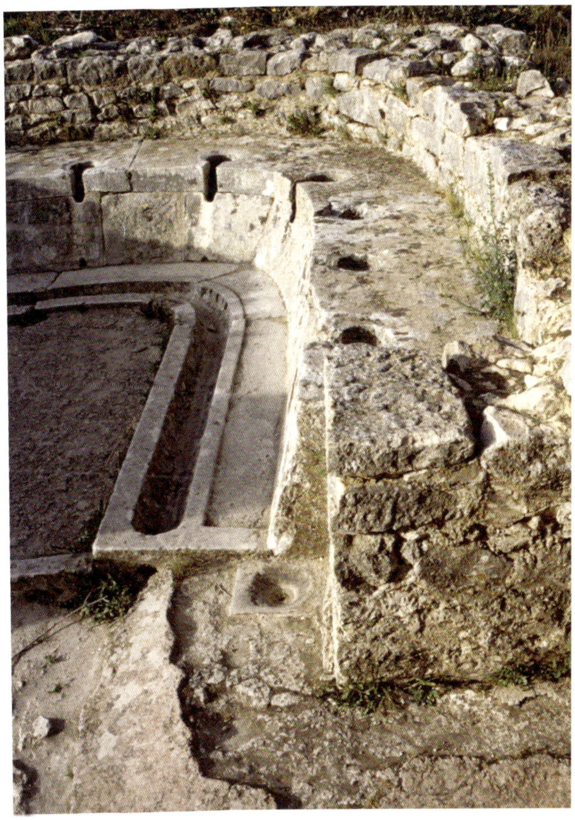

Fig. 7.16. Dougga, Baths of the Cyclops, detail of the water channel, latrines, drains for allowing spilled urine to enter the latrine drain, and possible rest for sponge stick (photo A. Wilson).

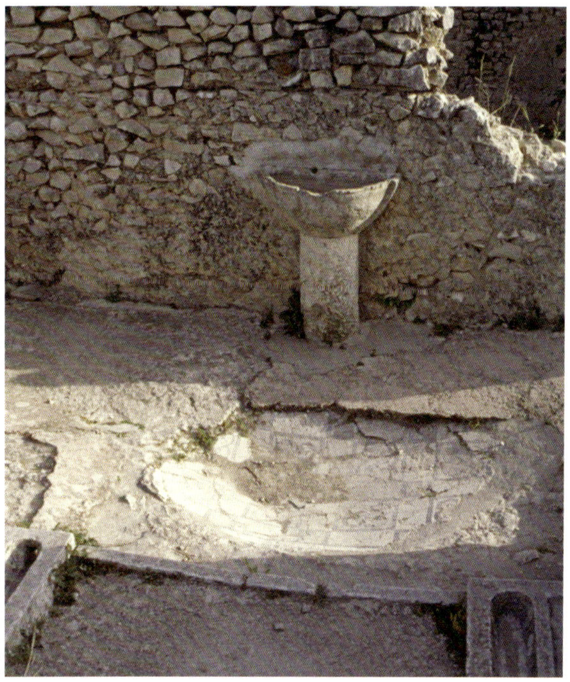

Fig. 7.17. Dougga, Baths of the Cyclops, latrines, washbasin (photo A. Wilson).

Notes

1 I am grateful to all those who have helped by providing references or examples: Jim Adams, Manfred Flieger, Barry Hobson, Manfred Horstmanhoff, Stefanie Hoss, Gemma Jansen, Andrew Jones, Beatrix Petznek, Günther Thüry and Gilbert Wiplinger.

2 E.g. *Gospel of Luke* 2.7.

3 Ancient detergents included vegetable alkali from plant ashes, soda, natron and fuller's earth: Forbes 1965, 186-188.

4 Lynch/Papadopoulos 2006.

5 On chamberpots and pisspots, see Daremberg-Saglio s.vv. *amis, matula*; Hilgers 1969, nos 210 (*lasanum*), 230 (*matella*), 231 (*matellio*), 232 (*matula*); Morris 1985, 402-403; Mattelaer 1999.

6 Kolling 2000; Blümner 1911, 147-148; Binsfeld 1994.

7 Binsfeld 1994, 130 n. 7 says there is no inn near the findspot of the graffito, but has the wrong location for the findspot (VIII 6, 6 instead of VIII 7, 6; Eschebach and Müller-Trollius 1993, 388, note an inn at VIII 7, 1-4 nearby.

8 Cf. also Martial, *Ep.* 6.89.1; 10.11.3-4.

9 Wilson 1995.

10 Howell's commentary (1989, 187-188) usefully collects the ancient references to chamberpots of precious metals, summarised below. Cf. also Martial, *Ep.* 11.11.5-6:
Te potare decet gemma qui Mentora frangis
In scaphium moechae, Sardanapalle, tuae.
It is for you, Sardanapallus, to drink from jewels, you who break a [work of art by] Mentor to make a chamberpot for your mistress (Loeb trans., adapted).

11 For *[vasa] murrina* as fluorspar, see Loewental/Harden/Bromehead 1949.

12 E.g. Tertullian, *De cultu feminarum* 1.5.2: *viderit, si etiam ad spurca instrumentis auri et argenti demens copia deseruit.*

13 Cf. also discussion of these passages in Thüry 2001, 15, 17, 25-26 and n. 35 and 48.

14 Arangio-Ruiz 1943, 582-585 (no 185).

15 Annese et al. 2000, 252-255.

16 This contribution was translated from German by Stefanie Hoss. The excavations took place during the project 'Carnuntum-Zivilstadt', directed by F. Humer in the Open-Air-Museum Petronell. The project was financed by the Government of the State of Lower Austria - Department for Cultural Affairs and the Archaeological Park, Carnuntum. For the excavations see also chapter 2, pp. 18-20.

17 In many cases the chamberpots are classified and published as storage or cooking vessels. It will be important for future ceramics publications to review the new and published material to show both the existence of the chamberpots and to further typological studies on them.

18 Further and more detailed comparisons see Petznek/Radbauer 2008, 51-91.

19 Gregory of Tours, *History of the Franks* 2.23. Gregory thinks that the priest's death by prolapse of the bowel shows that he must have been an Arian heretic, as Arius died in a public lavatory at Constantinople in the same manner. This theme of heretics dying on the toilet goes back to Eusebius and has a long tradition in medieval Christian writings - see Johnson 1998, 275-278; cf. Hoss, here pp. 48-49.

20 Mertens 1995, 218-219. I thank Gemma Jansen for this reference.

21 Some of the largest public latrines include Athens (Agora): 68 seats; Alexandria: 70; Kos: 71; and Apamea: 80. I am grateful to Richard Neudecker for these examples.

22 I thank Stefanie Hoss and Gemma Jansen for this reference.

23 *CIL* 8.6982 = *ILS* 4921b.

24 Three sides: Baths of the Cyclops at Thugga, Large Baths at Thaenae (Nielsen 1990, 171 fig. 190). Four sides: Large South Baths at Cuicul (Nielsen 1990, 174 fig. 194).

25 Memmian Baths at Bulla Regia, West Baths at Gigthis, Antonine Baths at Carthage, Summer Baths at Thuburbo Maius (Nielsen 1990, 161 fig. 176, 164 fig. 180).

26 Personal observation. The baths at Sabratha are those mentioned by Ward 1970, 26 and Haynes 1981, 133, though without detail on the latrines.

27 Gemma Jansen, personal comment, whom I thank for this information.

28 Stones: Aristophanes, *Wealth* 817-818; *Peace* 1224-1230 and scholiast on 1230; Athenaeus, *Deipnosophistae* 13.578e and 13.584c; cf. M. Gilleland, 'Ancient tersive materials' at http://laudatortemporisacti.blogspot.com/2006_09_01_archive.html (checked 1st January 2008). Potsherds: Papadopoulous 2002, although his suggestion that trimmed ceramic disks or ostraka may have been used as wipes is entirely speculative.

29 yT *Shabbat* 82a (11c 2-20).

30 Andrew Jones, personal comment.

31 Contra Scobie 1986, 411, who thought it might have served to carry away spilt urine. Cf. Wilson 2000b, 309.

32 E.g. at Ordona (Mertens 195, 219-220; Annese et al. 2000, 253) and Ephesus, Hanghaus 2, Wohneinheit 4, Latrine 4a (Outschar/Thüry 1997). I thank Gilbert Wiplinger and Gemma Jansen for these references.

33 Gilbert Wiplinger, personal comment.

34 Hodge 1992, 271 and 454 n. 77, seems to regard sponges as not being widely used and believes, curiously, that the gutter was both for washing hands, despite the provision of wash-basins, and for carrying away spillages, two functions which would appear to be mutually exclusive. Scobie (1986, 411) suggests that the gutter might have served to carry away spilt urine.

35 The *Mulomedicina Chironis* uses the term *solispungium*, (Oder 1901, 196 line 17 §614) but the emendation to *xylospongium* is assured since Chiron's source, Apsyrtus, for this section uses the correct Greek word (Oder/Hoppe 1924, 269 line 11). Pelagonius (348; cf. also 486), who used Chiron's *Mulomedicina* in turn as one of his main sources, makes clear what the instrument is in his rephrasing as *peniculum in fuste ligato* (a brush tied to a stick), and he is followed by Vegetius (*Mulomedicina* 2.135.3), *penicillo in fuste ligato.* I am grateful to J. Adams and M. Fleiger for these references.

36 *AE* 1941, 5.

37 For this interpretation, see M. Gilleland, 'Sponge on a stick' at http://laudatortemporisacti.blogspot.com/2006_09_01_archive.html (checked 1st January 2008). On these decorations see Koloski-Ostrow and Moormann (chapter 11, Case Study, pp. 178-181).

38 J.N. Adams, personal comment, whom I thank for this interpretation and for much helpful discussion of this passage. On ellipsis generally, see Löfstedt 1933, 233-274.

39 *P. Mich.* 471, 29. See Youtie/Winter 1951, 39-40.

40 Matt. 27.48; Mark 15.36; John 19.29-30.

41 Buckland 1976, 14-15; he says of the freshwater sponge *Spongilla lacustris* 'this small fragile species is wholly unsuitable for toilet use'.

42 Wilson 2000b, 309 and 310, fig. 3.

43 Jansen 1997, 125-126, 130; 2002a, 60 n. 295, 109, 158 and n. 227.

44 Jansen 2002a, 60 fig. II.79.

45 Shop or Tavern (*caupona*) of Euxinos (Jansen 1997, 126, fig 10.5) and houses at I 12, 9.14 and house I 12, 10.11. (Jansen 1997, 125, 130; 2002a, 60 n. 295).

46 Jansen 2002a, 109.

47 Jansen 2002a, 158 and n. 227: House of Fortuna Annonaria, Shop or Tavern (*caupona*) of Fortunatus, III vii, 5 (apartment building next to the Thunder-bolt House (Domus Fulminata) - Jansen 2000d, 123 fig. 13), House of the Protirus (Domus del Protiro), and Schola of Trajan.

48 Wilson 2000b, 309.

49 Jansen 1997, 127, figs 10.1, 10.2; 2002a, 60.

50 Small/Buck 1994, 47-49 and 305-306 figs 22-23, with reinterpretation in Wilson 2002, 11 n. 56.

51 Gemma Jansen *pers. comm.*

52 Mygind 1921, 314; Jansen 1997, 127.

53 E.g. at Pompeii, in House V 4, 6-7. See also Mygind 1921, 314-315.

54 E.g. Wheeler chapter 2.2, p. 20 for sand dumped in a latrine in Portsmouth.

55 B. Petznek, personal comment.

56 Basic description in Ballu 1897, 112-114; cf. also Neudecker 1994, 113-114. The additional information and interpretations presented here derive from a visit in March 1990, and from re-examination of photographs taken at the time. Three seats have been reconstructed since the original excavation (Courtois 1951, 27); Ballu's early photo shows no seating still in place.

57 *AE* 1985, 875a and b.

58 Ballu 1911, 76 and photo facing.

59 Ballu 1897, 112 n. 1; Wilson 2000b, 309.

60 26: Ballu 1897; 25: Courtois 1951, 27 and Neudecker 1994, 113; 24: Lassus 1969, 33.

61 Ballu 1897, fig. 6.

62 Poinssot 1983, 56-57; Neudecker 1994, 43 and Abb. 15.

63 Wilson 2000b, 309-310.

8

Location and Context of Toilets

8.1 Location and Context of Public Latrines
(Ann Olga Koloski-Ostrow)

From the middle of the 1st century AD to the 5th century AD, beautifully preserved public latrines can be found in Roman Italy (especially in Pompeii, Herculaneum, and Ostia), western Europe (including England, France, the Netherlands, and Germany), North Africa, Asia Minor, and the Near East. We can say with some certainty that Roman public sanitary facilities of different levels of technical achievement and design already began to flourish from the 2nd century BC onwards in a fairly wide variety of settings in and around the Mediterranean basin: in towns, cities, 'road stations' along isolated highways, suburban and country villas, spas, imperial enclaves, far-flung colonies, and military camps on the expanding Roman borders. The quality of the ruins, of course, varies considerably from site to site and period to period. When we consider the location of toilets specifically in urban settings, we find them most commonly sited near market places, fora, or in or near pubic baths. Somewhat less frequently they are also found in or near theaters, amphitheaters, *palaestrae*,[1] or along streets of a city or town, and not only the main streets.[2]

Foricae, or multi-seat facilities, generally open in plan, as we have seen earlier (chapter 5.1, pp. 53-55), were themselves public buildings or often attached to public buildings, although sometimes they might be privately owned. This type of public toilet (whether peristyle, square, rectangular, semicircular, or irregular in design)[3] offered some privacy from the truly public areas of the city, such as the streets and open markets, for an activity that was abhorrent to the public at large.

No Roman of Rome, Ostia, Pompeii, or any other Roman city would have enjoyed the stench or the sight of human excrement, offal, animal dung, and various other forms of offensive garbage strewn about the streets. While the arrival of public latrines in Roman Italy probably did improve the sanitary conditions of cities to some extent, we must not automatically assume that sanitary improvement was the one, the only, or the main Roman motive behind the construction of toilets. Perhaps the toilets served a political function for the Romans as well. The 'public' aspect of public latrines, like the Latin word *publicus* itself, does imply a political aspect. As the Romans were masters of confining to restricted spaces or areas all behaviors that were unpleasant to the State or community, in this case, the dirty business of urinating and defecating, it is worth considering toilets in this political light as well (see further discussion in chapter 9.2, pp. 131-133).

The Roman adoption of many Greek toilet customs is clearly visible in the archaeological remains. In a late Hellenistic site on the island Thera, a latrine was found near the agora.[4] Because it accommodated about eight persons and was attached to a market hall, we can safely assume that it was installed for communal use. F. Hiller von Gaertringen's excavation report shows that all the other latrines found on Thera were built into private houses, although some of these did have seats for three people and had direct access from the street.[5] The market hall latrine itself was a dark and grim room, despite the marble slabs that decorated its floor. The only light source for the latrine came from the door, and it appears that there was no supply of fresh water for the facility. A similarly modest public arrangement has been found at Amorgos on the island of Paros, also Hellenistic in date.[6]

The Romans seemed to adopt similar notions about where to site public latrines in their cities. As we have seen, many Roman markets had a latrine inside them or nearby. In addition, Roman public latrines are also frequently, although not exclusively, found in the context of public baths, especially from the 1st century BC to the 2nd century AD. The Romans were very practical people with an appreciation for functionality. Sometimes latrines were positioned to be near a water supply (or a supply of recycled water, such as one would find in public baths where *frigidarium* and *caldarium* tubs needed to be emptied from time to time). The outflow could clean the channels or sewer trenches under the latrines. Sometimes latrines were sited near the warm rooms of a bath, which would be very convenient on a cold winter day.[7]

There is little direct evidence to explain the growing popularity of bath buildings and the bathing habit, especially in the first period of growth from ca 100 BC down to the age of Augustus, but some reasons proposed for this popularity can also be applied to the increased construction of public latrines.[8] First of all, life in a Roman town or city was considerably more communal, more in the 'public' eye than anything we

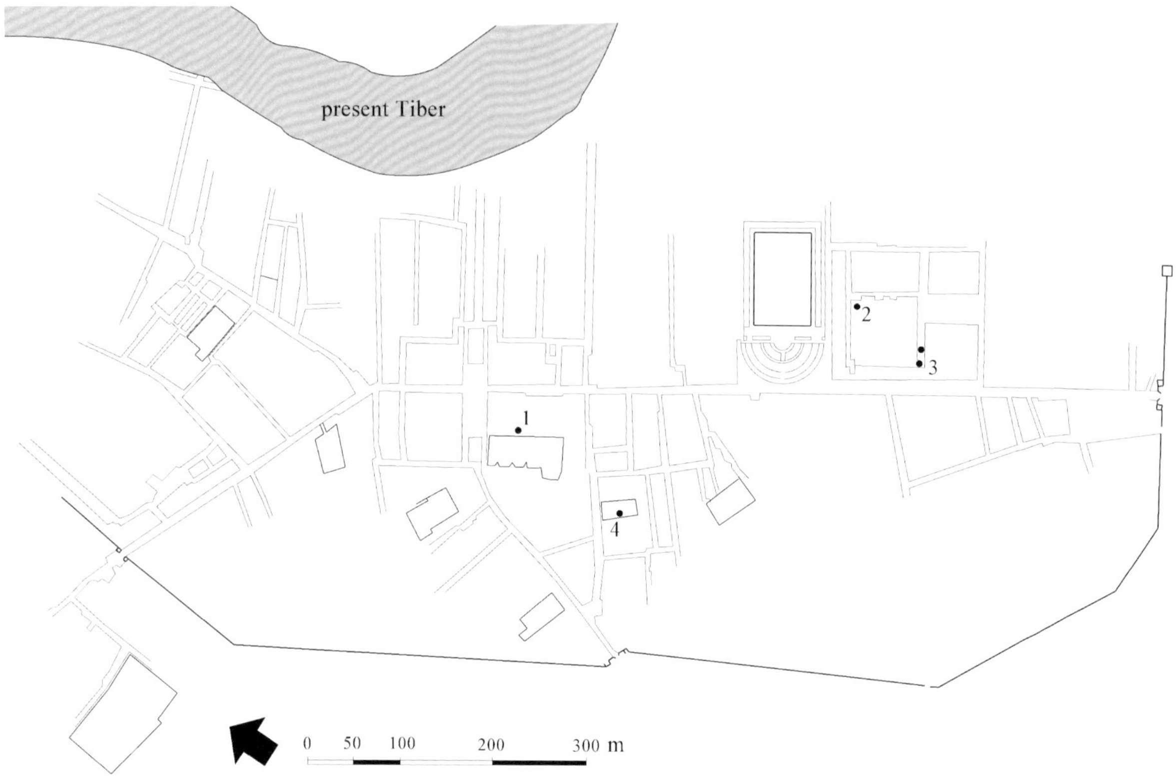

Fig. 8.1. Ostia, a few of the research related latrines in and near bath complexes: 1. Latrine of the Street of the Latrine in relation to the Forum Baths (I xii, 1), 2. Internal latrine of the Neptune Baths (II iv, 2), 3. External latrine of the Neptune Baths, 4. Latrine of the Baths of the Philosophers (V ii, 7) (drawing B. Maris).

can imagine in the modern western world. If we can understand this, the popularity of both baths and public latrines can be seen in a fresh light.

Thousands of Romans in any city would have been without all sorts of basic amenities that we take for granted, including kitchens, baths, and toilets. The plethora of *thermopolia*, simple eateries, for example, must have served as public kitchens for many people. Public baths substituted for non-existent private washing arrangements, and multi-seater latrines must have been attractive to those denizens cramped in tiny, impoverished apartments with no running water. In such crowded living quarters neither cesspits nor chamberpots could be emptied frequently enough, nor could their contents be given sufficient remove.

The rising population of Rome in this same period, combined with communal nature of many aspects of Roman life, would also have contributed to a greater demand for more public amenities, including baths and latrines. Squalor must have been everywhere, and the desire to escape from it never ceased.

Furthermore, just as Romans were trading and traveling to the eastern Mediterranean and bringing back new ideas for their cities, Hellenistic Greek city-dwellers were moving about as well, and in turn settling in Roman Italy. When this new ethnic population arrived in Rome, we must not imagine the acculturation of Greek taste only having an effect on the Roman elite.[9] The newcomers, especially the rich among them, would have exerted some pressure to see to it that their long-established urban institutions from the east were put in place in the west. The final factor that helps make the spread of public baths and latrines more understandable was the simultaneous improvement in building technology, most especially, the development of concrete (*opus caementicium*) that allowed for increasingly larger and more elaborate structures for baths and latrines.[10] It is the collective impact of these points that brings to light an understanding of why latrines (and baths) were constructed with more and more frequency at key locations within the urban landscape.

8.2. Location of Toilets within Baths
(Jeroen Van Vaerenbergh)

Although the following findings are the result of a specific study of the assemblage of latrines in and near the baths of Roman Italy,[11] they can to a great extent be applied to the overall picture of bath-connected latrines all over the Roman Empire.[12] The location of these latrines can tell us something about their accessibility, attitudes about discretion, the possibility of segregation of sexes, the potential existence of entrance fees, and the times of day for their use.

Accessibility

Most common are the toilets that were located at highly frequented spots, often accessible to both the bath visitors and a much larger public outside the bath complex, like passers-by and people who were living in the neighboring properties. This is most obvious with latrines located just outside bath complexes. A typical example is found in Ostia. The latrine of the Street of the Latrine[13] was situated at a busy intersection (*figs 1.1 and 8.1*); not only right across from the main entrance to the baths, but also near the forum in the middle of the lively city center. The accessibility of these toilets did not depend on the opening hours of the bath complex. On the basis of the archaeological evidence, it is difficult to determine if, in fact, they were accessible day and night. As remarked in the chapter on water supply (chapter 6, p. 85), if there were non-stop opening hours, this would have caused persistent flushing problems.

'Internal toilets' are a different case. The accessibility of these latrines depended on their precise location within the bath complex. Many toilets were situated along one of the entrances, which made them easy to reach from the street. Also, there were several latrines situated in the *palaestra*. It is difficult to say to what extent these courtyards were accessible to visitors who were not using the baths. The fact that many of these *palaestrae* had broad entrances and were equipped with shops, probably means that several of them were fairly easy to reach from outside the complex. The accessibility of the *palaestra* probably depended on the customs and morals of a certain period: whether the bath complex was exclusive or meant for the general public; and whether there were specific circumstances for particular users. For example, big crowd pleasers, like the impressive imperial baths of Rome,[14] provided one or more latrines accessible only to their own visitors.

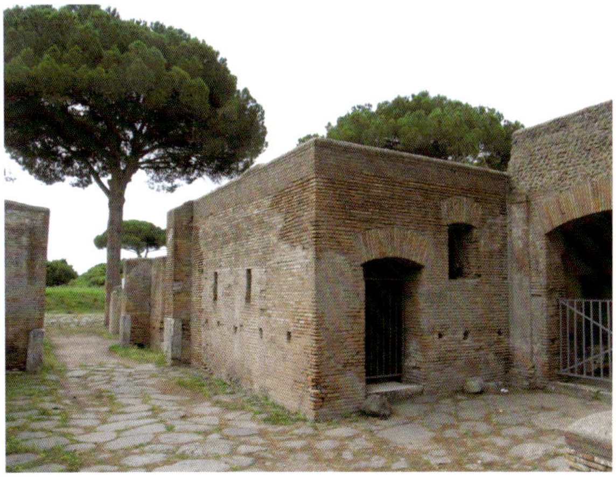

Fig. 8.2. Ostia, external latrine just outside one of the entrances of the Neptune Baths (II iv, 2) (photo J. Van Vaerenbergh).

We find a remarkable compromise in the large Baths of Neptune along the Decumanus in Ostia (*fig. 8.2*). In addition to an internal latrine,[15] we still find a second latrine just outside the complex,[16] with easier access for people who were in the neighborhood (*fig. 8.1 no 2 and 3*).

In general, we can say that at busy locations, the latrines were primarily aimed at toilet visitors from the surrounding area. The visitors to the baths were often merely a part of the intended public. Similar situations could even be found in some exclusive bath complexes, only meant for a select group of people.

A fine example of such a latrine can be found in the private Baths of the Philosopher in Ostia[17] (*fig. 8.1 no 4*). From its location in a crowded area of the city, we can see that the latrine of these baths lost its exclusiveness in favor of wider use by the inhabitants that lived in the adjoining insula. This situation certainly may not be generalized. Since most of the exclusive/private baths had a latrine that was only accessible to insiders, we can conclude that the Roman elite preferred a separate toilet for people with the same social background.

Discretion

It is obvious that the intended users for latrines were not the only concern of Roman designers. Finding a discrete location for a toilet was at least as important, and not an easy task when we think of the often crowded places where the latrines were situated. In the latrine of the *Praedia* of Iulia Felix in Pompeii,[18] we can see that not only was the door located at the end of a narrow corridor in the open air, but also its entrance was situated at a 90° angle off the corridor (in other words, staggered; *fig. 8.3*). This common arrangement made it unnecessary to close the latrine door, so more light and air could enter the room.

Instead of such a corridor, many latrines had a separate entrance room, a so-called vestibule, which prevented passers-by from peeking inside. Because of lack of space, such vestibules or corridors were not always possible. In the latrine of the Street of the Latrine in Ostia, the designers built revolving doors, which had the advantage of not being able to be left open.

It is clear that the Romans tried to screen the latrine users from the people who were outside the room. Although usually several people were using the toilet at the same time, their activities were still contained within the four walls of the room.

The Influence of Discrete Locations in Bath-Related Latrines on Social Attitudes

Even with these many privacy measures, some Romans were not satisfied: the most wealthy Romans could, and did, afford one-seat latrines in completely separate rooms.

In a luxurious spa, the so-called Taurine Baths in Civitavecchia, we can find several individual latrines up against the bathing rooms.[19] As far as we know, this is exceptional within the baths of Italy. Complete privacy, as we prefer today in the west, could be found only in the most exclusive Roman toilet facilities, but was mostly not feasible. Nevertheless, the spa in Civitavecchia also had a multiseat-latrine near one of the entrances to the baths. Apparently, a visit to a multi-seat latrine could still remain on one's agenda, even for those who had access to more private facilities. Perhaps this agrees with a gradual change in the mentality of the aristocracy in relation to public body care at the beginning of the imperial age. With the growing interest in body care becoming a part of the self-image of the elite Roman man, it seems that a visit to the toilet, also in public, became more and more a part of the elite way of life. As self-control was considered one of the biggest virtues of the Roman aristocrat, excessive use of public latrines was not considered appropriate. Therefore, it is conceivable that a visit by an elite to a public latrine was restricted, as much as possible, to certain times or spaces. For example, the visit to the baths was always at the end of the afternoon, a time of day usually reserved for public body care. Outside of this context, an aristocrat probably searched, where possible, for more private sanitary facilities.

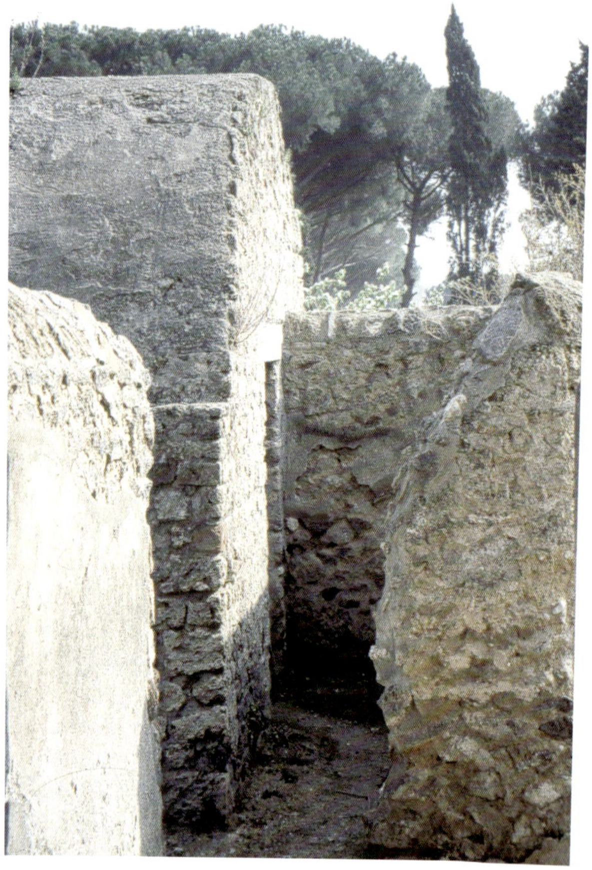

Fig. 8.3. Pompeii, Praedia of Iulia Felix (II, 4), narrow corridor giving access to the barrel-vaulted latrine (photo J. Van Vaerenbergh).

This explains why all the baths of the Hadrian's Villa, even those reserved for the emperor and his guests, were equipped with multi-seat latrines, while elsewhere in the villa, there is an abundance of private, single-seat latrines.[20] This is also the reason why almost all the exclusive and private baths are equipped with a multi-seat latrine, meant only for a select group of people, who had access to the baths.

To distinguish oneself even more from the majority of multi-seat latrines, characterized by a simple, functional interior of plastered walls and simple tiled floors, some of these elite toilets had a luxurious decor. The most excessive one is the latrine in the Small Baths of Hadrian's Villa,[21] adorned with multicolored *opus sectile* on the floor and elaborately cut floral inlays on the walls.

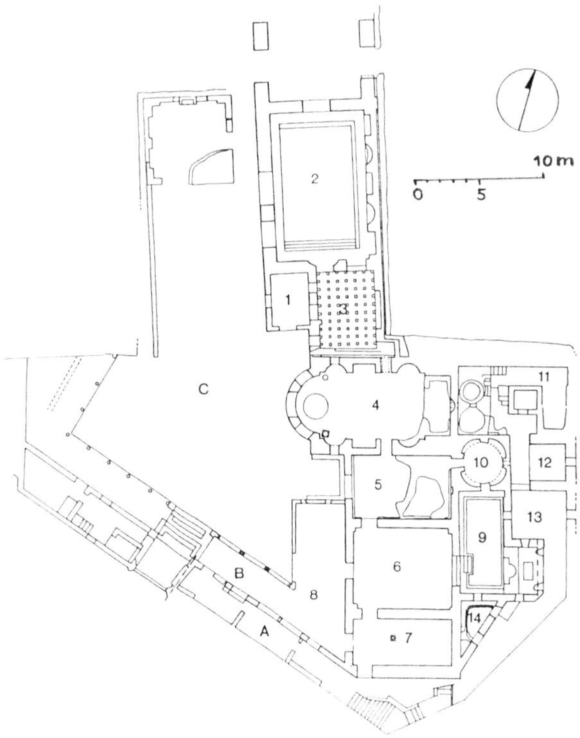

Fig. 8.4. Pompeii, Suburban Baths (VII 16, a), floorplan: praefurnia *(11), storage rooms (12 and 13) and latrine (14) (from Jacobelli 1995, 155 Fig.1).*

Such an arrangement, however, was exceptional, especially in the early cases at the beginning of the imperial age, as we find in Pompeii. All the latrines of the baths in Pompeii had, in contrast to the bathing rooms, an extremely simple design and were even kept completely outside of the main rooms in the bathing blocks.

This is even more prominent in exclusive baths, such as the luxurious Suburban Baths[22] of Pompeii, where we can find the latrine at a remote location, in the service area near the furnaces (*praefunia*) and storage rooms of the baths (*fig. 8.4*). The bathing rooms of this complex all have a very elaborate and colorful design, in contrast with the white plastered floor and walls of the latrine. It seems as if the designers of this bath complex tried to concentrate all smelly, filth-collecting utilities at one location.

One question we can pose is whether the Romans, in general, and the elites, in particular, at the beginning of the imperial age, were still less confident about using multi-seat latrines? Was such toilet use still a hidden activity? Mainly because of different privacy measures, such as small windows placed high up on the walls, hidden entrances, and sometimes closing doors, many toilets were poorly lit and difficult to ventilate (cf. chapter 7.4, pp. 99-100). Only in some cases, especially from the 2nd century AD on, did the Romans start to make bigger windows, for example, to improve circumstances. But even then it is not a general rule, as can be seen in the Hadrianic multi-seat latrine of the thermal baths in Civitavecchia, where the room was lit by just one small window. The external multi-seater of the Baths of Neptune in Ostia, from the same period, just had three little windows.

In contrast to what is often claimed, I think we can say that many of the researched latrines maintained an unpleasant atmosphere. It is striking that designers often gave more attention to privacy, with respect to the people outside, than to an attractive atmosphere inside. The popular picture of Romans having a cozy chat on the latrine must certainly be reconsidered.

Segregation of Sexes?

The question of whether both Roman men and women used public toilet facilities is not so easy to answer (cf. chapter 7.4, p. 101).[23] Although for the moment very superficial, the data of bath-related latrines can perhaps bring us a little bit closer to an answer.

Although it is tempting to interpret double toilet rooms within the same building as a clear sign of gender-segregated latrines, this was not necessarily the case. The fact that in the case study of the bath-related toilets of Roman Italy, these separated multi-seat latrines were almost non-existant proves that they were not that common and probably had nothing to do with separated use by male and female bath visitors.[24]

Most of all we have to ask ourselves if it was even socially acceptable for Roman women to use a public toilet. Without going into the issue too deeply, we can say that there is still a lot of discussion about how much Roman women appeared in public. Some scholars have the opinion that, throughout Roman times, there were social restrictions against elite women appearing in public, even in imperial times. On this assumption, a visit by women to public toilets must have been a socially risky business at the very least.[25] Others claim that from the 1st century AD onwards the emancipation of Roman women got the upper hand.[26]

By looking at the location of latrines within Roman bath complexes, a different and more complicated picture emerges. The earliest archaeological evidence of Roman bath complexes shows that until the beginning of the 1st century AD, where possible, there were in use segregated bathing rooms for men and women, with separate entrances. Examples can be found in Pompeii (the Stabian and Forum Baths) and Herculaneum (the Forum Baths). This segregation of sexes is also mentioned for other places in written sources.[27] At these baths, more resources were devoted to the part that was used by the men. Men had a larger set of baths and could make use of the *palaestra*. It is striking that the toilets of these baths all were connected to the entrance, which led to the men's part. Maybe this shows that, at that moment in time, going to a public latrine was still, to a great extent, a male activity.

During the 1st century AD, a new social development occurred related to public bathing that made separate bathing facilities disappear almost totally. As we also know from written sources, mixed bathing became very popular.[28] At least in the Bay of Naples this change already began before 79 AD, as the newly built Central Baths in Pompeii and the Suburban Baths in Herculaneum prove.[29] As a result, the toilets located within the walls of bath complexes also must have been freely accessible to women.

We can still ask ourselves if Roman women from the first century onwards actually made use of public latrines. When we think of the simple fact that men and women saw each other naked during bathing,[30] I believe that a visit to a mixed latrine probably would not have been that much of an issue, certainly when we consider that loose Roman garments, worn both by men and women, would have prevented everyone from seeing much of anyone's nakedness. This does not exclude the fact that, depending on social status, local or regional differences, changes in time, religious ideas and personal choices, there were probably still diverse attitudes about going to a public toilet.[31]

These considerations definitely need more research to clear up further the gender issue. For that matter, the determination of objects (earrings,...?) found in latrine deposits and the often neglected study of Roman graffiti in public toilets can probably be very useful.

Entrance Fees and Times of Use

Although these two topics, entrance fees and times of use, are crucial to understanding the function of bath-related[32] latrines within the social living space, they are difficult to detect in the archaeological evidence. Concerning entrance fees, we can make a distinction between latrines that are situated in the bath complex itself, and latrines just outside the walls of the complex.

The latrines within the building compound would depend completely on entrance fees for the bath complex itself. From written sources we know that for public baths, most of the time, one had to pay a small entrance fee.[33] Once paid, we assume that visitors could make use of most of the facilities offered within the complex, also the use of the toilets. We can ask ourselves if this fee also had to be paid when the latrine was situated along one of the entrances. This brings us to the question of the exact place where the entrance fee of the bath complex had to be paid, and if the use of separate toilets required a fee on its own. We also have to keep in mind that the visitors could have made use of special entrance tokens, so called *tesserae*, which they bought in advance.[34] Unfortunately, collecting money or tokens does not require a great deal of infrastructure, as present-day lavatory attendants still prove. Archaeological evidence for these activities, therefore, is almost impossible to detect.[35]

Regarding the times of use of the bath-related toilets, we already have mentioned the difficulties in determining non-stop opening hours for extramural latrines.[36] It is clear that toilets situated within the bath complex only were accessible when the complex itself was open, most of the time until sundown.[37] It seems as if a number of baths also were open in the evening or at night, as some written sources show.[38] Fragments of oil lamps found in the deposits of the final usage phase of the latrine in the Baths of the Swimmer in Ostia, could point to late opening hours of the latrine.[39]

Since most of the latrines were situated near the entrances of the bath complexes, we can assume that these facilities were mostly used at the beginning and/or the end of the 'daily' visit to the baths. In fact, two Roman writers speak indirectly of this matter. Galen warns 'warm natures' for bathing without first emptying one's bowels.[40] Plutarch indicates that hot baths can improve digestion.[41] As most Romans went to the baths in the afternoon, just after midday or just before dinner, going to the toilet must have been a common activity.

Baths and Latrines: the Perfect Complement

In general, we can conclude that interpreting all latrines is bound to different factors. Instead of pursuing the utopian image of the perfect latrine, the Romans looked for the most efficient solution for obtaining discrete latrines in highly frequented locations, fitted as well as possible, into the technical waterworks. Therefore, compromises were inevitable. Often this resulted in a rather unpleasant end result.

From this perspective we can say that the relation between latrines and bath complexes can be regarded as the perfect complement. The Romans killed two birds with one stone. First, they cited latrines to profit from the hydro-technical facilities of the baths, namely an assured water supply, drainage, and minimal water waste.

Second, the location of latrines took advantage of the large number of bath visitors, who were engaged in body care in any event.

Case Study: Public Latrines in *Augusta Emerita* (Mérida, Spain) *(Jesús Acero Pérez)*

The colony of *Augusta Emerita*, founded in 25 BC by Augustus and capital of the Roman province of Lusitania, is one of the most important towns in Hispania. Until recently, archaeological excavations have revealed a group of four public latrines, although the identification of some of them has not yet been confirmed. Three of them, related to the set of buildings for public spectacles comprising the theater and the amphitheater, are representative examples of latrines located in places with large crowds (*fig. 8.5*). Nevertheless, considering the fact that both the theater and the amphitheater were excavated during the first half of the 20th century, there are many unknown features regarding their latrines. We do not know the exact chronology of the latrines, some aspects of their configuration, or their exact mode of operation. For example, we have not determined the water supply of these latrines, but we certainly know that all of them are connected to the general sewer network of the city. Their location next to urban streets not only provided them with good access, but also made easier their drainage through the sewers under the streets.

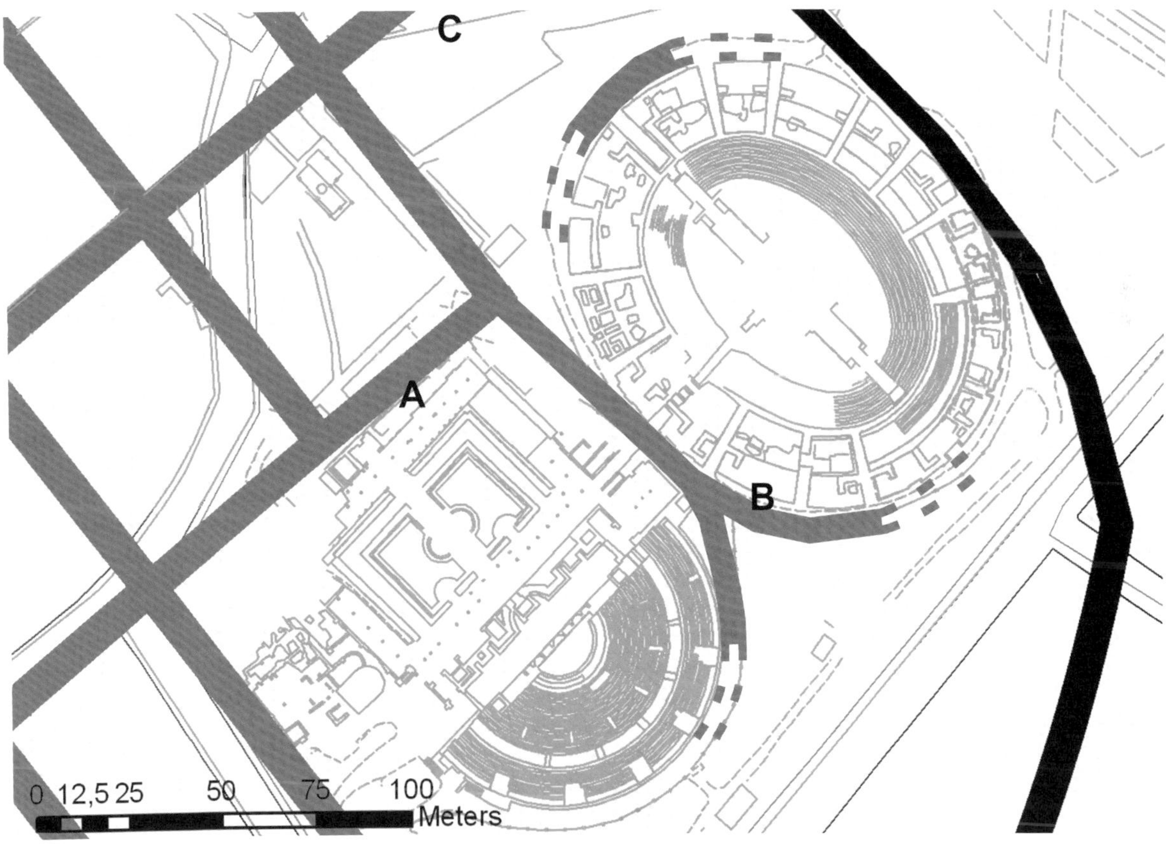

Fig. 8.5. Mérida, plan of the locations of latrines in the area of the buildings for public spectacles (drawing J. Acero, employing the urban GIS created by the Consorcio de la Ciudad de Mérida*).*

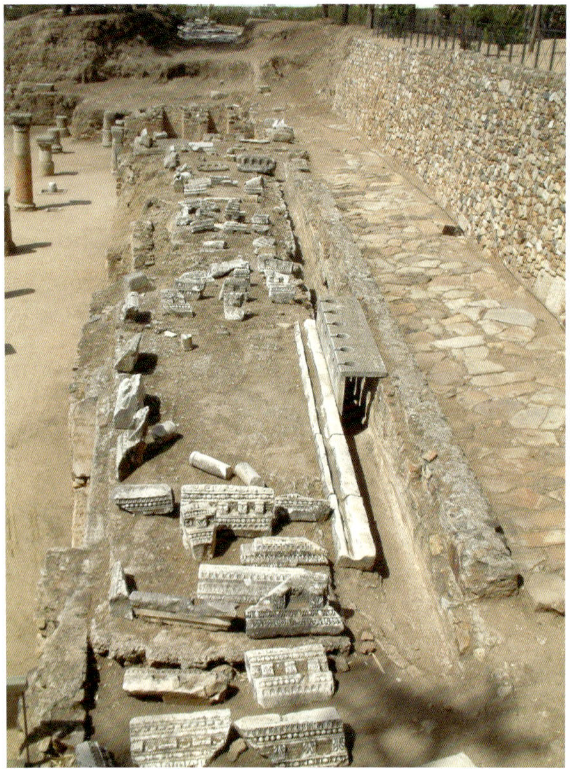

Fig. 8.6. Mérida, latrine A, placed in the porticus post scaenam *of the theater (photo J. Acero).*

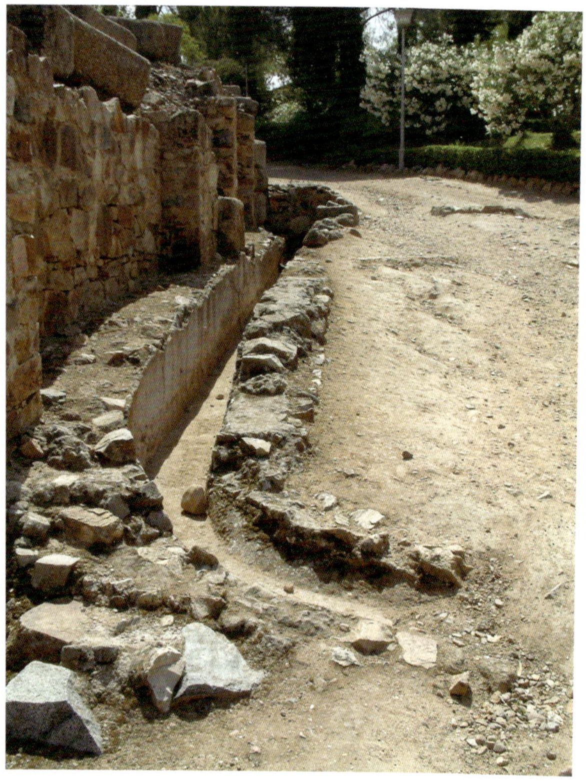

Fig. 8.7. Mérida, latrine B, in front of the amphitheater's façade (photo J. Acero).

The biggest latrine is situated at the back of the *porticus post scaenam* of the theater, alongside one of the streets giving access to this building, although the street and the latrine are at a much higher elevation than the level of the portico. For this reason, communication between the portico and the latrine was via stairs. The latrine consists of a long drainage channel with an estimated capacity of twenty-five users (*fig. 8.6*). Some time after its excavation, this channel was identified and reconstructed as a latrine by the architect J. Menéndez-Pidal,[42] following the model of the toilets of Dougga and Ostia. In this case, the sponge gutter and the seats were built in marble.

A possible latrine sits next to the amphitheater's façade, beside the main door of the building, of which a drainage channel with hydraulic mortar, part of a wall, and remains of the *opus signinum* floor are still visible at the present time.[43] This channel, with an extension of 11 m, maintains a slight curve towards the center of the street that surrounds the amphitheater, in the direction of the sewer that flowed under the street (*fig. 8.7*). According to J. R. Mélida,[44] director of the excavations of these public buildings at the beginning of the 20th century, on the other side of the Roman road there was another channel, parallel to the first, and that also curved towards the sewer. He believed that both channels were used to gather rain water in a terrain with an important natural slope. The characteristics of the present visible channel and Mélida's own description, however, suggest that it was a latrine, perhaps with an U-type plan. A precise excavation, of course, could validate this suggestion.[45]

Finally, a few years ago it was possible to excavate in an area close to a series of buildings for public spectacles, where a new latrine was identified (*fig. 8.8*), this time with a clear U-type plan, located in an open space that has been interpreted as a contiguous *palaestra* to the amphitheater.[46]

The remaining toilet is an archetypical example of a latrine that was documented within a private bath (*balneum*) dated to the 4th century AD, where it was used by the bath visitors. It had a capacity for three or four people. The latrine was cleaned easily by flushing water from the swimming pool of the *frigidarium* through a drainage channel that flowed towards the sewer under the street.[47] There might have been more examples all around the city, but, either they have not been found yet, or they have not been successfully interpreted. For example, we know about two big public baths, placed in the suburban area, where all the canonical parts of this type of establishment have been identified except the toilets. These most likely did exist, although these thermal complexes have not been fully excavated.

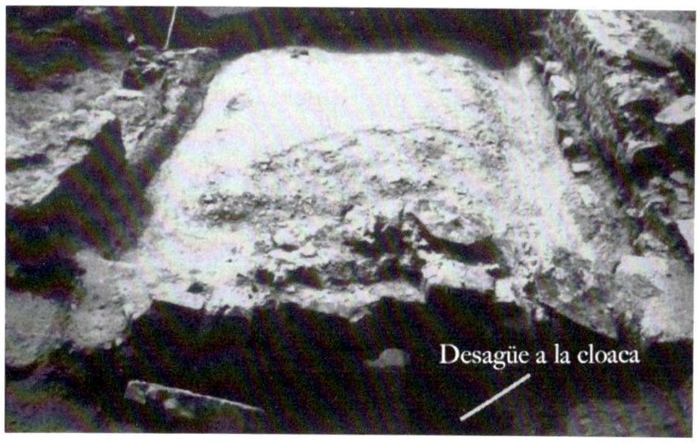

Fig. 8.8. Mérida, latrine C, located in a possible palaestra *next to the amphitheater (from M. Alba 2001, 72, fig. 18).*

Case Study: Toilets in Roman Spa Baths: The Taurine Baths *(Jens Köhler)*

Roman spas developed in the 1st and 2nd centuries AD from architecturally ill-defined structures set in remote, open-air areas, into monumental building complexes that needed the hygienic installations we call latrines, just as they were needed in conventional public baths.

But the peculiarities of health spas, especially regarding environment and use by men, highlight some major differences: For example, the high percentage of visitors who were sick required a larger number of toilets. In particular, for people with gastroenterological diseases, medical care in a spa was often recommended, and many salutary waters, if used for drinking, had diuretic effects. The risk involved concerning infections and contagious diseases, as treated in, e.g. the specialized 'baths of the lepers,' must have been known; but we do not know how this hygienic problem was kept under control either with ancient medical concepts, or from the resulting architectural solutions.

Most beneficial waters were, because of their high temperature and the tendency to create heavy incrustations, not adequate for the flushing of toilets. Roman engineers had to provide an independent supply of fresh water.

Only a few ancient spas are well preserved, and even fewer have been excavated. The poor documentation does not yet allow us to give a general overview on secondary installations, such as latrines. The Taurine Baths are a spa near *Centumcellae*, today Civitavecchia (*figs 8.9-10*).[48] The spring supplied calcareous, sulfurous water as hot as 47° C. An early imperial building was transformed in the Hadrianic period into a monumental health center, offering all the comforts of Roman imperial *thermae*, such as large heated halls and a library. The elaborate ornamentation of the interior and epigraphical evidence show that elite Romans frequented this spa.

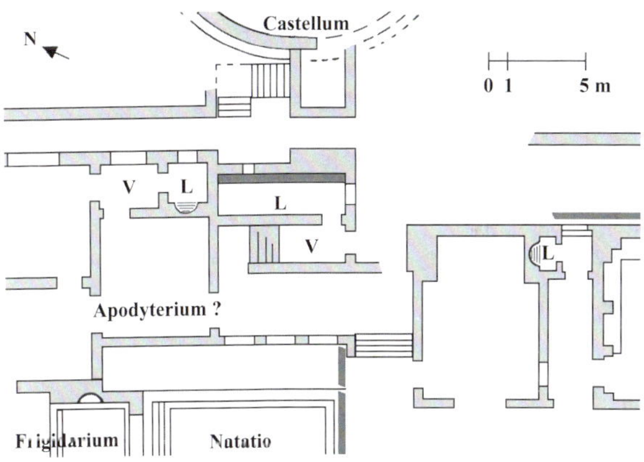

Fig. 8.9. Civitavecchia, Terme Taurine, sketch-plan showing the single-seater (left) and the multi-seater toilet (right), L = Latrine and V = Vestibule (drawing J. Köhler).

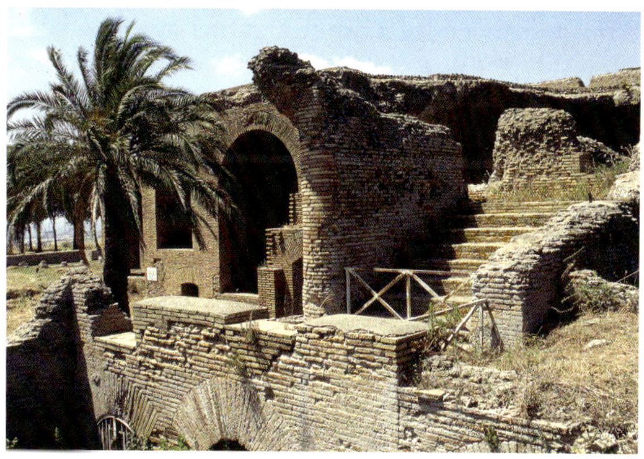

Fig. 8.10. Civitavecchia, Terme Taurine, staircase on top of the multi-seater latrine; in the back the huge frigidarium *window (photo J. Köhler).*

A total of seven toilets, two multi-seaters and five single-seaters, can be identified. Two latrines next to the main entrance illustrate the different types. A multi-seater is located under the staircase leading to the upper floor. One enters a small vestibule, with traces of a simple white mosaic floor, to reach the latrine (6.5 m x 1.9 m). The sewer and the holes to insert the supports for marble seats show that a bench for not more than eight users ran along the entire eastern wall. Adjacent to this room is a single-seater (1.9 m x 1.8 m), but with a separate entrance from the *apodyterium* (?). It has its own vestibule, a large window, and a semicircular niche for the seats. Some fragments of white marble slabs from the seats have been preserved. The toilet drained through the wall into the sewer of the multi-seater. Both latrines were flushed with fresh water, coming with high pressure from the nearby *castellum*, and both emptied, together with the waste water from the pools and with rain water, into the main sewer system. The two latrines shared the same water supply system, but they also suggest a social diversification between common people and elité users. This pattern is repeated in the southern part of the Taurine Baths: a narrow corridor leads to a central multi-seater below the probable hostel, whereas two single-seaters with niches flank the library.

CASE STUDY: STREET LATRINE IN THE CIVIL TOWN OF *CARNUNTUM* (*Silvia Radbauer*)

Die Straßenlatrine in dem römischen zivilen Stadtviertel von *Carnuntum* (Freilichtmuseum, Archäologischer Park Carnuntum, Niederösterreich) ist die einzige vollständig erhaltene Anlage in Westpannonien (*figs 8.11-12*).[49] Sie steht auf der nördlichen Wohnterrasse (*Insula* VI) in einer Nebenstraße, der sog. *Weststraße*, in der Nähe einer Straßenkreuzung und ist unmittelbar an die westliche Mauerfront der bislang noch nicht ausgegrabenen Bebauung angelehnt. Die Straßenlatrine war an dieser Stelle für Fußgänger gut zugänglich.

Die Erbauung der Straßenlatrine erfolgte im Zuge einer völligen Neugestaltung der Straßeninfrastruktur, die mit einem großen urbanistischen Ausbau (u.a. der Therme und der Wohnhausbebauung) gegen Ende des 2. bzw. Anfang des 3. Jahrhunderts in der Regierungszeit der Severer einherging. Dabei wurde erstmals eine Straßenpflasterung aus großen Kalksandsteinplatten verlegt und die Entwässerung auf größere Fließkanäle K 14 unter der Mitte der Straßen umgestellt, die die Abwässer von mehreren kleineren Seitenkanälen aus den umliegenden privaten und öffentlichen Gebäuden und Latrinen aufnahmen.[50] Die Anbindung der Straßenlatrine an die öffentliche Kanalisation garantierte eine zuverlässige Entsorgung der Fäkalien. Die Straßenlatrine blieb das gesamte 3. Jahrhundert in Verwendung und wurde mit der Aufgabe der gesamten Kanalisation in den letzten Jahrzehnten des 3. Jahrhunderts stillgelegt. Diese Datierung resultiert aus den mit Siedlungsmüll enthaltenen fundreichen Verfüllungen der Kanäle K 45 und K 14.

Als Fundament für die Straßenlatrine diente die Kanalsohle eines stillgelegten Kanalstranges der Frischwasserleitung, dessen Seitenwände für den Einbau entsprechend abgetragen wurden. Die Straßenlatrine war dreiteilig aufgebaut und bestand insgesamt aus zwei gleich großen übereinander gesetzten Kalksteinblöcken (0,74 x 0,80 x 0,48 m), auf denen oben eine 18 cm dicke Kalksteinplatte aufgelegt war. Bei den oberen beiden Teilen ist in der Mitte ein 24 cm großer runder Kanal ausgearbeitet, während der unterste Steinquader von der Mitte bis zum östlichen Rand eine schräge Abflussrinne aufweist. Durch diesen ausgearbeiteten Kanal wurden die Fäkalien in einen Holzkanal K 45 geleitet, der wiederum in den Hauptsammelkanal K 14 unter der Straßenmitte mündete. Der 1,65 x 0,48 x 0,05 m große Holzkanal K 45 war aus Nadelholz gefertigt und konnte für museale Zwecke konserviert und geborgen werden. Dicke Ablagerungsschichten von Urinstein wurden vor allem in der schrägen Abflussrinne der Latrine und an der Oberfläche des Holzkanals K 45 festgestellt (vgl. case study chapter 7, S. 97-98). Darüber hinaus kann bei dieser Straßenlatrine aufgrund der geringen fäkalen und sedimentären Ablagerungen sowie dem darin enthaltenen zeitlich eng geschlossenen Fundensemble aus dem Ende des 3. Jahrhunderts n. Chr. von einer konsequenten Wasserspülung und einer gelegentlichen Reinigung zur Instandhaltung ausgegangen werden. Die Wasserspülung erfolgte jedenfalls nicht über eine fixe Zuleitung. Auffällig waren in der Kanalverfüllung kleine Holzkohlestücke, die die Eigenschaft besitzen, Feuchtigkeit zu absorbieren und schlechte Gerüche zu neutralisieren.

Die 0,45 m über das Straßenpflaster hochgestellte Form der Latrine lässt keine gesicherten Rückschlüsse auf eine mögliche aufgehende Holzkonstruktion zu. Denn an den Außenwänden sind nur punktgespitzte Bearbeitungsspuren und Glättspuren an der Oberfläche vom Zuhauen der Steinblöcke sichtbar und auch das umliegende Straßenpflaster weist keine unmittelbaren Einarbeitungsspuren auf.

Zahlreiche Straßenlatrinen solcher Bauart, meist mit anderen externen Abfließ- und Beseitigungslösungen sind in römischen Städten der Nordprovinzen wie Augst (*Augusta Raurica*) sowie auch im gesamten Mittelmeerraum und Nahen Osten bezeugt.[51]

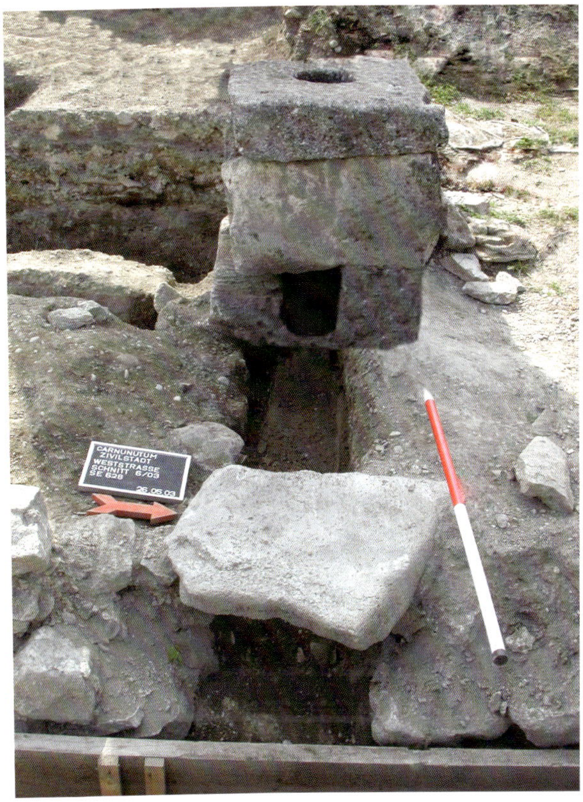

Fig. 8.11. Carnuntum, Weststraße, *Straßenlatrine mit Holzkanal unter der Pflasterstraße (photo S. Radbauer).*

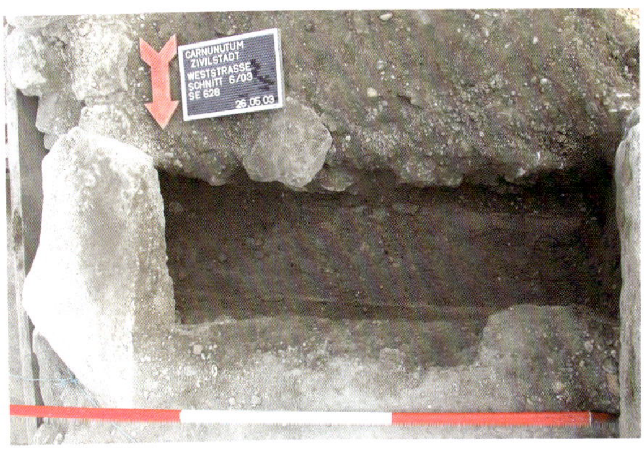

Fig. 8.12. Carnuntum, Weststraße, *Straßenlatrine, Detail von Holzkanal mit Urinsteinablagerungen (photo S. Radbauer).*

8.3. Location of Private Toilets

The Location of Latrines in Roman Houses at Pompeii (Barry Hobson)

In this chapter three different aspects of Roman life are considered to compare the provision of what might loosely be defined as 'private' as distinct from 'public' latrines. For the purposes of this section a private latrine will exist within a 'private' property and access to it will only be available to the people working or living there. The three types of properties are, firstly, houses and living accommodations, then workplaces (treated by Flohr, below, pp. 126-128) and, finally, army forts (see Goldwater, chapter 9.3, pp. 135-139), including buildings within the *vici* outside the fort. To a great extent the information that can be gathered from each of these three situations is flawed for reasons which will become apparent. All three, however, provide good evidence for the factors that might have governed where latrines were to be found and, perhaps, for whom they were available.

Pompeii has occupation evidence from around 500 BC, but the buildings can be dated from the 3rd century BC. To some degree, the development of latrine provisions may rely on cultural practices that were not necessarily Roman.

The *insulae* of Pompeii are subdivided into different numbers of properties. Although almost all of the *insulae* offer a variety of different types of property, the percentages of each type vary, and the question must be asked if this affected the provision of toilet facilities.

Private houses vary in size. Some, such as the house of the Faun, for example, occupy nearly a whole *insula*. Others are small with only two or three rooms. Does size determine whether or not the property has a latrine? There is considerable evidence for upper storey latrines that are likely to have been used by lower status groups, and perhaps smaller properties would not need their latrines on the ground floor.

Latrines are found in a number of different places within the houses. In many, the latrine is associated with the kitchen.[52] In some of the *insulae*, there is a preponderance of latrines situated just inside the entrances to the houses.[53] There

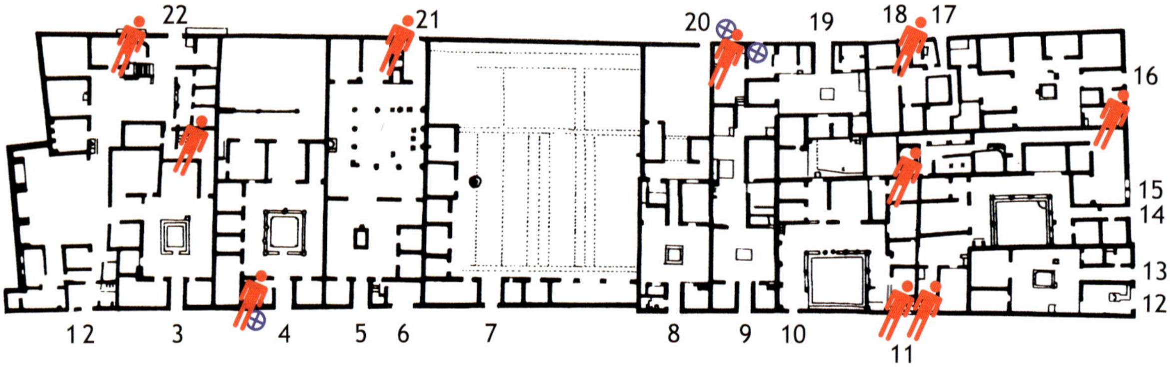

Fig. 8.13. Pompeii, VI 5, plan showing latrines and down-pipe (drawing B. Hobson).

may be a number of reasons for this, but one was almost certainly to allow the excrement to be disposed of through the walls into the cesspits that lie under the sidewalks in the street. Other reasons for building the latrine in this particular part of the house may be for the convenience of access, and also that there may have been fewer problems with the smell from the latrine, with the cesspit 'away' from the inside of the house. The plan of VI 5 shows eleven properties (*fig. 8.13*). Eight of the latrines are situated just inside the houses close to entrances. In contrast, VI 14 has virtually no latrines near to entrances, but has a number of down-pipes indicating upper storey latrines.

In the case of the larger houses the subdivision of the rooms and space within the house may indicate areas where slaves/servants worked. In a number of properties, these areas also appear to define the place where the latrine was sited. Such a house is VI 13, 12, 19. In the northeast of this property there is a well defined work area. A corridor separates these rooms from the rest of the house, and the latrine is at the end of the corridor by the 'tradesmen's' *entrance* 12. It would seem unlikely that well-to-do guests would use this facility. Another house (IX 5, 13, 14, 15) has its latrine well away from the main rooms, although, in this case, the corridor containing the work areas lies adjacent to the peristyle (*fig. 8.14*). A convenient location for the latrine is under staircases. One can be found inside the house at VI 4, 36.51 In one or two very large houses, the latrine is to be found in association with a bath suite, e.g. in the *Praedia* of Iulia Felix.[54] In this particular case, the latrine may not offer privacy (*fig. 8.3*), but it is likely that patrons were of a similar social status, and may even have known each other. There is a second latrine in this property associated with the kitchen, off the rear entrance (II 4, 10). Presumably this offered a facility for the workers who were tending to the needs of the users of the bathhouse.

The domestic latrines in the houses of Pompeii are, in general, only for one person, although in one or two of the very large houses the size of the seat may indicate that there were places for two persons.[55] Almost all of these are within servants' working areas and the graffiti associated with the latrine in the House of the Centenary (to the right of the entrance, IX 9, d) suggests that only the servants used this latrine.

In some situations the latrine appears to be associated with the garden. In II 8, 1, a property that almost certainly has a dining area in the garden, the latrine is up against the south wall, well away from all other buildings. In I 11, 10, 11, and 12, the latrine, which is directly available from the garden, is back-to-back with the latrine within the house.

The destruction of the upper stories of Pompeii in the eruption of AD 79 has left many questions unanswered about the usage of the upper floors. Latrines in upper stories were treated in an article discussing private latrines in Pompeii.[56] Many terracotta pipes run through the walls of the buildings, and the upper ends of the vast majority are broken and give no hint from where they originate. Although their existence is said to confirm upper floors,[57] it has been suggested that these may have carried water from roofs. Recent evidence confirms that they carried excrement from latrines.[58] Architectural confirmation for these latrines is sparse. Fourteen have been found so far.[59] Figure 8.15 shows the niche into which the wooden seat was placed. The chronology for the development of latrines suggests that these upper storey latrines were installed in the 1st century AD.

A property called the School House (VII 12, 14) has a narrow room with two down-pipes. One of these is coming from under the seat of the first-

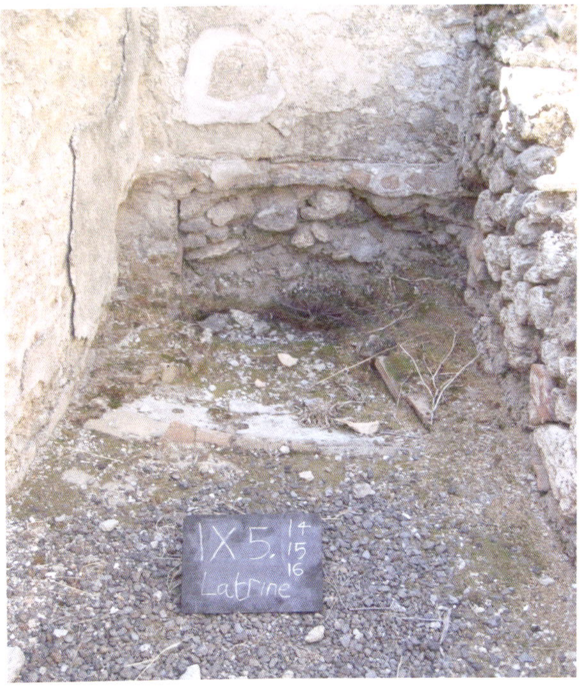

Fig. 8.14. Pompeii, IX 5, 13-15, latrine (photo B. Hobson).

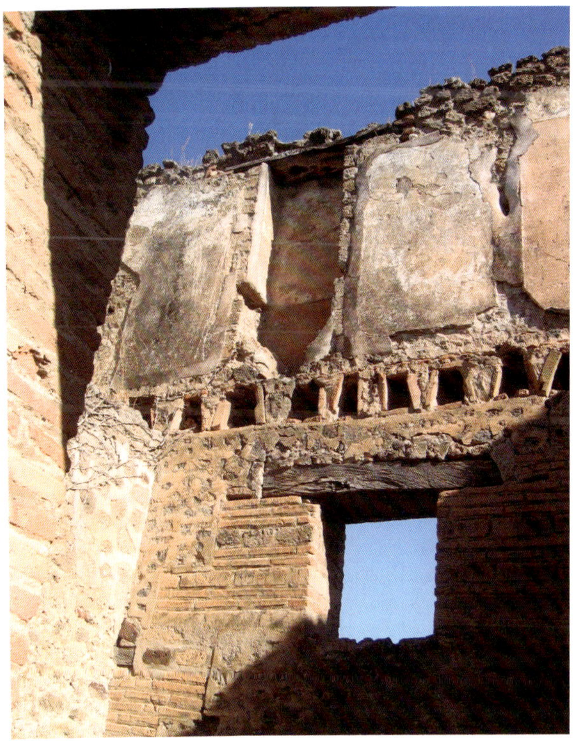

Fig. 8.15. Pompeii, VII 2, 18, latrine on upper floor (photo B. Hobson).

storey latrine, and the other appears, from the scar in the wall, to be coming from a second-storey latrine. This interpretation may explain a number of dual down-pipes running together in walls in other parts of the city.[60]

There appears to have been a profusion of public latrines in Ostia, but perhaps these were used only by males. In Pompeii there are only a small number of multi-seat latrines, all of which may not have been for public use, and at least one of which was probably not functioning at the time of the eruption.[61] What facilities were available in Roman towns for females, and were there semi-private public latrines, that is, latrines blocked to general use for some hours and open to all at other hours? There are a few 'private' latrines that are directly accessible from the street. In most case these are associated with staircases leading to upper storey accommodations (e.g. VII 9, 64). Would access be allowed to a latrine in a private house, or perhaps more likely a latrine in a bar?

Taverns and eateries (*thermopolia*) throng the streets of Pompeii. As one entered the city by the Stabian Gate or the Herculaneum Gate bars would have been offering food and drink all along the way. VI 1 has two bars on the Consolare Street: The Bar of Acisculus (VI 1, 17) and the Bar of Phoebus (VI 1, 18, 20). Both of these bars had latrines at the rear of the property. The one in VI 1, 17 only had access through the bar and past the cooking area (Room 3). In the case of VI 1, 18, 20, there was a rear entrance from the narrow Narcissus Street, and the latrine was immediately to the right (Room 3). In the property I 9, 3, 4, entrance 3 leads into the 'house,' whereas entrance 4 is a bar. The latrine in this property is at the rear of the property through the garden beyond room 9. This situation would make it most unlikely that the latrine was available to passers-by.

There are 30 locations in Pompeii for commercial bread making (see Flohr, below). The latrine in V 1, 14, 15, 16 is situated well away from the living rooms at the rear of the property (*fig. 8.16*). Similarly, the latrine in a house that includes a bakery (I 12, 1, 2) is almost as far from the living accommodation as it is possible to get. The owner of the bakery at VII 1, 37, 38 appears to have acquired a portion of another property, VII 1, 30, in order to construct a latrine for the workers. This latrine is at ground level (*fig. 8.17*). Despite there being a staircase to upper floor accommodation, there is no evidence of down-pipes.

There are obviously a number of reasons for having the latrine in these situations. Smell has already been mentioned. Privacy, social status, and/or gender may also be factors. The latrine in the House of the Centenary, mentioned above, is notable for offering information of interest on two of these factors. The latrine is in the service area of the house, by a rear entrance, with disposal of excreta out through the wall and under the sidewalk, and flushing water onto the street.

> *Marthae hoc trichilinium est, nam in tricliino cacat*
> This is Martha's *triclinium*: in fact, she poops in the triclinium.

This graffito (*fig. 8.18*) on the wall of the latrine refers to Martha, probably from Judea, who defecates in this area. She is a slave (or a servant) with notions above her station, since she is being compared to the elites who defecate in the *triclinium*, probably into chamber pots. This brief look at the location of latrines in one city reinforces the fact that only by looking at cultural aspects of Roman life can we interpret the reasons for the location of their latrines.

Latrines and Workshops (Miko Flohr)

Another place where toilets are likely to be located is in buildings that contained a workshop. Craftsmen worked long days, during which one or more visits to the toilet might be needed. The position of toilets in these buildings tells a story about the functioning of workshops and about the toilet behavior of craftsmen during the work day. Unfortunately, ancient workshops have not received much attention from classical archaeologists, and there are very few systematic and detailed studies of specific workshop types and their material remains. At this moment, there are only two ancient sites at which the workshops have been studied sufficiently to allow for a comprehensive discussion of their relation to toilet facilities. These are Ostia and Pompeii. Though these sites are near to each other both geographically and chronologically, the scale and nature of economic activities in both cities are so different that they together cover a fairly wide spectrum of the contexts in which we might expect ancient workshops to occur. Hence, these sites can be used to build up the picture, which then will be contextualized by parallels from some sites in other parts of the ancient world. Many workshops, especially the smaller ones, were situated in *tabernae*. As these have been discussed above by Hobson, they will not be treated here. There were, however, also workshops in other contexts deserving some special attention.

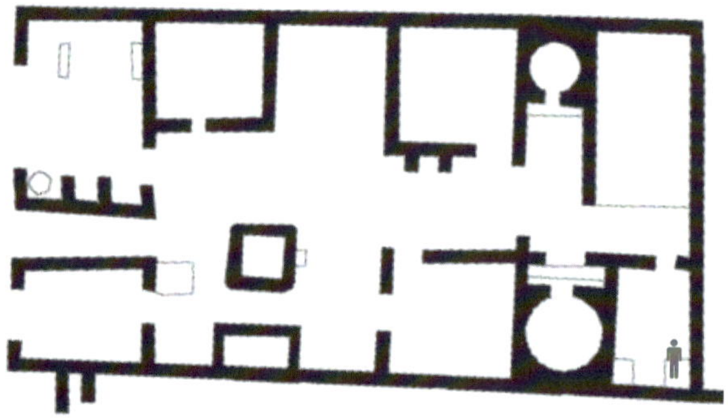

Fig. 8.16. Pompeii, V 1, 14-16, plan of the bakery with toilet location (drawing B. Hobson).

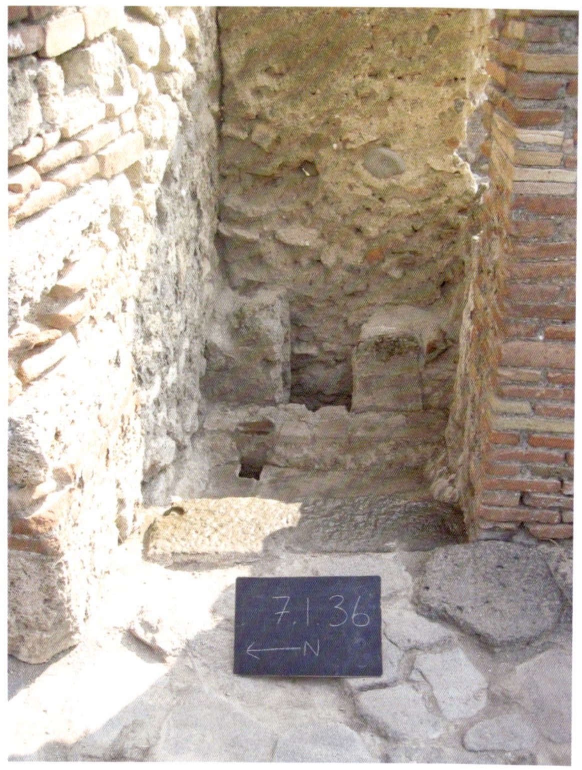

Fig. 8.17. Pompeii, VII 1, 36, latrine (photo B. Hobson).

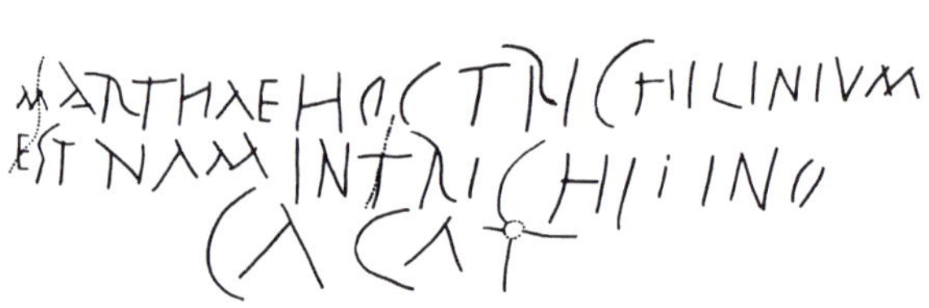

Fig. 8.18. Pompeii, House of the Centenary (IX 8, 3, 6, a), graffito in latrine: Marthae hoc trichilinium est nam in trichliino cacat.

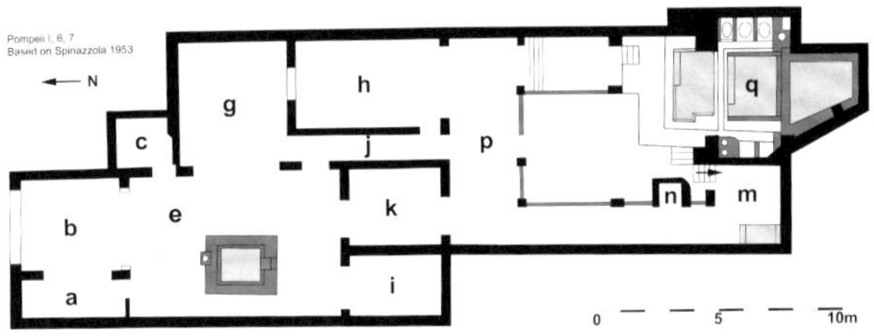

Fig. 8.19. Pompeii, fullonica *of Stephanus (I 6, 7), with workshop (q), kitchen (m) and latrine (n) (drawing M. Flohr).*

Pompeii

Pompeii has brought to light a large number of well-preserved workshops. 23 mills-bakeries can be identified, along with seven bakeries without mills, fourteen *lanifricariae*, whose use is unknown, ten fulleries, six textile dyeing establishments, and a tannery. Only nineteen of these were situated in *tabernae*. Of the others, most were located in *atrium* houses that combined domestic and commercial functions under one roof.[62] Many of these complexes had toilets, just like other houses, and mostly in similar locations, that is, in the kitchen or related to service areas.[63] This means that they often also were near the workshop, which was often associated with the kitchen. For example, in the *fullonica* of Stephanus, the two-seater toilet is directly next to the kitchen, and only a few steps away from the main working area (*fig. 8.19*). In the House of the Oven (VI 3, 3, 27-28), the toilet is in the kitchen that was only accessible from the workshop and the first floor. Variation, however, was possible. Toilets were in different locations as well. In the large house, VII 2, 3, 6, the kitchen was located in the *atrium* zone, the latrine was in one of the service rooms off the peristyle in the southern part of the house, and the workshop, a large bakery, was situated in a large annex west of the *atrium*-peristyle complex. In house VII 1, 36-37, which contained a bakery, but did not have a kitchen, a one-seater latrine was situated directly next to the mill room.

A second group of workshops were situated in complexes of a layout that does not fall under the two categories just mentioned. Many of these resembled *atrium* houses and had residential quarters, although they were spatially organized in a different way. A small group of six large mills-bakeries, one *fullonica* and a dyeing workshop, however, did not have living space.[64] Of these eight workshops, five had a latrine of which the remains are still visible or have been identified by their excavators.[65] These toilets were mostly situated away from the areas were many people worked together, in a corridor, such as in bakery IX 5, 4, or, more often, in a remote part of the complex, such as in bakery IX 1, 3, 33, where the latrine is just next to the back door. Thus, at Pompeii, large workshops, either in houses or in other complexes, often had toilet facilities so that workers did not have to go to other places to relieve themselves.

Ostia

The situation at Ostia was different. While the Pompeian evidence covered a spectrum of small to medium-sized workshops that were predominantly functioning in a domestic context, Ostia shows a sharp dichotomy between small shops and workshops in independent *tabernae*, on the one hand, and large industrial factories, on the other hand. Only the second group deserves some discussion here. Compared to Pompeii, the number and variety of the archaeologically discernible workshops is lower. Only two types can be recognized: *fullonicae* (fulleries) and mills/bakeries. Three large fulleries have been found and two complete bakeries. All these workshops have been studied relatively thoroughly.[66] The complexes mainly consisted of working rooms and lacked connections to living spaces, either on the same level or on a second floor. People working there seem to have arrived when the work day started and must have left when it ended. Remarkably, none of these workshops contained traces of toilets, even though the number of workers in each is likely to have been between thirty and forty at peak hours (*fig. 8.20*). Arguably, we can not always be sure whether there was a toilet that cannot be traced any more, but at least in the case of the three large fulleries, the presence of toilet facilities can be excluded.[67] This is extremely remarkable because if there was kind of workshop that could easily have a well-flushed toilet installed, then it was the large Ostian *fullonica* with its enormous rinsing basins.[68] The lack of a latrine meant that workers, if they needed to, would have had to go to public latrines nearby, which may suggest that these people were generally expected to relieve themselves outside of work hours. Nevertheless, it likely occurred regularly that someone had to leave the workroom for a short visit to a latrine elsewhere.

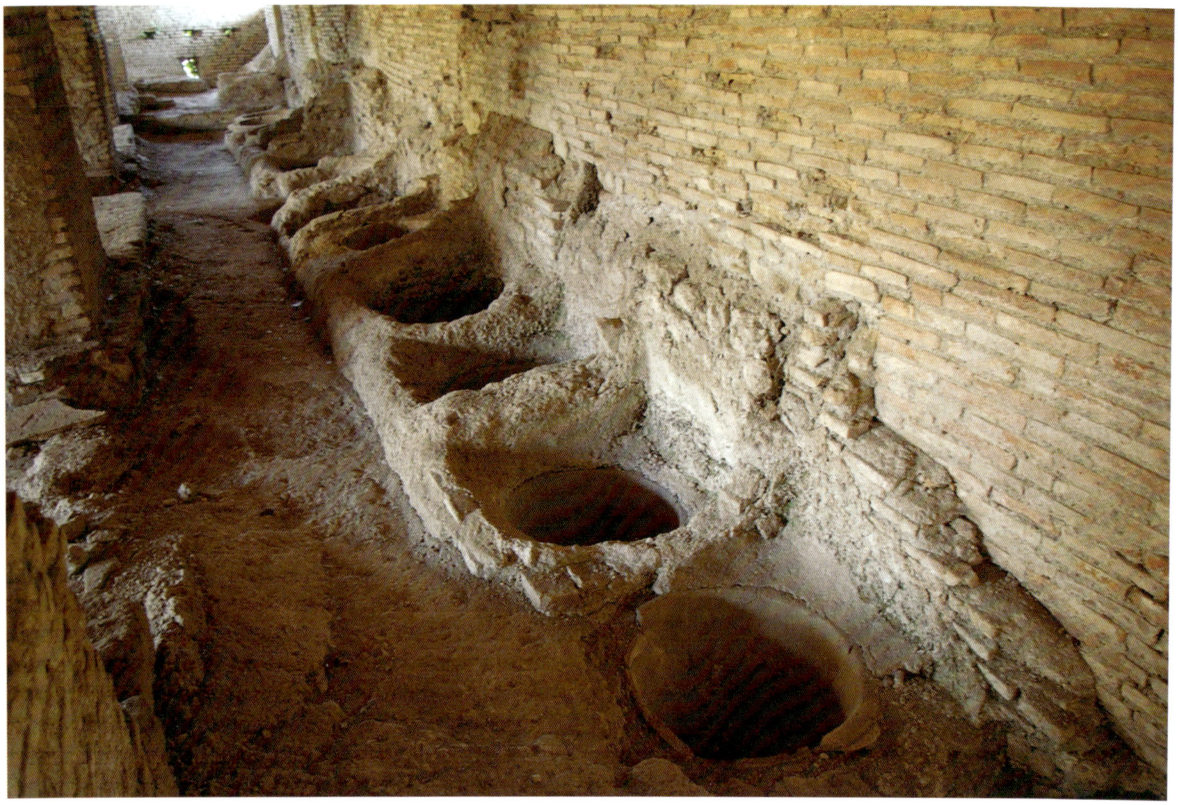

Fig. 8.20. Ostia, fullonica *V viii, 3: though there was space for more than forty workers, there was no toilet (photo M. Flohr).*

Parallels

The situation in Ostia differs sharply from that in Pompeii, and it appears to be rather exceptional compared to other Mediterranean sites as well. Even the large non-domestic workshops from Pompeii are unparalleled elsewhere: the common location for workshops was in *tabernae* or in houses and the scale was smaller than in imperial Italy. A good example is the situation at Delos. This site only knew small-to medium-sized workshops in shops or houses.[69] As to those in houses, recent study by Brun has revealed a perfume workshop in a peristyle house in the Stadium Quarter (house Ib) and a workshop devoted to the production of olive oil in a complex in the Theater Quarter (house 3O) that presumably originally had had domestic functions.[70] Both complexes had a toilet in a position where the toilets of Delos usually were situated, which is near one of the entrances directly next to the street.[71] Here, just as in Pompeian *atrium* houses, the location of the toilet is in the first place dictated by the way houses were commonly organized, even though, in both cases the distance between workroom and toilets is short. As at Pompeii, workers could satisfy their toilet needs in most cases within the walls of the complex where the workshop was situated.

Notes

1 Cf., for example, the multi-seat toilets in the large theater, in the peristyle next to the large theater, and in the large *palaestra* near the amphitheater of Pompeii.

2 Ostia has many good examples of this latter type of toilet, usually in the ground floors of *insulae*.

3 I am grateful to Antonella Merletto for classifying these design types.

4 Neudecker 1991, 14 with n. 32. Cf. *Thera* I, 164-167; 174-176. See also, Monika Trümper (chapter 3.3) for further discussion of Hellenistic latrines.

5 *Thera* I, 174-176.

6 Neudecker 1991, 14 with n. 35. I was not able to locate L. Marangou, *Anaskafi Minoas Amorgou* (1986) to see the original publication of this latrine, but I thank A. Merletto for the reference.

7 I am grateful to A. Merletto for telling me about several specific latrines in baths sited near warm rooms or heat sources. For latrines near one or two *praefurnia*: latrine in the women's baths of Augusta Raurica (Laur-Bélart

1948, 95); latrine in a public building in the Forum Claudii Vallensium (Wiblé 1977, 199-214); and latrine in the Forum Baths of Belalis Major (Mahjoubi 1978, 198). For a latrine next to a room with a hypocaust: see Capitolium Baths at Cuicul (Ballu 1926, CLXI). For a latrine next to the sudatorium: latrine in Baths of the North Gymnasium in Pergamon (Schatzmann 1923, 91; and latrine in the small town baths of Les Fontaines Salées (Luis 1943, 27). For a latrine near a *caldarium*: see the latrine in the North-East Baths at Epidaurus (Ginouvès 1955, 141).

8 Cf. Fagan 1999, 75-84.

9 Fagan 1999, 83, with n. 30: While Hellenization had been in progress since the 3rd century, and while admittedly, the majority of Romans were excluded from the brunt of the cultural explosion (because they could not read, write, nor buy expensive decorations for their humble habitations), Fagan would not have us forget the 'new and interesting patterns of behavior...passing between foreigner and Roman' in the seething streets of the Subura as well. His n. 30 also includes a vast array of inscriptions from Rome bearing Greek names, which attest to the presence of easterners in the city.

10 Cf. Blake 1947, 324-352; Anderson 1997, 145-151. Fagan 1999, 83, n. 31 considers this development further.

11 Van Vaerenbergh 2001. For a summery of this comprehensive study: Van Vaerenbergh 2006, 453-459.

12 Nielsen 1990; Yegül 1992 (specifically on latrines: 411, 413); Neudecker 1994, 83-91.

13 Neudecker 1994, 109, 130, 162, n. 190.

14 Although the impressive imperial baths of Rome are fairly well documented, there are still difficulties with locating the latrines. Only in the Baths of Diocletian can we definitely locate the latrine(s) in the *exedra(e)* in the northeast wall of the *palaestra* (Tagliamonte 1998, 34). In comparison to these latrines and toilets in similar bath complexes, as in the Antonine Baths of Carthage (Lézine 1969), can we probably find the latrines of the other imperial baths in Rome in some of the big *exedrae* adjoining the *palaestrae*.

15 Neudecker 1994, 108, 161-162 n. 273, 279.

16 Becatti 1961, 59-60, pl. 74 (118); Neudecker 1994, 60, 90, 108, 161-162, n. 273, 279. It was Becatti who pointed out that this room was a latrine. Other authors had given it a different function. Several recent authors have therefore overlooked this latrine. The presence of a gutter against the south and west wall, a sponge basin near the door, and a mosaic with a Nile scene are proof of its latrine function.

17 Boersma 1985, 392-393.

18 Parslow 1998, 206.

19 Köhler 2000, 190, n. 55.

20 Jansen 2002b, 76-83; 2003, 137-152; 2007, 165-181.

21 Jansen 2003, 142; 2007. Recent in-depth research (October 2003) of the latrine of the Small Baths has shown that there is still a lot more to say about this latrine. The rich decoration is just one of the new finds. An article (Van Vaerenbergh, forthcoming) will be published within the framework of the multidisciplinary Ri.V.A.-project, which restudies Hadrian's Villa. The findings of this excavation have been studied by A. Blanco (Blanco 2007).

22 Jacobelli 1987, 153-154; 1988, 206; Manderscheid 1993, 339-340.

23 Neudecker 1994, 64-65.

24 Comparison to similar bath complexes (note 4) suggests that the great imperial public baths of Rome, had two impressive latrines, which probably only reflect the greatness of the baths and its symmetrical plan. The mirrored layout of the baths of the Arvales-brotherhood at La Magliana also suggests the existence of two toilet rooms. It is striking that these baths were only used by a male public. Numerous baths had a symmetrical/axial layouts.

25 Neudecker 1994, 64-65; MacMullen 1980, 208-209.

26 Bowen Ward 1992, 125-147; Cantarella 1987, 135-150. The emancipation already had its roots in the second century BC.

27 Varro *L.L.* 9.68; and others. More detailed information on the early development of Roman Baths: Bowen Ward 1992, 126-131.

28 More detailed information on changes in bath architecture and women bathing with men: Bowen Ward 1992, 126-142.

29 Is it a coincidence that the first public latrine at the Forum of Pompeii (Neudecker 1994, 163) was constructed at this same moment?

30 Bowen Ward 1992, 135-139, 147 ('public baths as a locus for nudity').

31 The only evidence of alternating use by men and women of the same set of baths can be found in Vipasca (Portugal) (*CIL* 2.5181). Roman Christian writers criticized the fact that men and women, also Christians, bathed together. Therefore Christian women were encouraged to bath in an orderly, modest and moderate manner; only for reasons of cleanliness, not for pleasure. Just in the late 4th and 5th centures AD individual and segregated bathing became more common. It was also at this time that the *History Augusta* was written. The Christian author 'made up' contrasting biographies of 'good emperors' (Hadrian, for example) who forbade mixed bathing, and 'bad emperors', who allowed it. More detailed information on Christian attitudes: Bowen Ward 1992, 142-146.

32 Nielsen 1990; Yegül 1992.

33 At first an entrance fee of one *quadrans* was customary (Cic. *Cael.* 62; Sen. *Ep.* 86.8; Mart. *Epig.* 8.42, 3.7.3; Juv. *Sat.* 6.447; Hor. *Sat.* 1.3.137). In Diocletian's time, we know from the Price Edict one had to pay two *denarii* (inflation). On special occasions (gift of the emperor or of a local aristocrat, etc.) public baths were free. Probably one had to pay more when visiting baths with a private owner, since he or she would likely be interested in greater profits.

34 Nielsen 1990, 134.

35 Little rooms near the entrances of the Stabian and Central Baths in Pompeii and the Baths of the Swimmer in Ostia are often labeled as places where the visitors had to pay an entrance fee. For the moment such suggestions are still doubtful. Maybe we have to be more attentive to the possibility of finding spare tokens and coins in the toilet deposits, which did not make it into the hands of a toilet attendant.

36 Opening hours have already been briefly discussed in chapter 6 on bath-related water supply and accessibility.

37 We can assume that most baths were closed at sundown. For example, Christian sources like the *Didascalia* from Syria, written prior to AD 250, attempts to persuade Christian women to go to the mixed baths after the tenth hour (certainly in winter it gets dark), when fewer people (men) would be present (*Didascalia* 3.1.9 f.). Martial wrote that the tenth hour was a little bit late to be at the baths (Mart., *Epig.* 3.36).

38 Emperor Tacitus ordered that all baths had to be closed

at sundown (*S.H.A. Tacitus* 10.2). This, in fact, shows that some baths had nightly opening hours. In contrast, it is said that emperor Alexander Severus provided lamp oil to make sure that the baths could stay open at night (*S.H.A. Alex. Sev.* 24.6). These sources probably tell us more about the time when these biographies were written (end of the 4th century AD). It shows how these emperors then were looked at from a Christian point of view (that is, as good or evil). Cf. n. 31.

39 Carandini et al. 1973, 30, 78-82 (Strato IIIA), 87-89 (Strato IVA). For the moment we have to be careful with this interpretation, because the fragments could have been transported by the water from other locations, or could have been sunk down from the deposit fill. Comparison with findings from other latrine deposits is necessary.

40 Gal., *De san. tuenda* 5.12.14.

41 Plut., *Mor.* 131C.

42 Menéndez-Pidal 1976, 211; see also Álvarez 1983, 307.

43 Alba 2001, 72.

44 Mélida 1921, 10.

45 During the process of publishing this text, it was possible to carry out archaeological excavations on the referred latrines, within the Research Project '*El teatro y anfiteatro de Augusta Emerita: documentación, investigación y presentación de dos edificios de espectáculo de época romana*' (3PR05A104), developed by the *Instituto de Arqueología de Mérida* and the *Consorcio de la Ciudad Monumental de Mérida*. Due to these interventions, it was possible to confirm the stated hypothesis and to obtain interesting data about its construction and evolution, which are being studied and will be published in the near future on a monograph that will include the results obtained throughout this Project.

46 Alba 2001, 72.

47 I would like to thank G. Sánchez, archaeologist at the *Consorcio de la Ciudad de Mérida*, for providing me with this unpublished information.

48 Bastianelli 1942; Köhler 2000; Köhler/Rapone 2002.

49 The excavations took place during the project 'Carnuntum - Zivilstadt', directed by F. Humer in the Open-Air-Museum Petronell. The project was financed by the Government of the State of Lower Austria - Department for Culture Affairs and the Archaeological Park Carnuntum.

50 Radbauer/Humer 2005, 903-906.

51 Hänggi 1989, 73-96.

52 E.g., I 7, 1; I 7, 7; I 12, 1, 2; II 2, 1, 2; II 4, 10; V 4, 3; VI 1, 6, 7, 8; VI 1, 17; VI 2, 17; VI 2, 27; VI 5, 9, 19; VI 6, 1, 8, 22; VI 7, 23; VI 7, 25; VI 9, 3, 12; VI 10, 14; VI 15, 7, 8, 9; VI 16, 36, 37; VII 6, 30, 37; VII 12, 30-32; VIII 3, 17; IX 3, 14.

53 E.g., I 6, 15; I 11, 1, 2; I 11, 8; I 12, 11; I 14, 2; I 14, 8, 9; II 1, 7, 8, 9; II 4, 10; II 8, 1; V 1, 23, 25, 26, 10; V 4, 1, 2; VI 1, 5; VI 1, 9, 10, 23; VI 1, 18, 20; VI 2, 16, 21; VI 2, 26; VI 5, 1, 3, 22; VI 5, 4; VI 5, 5, 6, 21; VI 5, 8, 20; VI 5, 9, 19; VI 5, 10; VI 5, 11, 14; VI 5, 16, 17, 18; VI 6, 1, 8, 22; VI 7, 4, 5, 6; VI 7, 15; VI 7, 20, 21, 22; VI 9, 3, 12; VI 9, 6, 9; VI 11, 8; VI 13, 10, 11; VI 13, 12, 19; VI 15, 4, 5, 24, 25; VI 16, 17; VIII 3, 12; VIII 3, 14; VIII 3, 17; IX 2, 19, 21; IX 5, 11, 13; IX 6, 1, a; IX 7, 21, 22; IX 8, 1; IX 8, 3, 6, a; IX 9, 1.

54 Others at I 6, 1; V 2, 4; VI 7, 8-12; VI 14, 40.

55 Also Casa del Labirinto VI 11, 9, 10.

56 E.g. House of the Faun VI 12, 2, 7; House of the Centenary IX 8, 3, 6, a: Also IX 1, 20, 30.

57 Jansen 1997, 125.

58 Pirson 1999, 170.

59 Love 2007.

60 In Regio V there are three: V 1, 8; V 1, 30; V 3, 10. Regio VII has three: VII 2, 18; VII 2, 20; VII 12, 14. There are two in Regio VIII, viz. VIII 4, 37 and VII 6, 7. and six in Regio IX: IX, 2, 7,8; IX 2, 19, 21; IX 3, 4; IX 3, 17; IX 5, 21; IX 13, 1.

61 Also VIII 4, 37; IX 1, 9.

62 Forum; Forum Baths; Central Baths; *Praedia* of Iulia Felix; Gladiator latrine, Large Theater; Grand Palaestra latrine.

63 Flohr 2007.

64 Flohr 2007, 139-140, 142-144.

65 Mills-bakeries I 3, 27, I 4, 12-17, VI 6, 17-20, IX 1, 3.33, IX 3, 10-12 and IX 5, 4; *fullonica* VI 16, 3, 4; dyeing workshop I 8, 19. Cf. Flohr 2007.

66 The latrines are still visible in IX 1, 3, 33 and IX 3, 10-12 (cf. Jansen 2002a, 87-88) and they have been recorded in I 3, 27 (Eschebach 1993, 25), I 8, 19 (Eschebach 1993, 47) and IX 5, 4 (*NSc* 1878, 41). Mills-bakeries I 4, 12-17 and VI 6, 17-20 and *fullonica* VI 16, 3, 4 did not have a latrine.

67 For the fulleries see Pietrogrande 1978 and De Ruyt 2001, for the mills-bakeries Bakker 1999.

68 *Fullonicae* II xi, 1, III ii, and VI xiii, 5. There might be some kind of portable urinating facility in these *fullonicae*, serving to assemble urine later to be used in the production process (see chapter 10), but there was no possibility to defecate.

69 Flohr 2006.

70 For a recent overview of workshops in Delos see Brumet 1998.

71 Brun-Brumet 1997, 573-613; Brun 1999, 103.

72 See above, Trümper, chapter 3.4, pp. 37-39.

Users of the Toilets: Social Differences

9.1. Einführung (*Richard Neudecker*)

Der Mensch ist ein soziales Wesen. Auch seine einfachsten täglichen Verrichtungen verraten etwas davon. Der Gang zur Latrine ist in zweierlei Weise sozial bestimmt: zum einen kann die Latrine selbst zum Raum mit sozialer Funktion werden, zum anderen können die unterschiedlichen Erscheinungsformen aller Latrinen eine Strukturierung der Gesellschaft widerspiegeln. In diesem Abschnitt wird es darum gehen, ob und gegebenenfalls in welcher Weise für unterscheidbare Benutzergruppen auch verschiedenartige Latrinen vorgesehen waren; die Benutzergruppen müssen nicht ausschließlich sozial definiert sein, denkbar sind auch situationsbedingte Festlegungen. Die Untersuchung kann von Lage und Kontext der Latrine ausgehen sowie von der jeweiligen Gestaltung und Ausgestaltung. Eine solche Betrachtung ist vielversprechend, denn ähnlich wie in der bürgerlichen Stadtkultur des 19. und frühen 20. Jahrhunderts waren in der Antike öffentliche Räume in den Diskurs um Rang und Status nicht nur eingebunden, sondern ein wesentlicher Ort zu ihrer Festigung.

Eine Gliederung des Stadtareals in öffentliche und private Räume bietet sich aus unserer modernen Perspektive an. Dabei ist freilich zu beachten, daß Öffentlichkeit in der Antike nicht als Gegensatz zu einer Privatheit oder gar häuslichen Intimität empfunden wurde. Öffentlichkeit bildete sich in Räumen und Situationen, in denen der Mensch sein Verhalten gezielt auf eine Vielzahl von Mitmenschen ausrichtete, weil dort sein Status stetig erneuert und bestätigt wurde. Diese Öffentlichkeit war aber keine generelle, sondern erfuhr schrittweise Eingrenzungen. Ein Beispiel ist das Wohnhaus, das im vordersten Bereich um das Atrium einen selektierten öffentlichen Zutritt vorsah. Doch mit jedem Schritt in das Haus hinein zu unterschiedlichen Empfangsräumen und Gärten bis hin zu den *cubicula* wurde die Zugänglichkeit exklusiver, die Öffentlichkeit reduzierter. Was sich bei dieser Abstufung änderte, waren die Formen des sozialen Kontaktes.[1] Ein Kernbereich echter Intimität war also minimal.

Die Latrine ist innerhalb dieser verschiedenartigen Räumlichkeiten ein sozialer Ort immer dort, wo man Vorrichtungen geschaffen hat, die über das zur Defäkation Notwendige hinausreichen. Wohnarchitektur, von der Insula bis zur Luxusvilla, enthält vom Nachtgeschirr und Abtritt in der Küche bis hin zu feinen und weniger feinen Mehrsitzern ein weites Spektrum an Latrinen, das sich mit sozialen Strukturen im Haus vergleichen läßt. Von diesen häuslichen Latrinen wird Ann Olga Koloski-Ostrow sprechen (unten S. 139-141). Eine besonders vielfältige Mischung abgestufter Öffentlichkeiten weisen Herrschersitze wie der Palatin und Kaiservillen auf. Die Villa Hadriana bietet sich für eine Fallstudie über soziale Zuordnungen von Latrinen an. Eine wenig differenzierte, aber deutlich erweiterte Öffentlichkeit kennzeichnet hingegen Bauten für sozial eng umschriebene Gruppen, wie die *collegia*, oder für eine situationsbedingte Gemeinschaft, wie Militärbauten. In solchen Bereichen kann selbst eine mangelhafte oder gar fehlende Ausstattung mit Latrinen aufschlußreich sein.

Große Gemeinschaftslatrinen kennen wir vor allem von zentralen Stadträumen mit einer scheinbar unbegrenzten Öffentlichkeit in, an und zwischen den urbanen Großbauten. Tatsächlich sind Theater und Circus uneingeschränkt offen. Soziale Regulierungen des Publikums finden sich aber bereits auf den *fora*, und bei den unterschiedlichen Bädern nehmen sie zu. So bildet der ganze Stadtraum ein kompliziert verzahntes Mosaik von sozial konnotierten Orten und Bezirken. Wenn darin die Latrinen einbegriffen sind, dann können sie nicht so uniform und gleichmäßig verteilt sein, als stellten sie einzig die hygienische Infrastruktur eines Stadtareals dar.

In den folgenden Abschnitten wird es darum gehen, wie sich in spezifischen Räumen die Latrinen jeweils auf soziale Funktionen beziehen lassen, d.h. was sie über Benutzer aussagen.

9.2. Öffentliche Latrinen

Bereits der gröbste Überblick über öffentliche Latrinen ist erhellend.[2] Denn sie fehlen im direkten baulichen Zusammenhang von Theater, Circus und Stadion. Bei Veranstaltungen, die viele Stunden, oft den ganzen Tag dauerten, muß freilich für Hygiene gesorgt worden sein. Offensichtlich handelte es sich um ephemere Strukturen, die einzig der Notdurft dienten.[3] Eine wesentliche Bedeutung solcher Veranstaltungen lag in der Vorführung und Versicherung sozialer Gruppenidentitäten; die regulierte Sitzordnung ließ das Trennende, aber auch das Gemeinsame zum Erlebnis werden. Hier bestätigt das Fehlen von sozial konnotierten Latrinen indirekt, daß in andersartigen Arealen ein sozialer Aspekt den dort vorhandenen Latrinen eben anhaftete.

Allerdings finden sich Großlatrinen, sogar Prachtlatrinen, gelegentlich recht nahe an Theatern. Dann aber lassen sie sich, wie in Side,[4] in Timgad[5] und in Minturnae,[6] auf die Nachbarschaft von Forum oder Agora beziehen. Unmittelbar an der römischen Agora liegt eine prachtvolle Großlatrine in Athen,[7] eine figürlich ausgemalte Latrine befindet sich im Zugangskorridor des Forums von Bolsena,[8] weitere Beispiele liefern Conimbriga[9] und Ephesus;[10] eine Großlatrine am Forum Iulium in Rom ist auch vom Forum Romanum nicht weit entfernt.[11] All ihre Benutzer darf man in jenen Forumsbauten vermuten, die einer sozial distinguierenden Tätigkeit dienten, in der Regel sind das Basiliken und Heiligtümer mit juridischen Funktionen: Advokaten, Richter, Praetoren, Prozessierende, sowie Bankleute und deren Geschäftspartner, somit eine gehobene Bevölkerungsgruppe, die sich den halben Tag und länger hier aufhielt. Ein kommunikativer Ort mit einer dem Status angemessenen Ausstattungsqualität dürfte dem Tenor des sozialen Lebens hier bestens entsprochen haben. Der Zutritt zu diesen Großlatrinen war durch Usus und visuelle Hinweise geregelt. Zu allen derartigen Latrinen führen Vestibüle, in denen die Sklaven der sitzenden *domini* für eine Regulierung sorgen konnten.

Der Tag der *domini* verlief zwischen den Business-Räumen der Stadtzentren und den Bädern. In oder an Thermen fanden sich in jeder Stadt mit größter Wahrscheinlichkeit große öffentliche Latrinen - nicht unwichtig für Ortsfremde - und nicht nur, weil damit ein Funktionieren der Hydraulik garantiert war, sondern auch, weil das Bad und die Verdauungsvorgänge einem gemeinsamen Diskurs um Körper und Verhalten angehörten; die Kommunikation darüber fand nicht nur in den Badesälen, sondern auch in den Latrinen statt. An vielen Thermengrundrissen fällt auf, wie groß die Latrinen im Verhältnis zu Baderäumen waren. Bei den Kaiserthermen Roms mit Tausenden von Besuchern während weniger Stunden mußten daher auch entsprechend viele Latrinenplätze eingerichtet sein. An den Traiansthermen, den Caracallathermen und den Diokletiansthermen sind sie in weiten Exedren im Randbereich positioniert, dort, wo die kulturellen Zusatzfunktionen der Thermen zu finden waren.[12] Wer das Angebot zu gymnastischen und kulturellen Aktivitäten der Thermen nutzte und somit auch über mehr Zeit verfügte, befand sich häufig auch näher an den Latrinen. Auch dies ist ein sozialer Indikator für das Publikum solcher Latrinen.

Thermen sind diejenigen öffentlichen Räume, unter deren Publikum am wenigsten mit Frauen gerechnet wurde. Dennoch weisen einige Thermen wie die Hadriansbäder in Leptis Magna je zwei sehr prächtig ausgestattete Latrinen auf, die jeweils einer der beiden parallelen Badetrakte angegliedert sind. Die Verdoppelung der Funktionsbereiche kann auf temporär reduzierten bzw. erweiterten Besucherandrang zurückgeführt werden, sie ist kein Hinweis auf parallele Einrichtungen für Frauen und bestätigt damit, daß die inszenierte Körpersorge etwas mit Männlichkeit zu tun hatte.[13]

Die besondere Bedeutung öffentlicher, meist recht gut ausgestatteter Großlatrinen in einem Sektor des öffentlichen Raums, welcher dem Otium zugerechnet wurde, reichte über die Thermen hinaus. In der einmaligen Urbanistik des kaiserzeitlichen Rom entwickelte sich um die Bäder des Marsfeldes eine Freizeitkultur von betuchten Müßiggängern und solchen, die Anschluß an diese Kultur suchten. Es ist deshalb nicht erstaunlich, daß einzig hier auch abseits von den zentralen Fora eine Häufung von drei Großlatrinen am Rande der Monumente des Pompeius und der Crypta Balbi zu verzeichnen ist.[14] Ihr Publikum ist einer entsprechend gehobenen Bevölkerungsgruppe zuzurechnen.

Die Positionierung dieser gut ausgestatteten Großlatrinen im städtischen Raum beweist, daß ihnen eine über Bedürfnisanstalten hinausreichende und daher soziokulturelle Bedeutung zukam. Der bereits genannte Diskurs um den Körper entstand zunächst unter den Angehörigen der oberen sozialen Gruppen. Weil dieser Diskurs sich nicht auf die Körperfunktionen beschränkte, sondern das ganze Verhalten mit einschloß, wurde er zum Bezugssystem für die soziale Position. Aus der Vielzahl von einfach ausgestatteten Großlatrinen ragen die wahren Prachtlatrinen der hohen Kaiserzeit hervor. Sie sind ein Phänomen, das auf eine soziale Zuordnung von Latrinenbesuchern zurückzuführen ist. Wie in der römischen Architektur grundsätzlich die Zugänglichkeit durch visuelle Zeichen, vor allem Bauformen und Ausstattung, geregelt wurde, so verweist auch bei den öffentlichen Latrinen das Niveau an Luxus auf diejenige soziale Gruppe, für die der Zutritt vorgesehen war. Um allzu restriktive Regelungen wird es sich nicht gehandelt haben, so fehlen etwa inschriftliche Hinweise vollkommen. Doch die Marmorsäulen, figürlichen Mosaiken und Wandmalereien schufen eine ästhetische Umgebung, die sich ohne Zweifel auf die oberste Schicht bezog. Die Grundrisse signalisierten eine Sphäre des Otium, vor allem die Exedren, die noch dazu an Gesprächsrunden in Villengärten erinnerten. Dies fand alles unter Leuten statt, deren Zeitplan von Körpersorge bestimmt werden konnte. Auch das ist eine soziale Distinktion. Die Mehrzahl öffentlicher Großlatrinen freilich begnügte sich mit einfacheren Annehmlichkeiten wie Wasserbecken, Belüftung und Vestibül. Mag auch der Diskurs um den Körper und der Wunsch nach Latrinenkommunikation im Lauf des 3. Jahrhunderts n.Chr. nach unten durchgesickert sein, so war es doch immer der Ausstattungsluxus, der die Benutzerkreise einer Latrine definierte. Bemerkenswert ist, daß im öffentlichen Raum solche Großlatrinen fehlen, die durch jeglichen Mangel an Bequemlichkeit für die niedrigste, aber zahlreichste Schicht der Stadtbevölkerung vorgesehen war. Für die gesamte hygienische Versorgung einer Stadt sind daher alle jene Latrinen mit einzubeziehen, die in Winkeln der Wohnhäuser eingerichtet waren. Sobald es sich dort aber um mehrsitzige Latrinen handelt, liegen sie nicht selten im Eingangsbereich. In Timgad wurden gleich mehrere solcher Latrinen auf öffentlichen Grund vor die Wohnhäuser gesetzt, so daß man eine geplante Mitnutzung durch 'Laufkundschaft' vermuten möchte.[15]

Die uns erhaltenen öffentlichen Großlatrinen im Stadtraum teilen uns nicht direkt mit, wer sie tatsächlich benutzte. Doch indirekt, nämlich durch die Sprache der Architekturausstattung und durch den Kontext, können wir zumindest soziale Differenzierungen des vorgesehenen Publikums ablesen.

Collegia

In einem Bereich eingeschränkter Öffentlichkeit stehen die Versammlungsbauten der städtischen Vereine, des *corpus sodalicium*. Sie sind eine Form des sozialen Zusammenschlusses meist nach berufsständischem Kriterium. Unter den Handwerkern, Schiffsleuten und *negotiantes* verschiedenster Güter können wir eine sozial definierte Gruppe von möglicherweise gemeinschaftlichen Latrinengängern erwarten.

Bei allen Schwierigkeiten der Identifizierung ihrer Vereinsbauten, der *scholae*, sind zumindest Bankettsäle in Verbindung mit Kultbauten ein brauchbares Indiz.[16] Denn über die Aktivitäten in den Räumen sind wir ausreichend informiert. Es handelt sich um regelmäßige administrative Versammlungen sowie um festliche Kultfeiern, beides von Banketten begleitet, die als 'Freß- und Saufgelage' charakterisiert wurden (Tert. *Apol.* 39.6). Primär ging es also um die Pflege sozialer Beziehungen. Überblickt man die knapp 80 zuletzt zusammengestellten *scholae*, in der Mehrzahl in Rom und in Ostia, insbesondere unter dem Blickwinkel der Gelageteilnehmer, so fällt der fast vollständige Mangel an Latrinen auf.

Eine der nach Größe und Ausstattungspracht eindrucksvollsten Anlagen ist die sog. Schola del Traiano in Ostia.[17] Nicht allzu fern vom Speisesaal befindet sich an der Außenmauer des umlaufenden Korridors eine viersitzige Latrine (*Abb. 9.1*).[18] Angesichts der Größe der *schola* kann sie nur als das Minimum an Hygieneeinrichtung bezeichnet werden. Das gesellschaftliche Leben der *navicularii* oder *fabri navales* bei den *convivia* war sicher ausgeprägt. Darüber hinaus einen weiteren Kommunikationsort einzurichten, bestand offensichtlich kein Bedarf, hingegen der Wunsch, dem zwangsläufigen Latrinengang ein ansprechendes Ambiente zu bieten. Was das *collegium* an Marmorausstattung für die Bankette und Kultereignisse aufwendete, setzte sich in der Latrine fort und unterstrich den Anspruch der Mitglieder auf gehobenen Stand.

An die Aula und den Kultbau der *mensores frumentarii* in Ostia grenzt ein Wirtschaftshof mit einer Gemeinschaftslatrine an (*Abb. 9.1*).[19] Vom Versammlungsraum aus liegt sie am entferntesten Ende. Eher mag sie den Sklaven der *mensores* gedient haben, und entsprechend minimal ist sie auch ausgestattet. Nicht anders verhält es sich mit einem kleinen Klo unter einer Treppe in der Casa dei Triclini ebenfalls in Ostia, die im 2. Jahrhundert n.Chr. von den *fabri tignarii* als Vereinsbau genutzt wurde.[20] Später, im 3. Jahrhundert n.Chr., wurde am Südosteck des Blocks eine große Doppellatrine eingebaut, die aber nur von außen und somit öffentlich, und zwar bevorzugt von den Gästen der Terme del Foro, aufgesucht werden konnte. Trotzdem kann man sich vorstellen, daß die *fabri* auch das Bad gemeinsam besuchten und somit der Latrinengang in ihre Agenda dennoch aufgenommen war.

Tatsächlich finden Vereinsmitglieder des öfteren öffentliche Latrinen in nächster Nähe. Eine solche liegt an der sogenannten Palästra derselben Terme del Foro in Ostia, an deren Südrand ein Vereinsbau - allerdings erst im frühen 4. Jahrhundert - plausibel identifiziert wird (*Abb. 9.2*).[21]

Diese Nachbarschaft mag insofern ungeplant sein, als Vereinshäuser ebenso wie öffentliche Latrinen eben meist nahe den Stadtzentren liegen. Zufällig ist sie dennoch nicht. Jene öffentlichen

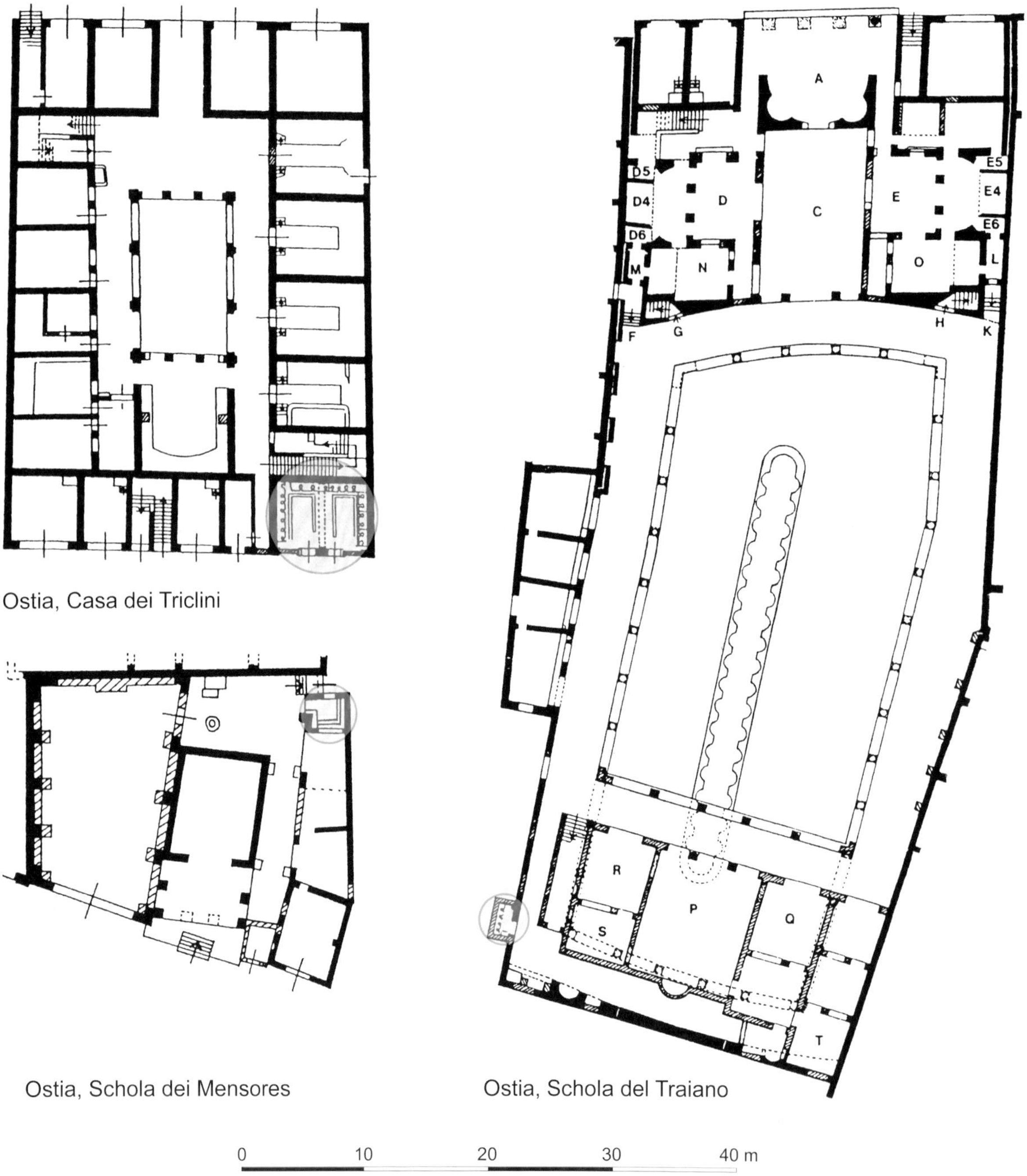

Fig. 9.1. Ostia, Casa dei Triclini, Schola dei Mensores und Schola del Traiano mit Toiletten (Zeichnung M. Schützenberger nach Bollmann 1998, Abb. 1. 13. 30).

Latrinen - es sind stets relativ einfache Anlagen - fanden einen gut Teil ihres Publikums eben in denjenigen sozialen Gruppen zwischen *plebs* und *decuriones*, die in den *scholae* zusammenfanden. In Ephesus hatten sie vielleicht sogar eine Sitzplatzreservierung in den öffentlichen Latrinen der Thermen.[22] Der Gang zum Vereinshaus geschah sicher im Rahmen eines aktiven, gesellschaftlichen Verweilens im umgebenden öffentlichen Stadtraum und kann auch einen Abstecher in eine kommunikationsfördernde öffentliche Latrine vorgesehen haben.

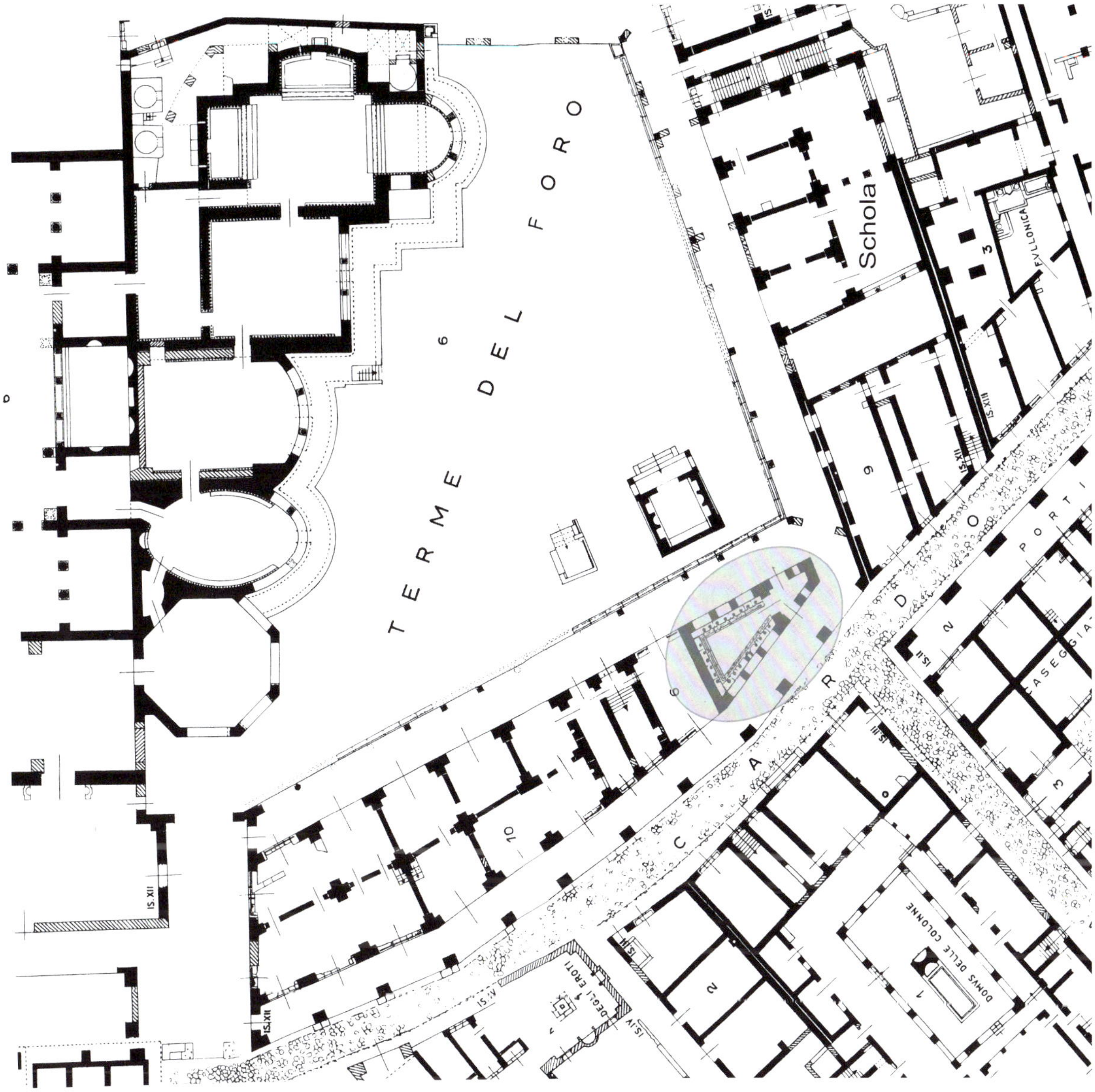

Fig. 9.2. Ostia, sog. Palästra delle Terme del Foro mit Schola und Toiletten (Zeichnung M. Schützenberger nach G. Calza, Ostia, 1. Topografia generale (Roma 1953)).

Damit bestätigt sich zugleich, daß die besondere Erscheinung der öffentlichen Prachtlatrine auf ein sehr viel gehobeneres soziales Ambiente bezogen ist. Ein *collegium* besonderer Art bilden die *Fratres Arvales*, deren Kultaufgaben man als standesgemäße Berufstätigkeit von *senatores* und *equites* werten kann. Ihr Versammlungsgebäude bei Rom verfügt dementsprechend über eine vereinseigene Therme mit eigener Gemeinschaftslatrine; der Luxus ihrer Ausstattung ist standesgemäß.[23]

9.3 The Roman Military in Britain
(Adam Goldwater)

> 'Roman plumbing excites the popular imagination partly because of the special British fascination with, and horror, of the lavatorial habits of other nations.'[24]

This section outlines the physical evidence for latrines constructed by the Roman military and outlines the evidence for their presence on military sites in Roman Britain.

Britain was a frontier province of the Roman Empire, beginning as such, and remaining so until the troops were recalled in the early 5th century AD. During this period of nearly 400 years, about thirty legions (of which three were permanently stationed in Britain) served in the Province - a nominal strength of around 50,000 citizen legionaries, in addition to officers. Add to this the auxiliary troops divided into cohorts of infantry, cavalry and mixed units, giving an overall approximate garrison of about 30,000-40,000 men. As such the Roman military was proportionately more important to Britain than any other single province[25] holding a huge standing garrison. With a military strength of around 50,000 men,[26] it amounted to nearly one-eighth of the entire armed strength of the empire. These troops had to be accommodated, fed, provided for, and equipped. Not only that, but they had to be provided with basic sanitary provisions.

It was certainly recognized by the military that a well organized and competent sanitary system was essential for the general well-being of the troops. They demonstrated their engineering abilities by developing water supply, drainage, and sanitary provisions into integrated systems. Evidence for the existence of latrines in Roman Britain has been summarized by Collingwood,[27] and Johnson,[28] but to date no comparable treatment of the latrines servicing military sites has been published, and their prevalence has, in consequence, been seriously underestimated. It is the purpose of this study to inspire further re-analysis of sites that have produced evidence, albeit often circumstantial, pointing to the presence of latrine facilities. There are numerous sites that reveal details of latrines, but there are many more that have shown none - the missing information was either not recorded during excavations, because the evidence had been completely destroyed beforehand, or the excavators were not particularly looking for them. As such, most general studies of Roman military architecture or Roman Britain have little to say about latrines. Sanitation, however, was certainly a vital part of military planning, and must have been given some priority in the laying out of military sites.

The Ordnance Survey Map of Roman Britain, 1991, lists 235 Roman forts and 75 fortlets,[29] shows nine legionary fortresses (ten if Inchtuthil is included), and sixteen vexillation fortresses in addition to six other sites. With allowances for new discoveries this gives a total of about 350 military establishments known in Roman Britain. Only about 40% of these forts (137) have yielded specific evidence of latrine and latrine-related features. For the purpose of this study I have grouped latrines into the following categories and illustrated with appropriate examples. This is not meant to be an exhaustive list, but a way of demonstrating the variety of latrine evidence available in the archaeological record.

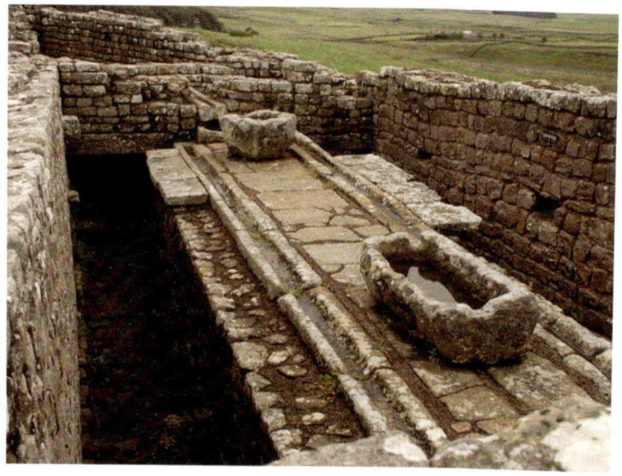

Fig. 9.3. Vercovicium Roman Fort (Housesteads, Northumberland), Communal latrine (photo A. Goldwater).

Communal Latrines

The best surviving example of a latrine can be found at Housesteads Roman Fort, on Hadrian's Wall (*fig. 9.3*). Consisting of a deep sewer flowing around a central platform leading to an outflow through the fort defenses, it is situated at the lowest point of the fort so run-off water was (and still is) channeled into drains to flush the waste through the sewers out of the fort. The central raised platform is paved with flag stones. Entered from one end of the building, the remaining sides of the structure would have been taken up by a row of seats - the sockets for such a framework are still evident. There appears to be no arrangement for privacy. Extra water for flushing cisterns was provided to supplement what was already provided by run-off, or to supply water to the 'sponge gutter'. Of the permanent stone military establishments in Britain other, well preserved, excavated examples are found at Caerleon,[30] Castlecary,[31] South Shields,[32] Vindolanda[33] and Bearsden.[34] All of these examples share similar plan, construction, and situation within the fort/fortress, along with similar internal features. Different styles of construction or more unusual plans, or utilization of different areas of the fort are found at Vindolanda (northeast corner turret),

Neath (southwest corner turret),[35] Piercebridge (semi-circular in plan),[36] Dover (plan with obtuse angles).[37] Included in these should be the difficult to interpret structure identified as a latrine at Old Kilpatrick (building XII).[38] All of these examples tend to share the same main feature - situated in the *intervallum* with the purpose of getting waste out of the fort as quickly as possible and as such are situated at the lowest point of the fort - Bar Hill, Housesteads, South Shields, Caerleon and the numerous examples now evident at Vindolanda exemplify this. A third communal latrine was discovered here during the 2005-2006 excavations, flushed by a stone-lined drain capped by large flag stones.[39] There always seems to be a latrine which does not fit the common plan - and this is at Piercebridge, where the waste does not flow through the fort wall in the northwest corner, but instead the sewer heads south and passes through the fort wall in the south corner. Although these are the most well preserved structures located within military establishments, they are not the only facilities, and a brief discussion of the evidence highlights the variety of sanitary provisions constructed by the army.

Private Latrines in Commanding Officer's Residences (praetorium)

Evidence of a private latrine of an officer that flushed by large stone drains can be found at Housesteads. Located within the west range of the building, the latrine consists of a deep stone lined drain round three sides of the room with a flagged centre. The drain runs along the outside face of the west wall of the house.[40] Similar facilities have been discovered at Vindolanda.[41]

The evidence for small latrines in *principia* (quarters for high ranking officers of the army) within forts is often associated with the remodelling of these buildings for the purpose of accommodation - as evident at Vindolanda where two small latrines were added to the southeast corner of the building, contemporary with the introduction of a hypocaust.[42] Similar facilities have been discovered at Chester in the southwest corner of the *principia*.[43]

Private Latrines in Centurion's/Officer's Quarters and Barracks

Frequently, centurion's quarters have a small latrine, usually found in one of the small rooms at the end of the quarters, and often constructed with access in mind to the fortress or fort drains running past the ends of the barrack blocks. This kind of arrangement is evident at the centurion's quarters at Abbey Green, Chester. When the block was rebuilt on stone sills in ca AD 100, the most westerly of those known contained a lead-lined latrine, found to be emptying directly into the main drain along the north side of the barracks.[44] Parallels occur in other provinces - the frequent occurrence of latrines in centurion's quarters at Bonn should be noted.[45]

These arrangements are not restricted to legionary fortresses. At Housesteads, the centurion of Barrack XIV was very well provided with facilities. His latrine was a three-sided structure of stone blocks. The outlet of the latrine led through the end wall to connect with the main drain of the fort. Another drain also flowed into the main drain, perhaps related to carrying away kitchen waste or rainfall, but it was not connected to flushing the latrine.[46]

Cesspit P1 at Chester is a trench 4.5 m long and 0.50 m wide and dug as a latrine during the early stone phases of the fortress (ca AD 120-160). It was dug in the middle of the centurion's quarters, and survived until at least the beginning of the 3rd century. What is most surprising about the trench is its size - perhaps demonstrating that a large number of people frequented the centurion's quarters. Rooms 3 and 4 had mortared floors, and were clearly separate from the latrine (and presumably its associated odors) by way of a transverse corridor perhaps forming at least part of the main entrance.[47] That this served the whole century of the garrison is further suggested by the considerably sized cesspit, P47, of contemporary date. This pit was excavated at the extreme north end of the veranda of the barracks, adjacent to the centurion's quarters. Post holes were discovered at the corners of the pit, in addition to a number of nails, suggesting a framework for a shed blocking the end of the veranda. This pit was most likely boarded over, and the gulley at its south end enabled containers of waste to be emptied into it. Similar timber-lined latrine pits were constructed and used in the ends of the two verandas excavated as part of the 2nd-century Princess Street barracks, and it appears that this placement of latrines in the verandas of barracks was common practice at Chester.[48] The juxtaposition of these pits suggests that this corner of the barracks was used for latrine and ablution purposes. Interestingly, these pits were located in the officer's quarters. The capacity would seem to be over generous for the needs of the officers and staff, and they also may have been used by men of the barracks.

Other latrines seem only to have served a single *contubernium* (tent). In the *arma* (room for storing weapons) of the barrack south of the *via sagularis* at Carrawburgh, a pit with a tongue-like projection had been dug into the floor. Possibly a latrine pit, the projection or gully is similar to the gully of P47 at Chester. If so, the pit would presumably have been covered by wooden boards.[49] Timber boarding and clay lining of some of these pits would presumably stop solids and liquids readily soaking away, and it is likely that solids would pile up and require periodic emptying - an obvious interpretation of the bucket or tub provisions at places such as the Lunt. The duty roster of Legio III Cyrenaica for the first ten days of October AD 90 or 96 records an unlucky M. Longinus clearing out the latrines.[50]

Hospital Latrines

Within a courtyard building interpreted as a hospital at Wallsend a latrine was discovered within the hospital, added to the fort AD 180/200. Consisting of four ranges of rooms surrounding a central courtyard, two water channels converge on a room in the southwest corner. A stone toilet seat was discovered in this room - the upright seat support and seat are extremely rare in Britain (*fig. 9.4*). A similar structure has been identified at Housesteads - within a courtyard building of similar plan. As we saw before, the room to the southwest was constructed with a deep stone-lined pit and accompanying drains was for ablutions or water treatment. The small latrine adjacent was flushed by its waste water. The drain traced from the southwest corner of the courtyard most likely collected surface water from the courtyard and eaves drips, aiding the flushing of the latrine.[51]

Urinals

Evidence of urinals has come from a number of establishments. In the northeast corner of *contubernium* 8 at Goss Street, Chester, the top half of an amphora, filled with cobbles, and presumably to enable drainage of liquids is preserved. Its use may have been confined to the men of that particular *contubernium*. A similar type of facility was discovered in *contubernium* 2 of barracks V at Caerleon, Myrtle Cottage Orchard. Here, a small recess 37 cm wide and 45 cm high was built into the south wall at ground level in the 3rd century. This particular 'urinal' had an external outlet onto the veranda paving and was fronted inside by a single upright slab. The simple eaves drip channel of the east wall of barracks 2 at Brough on Humber appears to have been used as a urinal for the whole block during period IIB of occupation.[52]

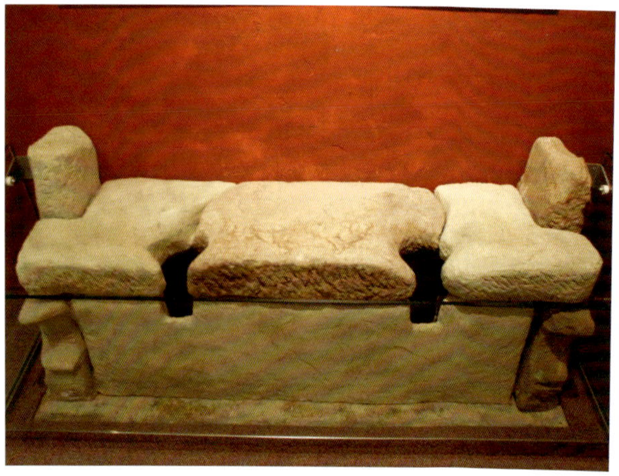

Fig. 9.4. Segedunum Roman Fort (Wallsend, Tyne and Wear), Hospital latrine (photo A. Goldwater).

Discussion

Noticeable is the substandard level of construction of latrines of a later period. A certain degree of knowledge of hydraulics and engineering would have been required to construct a fully functioning and efficient latrine system - something perhaps above the normal level of skills required by an ordinary member of the army, who could put up a barracks block, but maybe not a latrine. Indeed a particular problem seems to have been posed by these latrines, especially as barracks were often in need of constant maintenance and reconstruction. During the later 2nd century the north end of the Northgate Brewery barracks at Chester was in danger of collapsing into the latrine situated in the veranda.[53] Indeed, a similar sized cesspit under the northeast corner of Barracks IV at Nanstallon caused an inevitable collapse.[54] Initially, therefore, I would suggest that these structures were designed by someone with a knowledge of water hydraulics - an *architectus* - and this would explain the uniformity in 'type,' yet flexibility in 'detail' (with regard to site/location, etc.) of this standard military building. But outside periods of intense building activity, it is unlikely that there was a steady demand for buildings to be designed. Thus the *architectus* was probably present only at the genesis of the site - the initial planning and construction phases. When a barracks required rebuilding, the garrison probably did the best they could with the knowledge they had - knowledge clearly within defined parameters of what was required depending on the nature, size, shape, and the number of men using the barracks, and the extent of architectural elaboration deemed appropriate, but not much else. This is why some rebuilding of latrines at a later period is often shoddy compared to earlier work. The same could probably be said for many buildings in the fort. There is still a coherent system of planning in place, but what differs is the separation of 'architecture' from mere 'building'.

Latrine facilities found in the military context should be seen as a solution to a problem. Just as problems might have been encountered getting water into a fort or fortress, similar problems were encountered getting waste water out of the base as quickly as possible. These factors were unique to each and every site and should be considered just as important. In the excavations of Housesteads, Bosanquet[55] was able to identify the astonishingly well preserved latrine structure. In his report, and others like it, he wrote that such buildings are almost always found in Roman forts and called for little comment.

Especially in light of this new sanitation research, I would suggest that such comments by archaeologists are rather brusque. Rather more considered are the words of John Ward writing about his excavations at Gelligaer:[56]

> 'If a number of plans of Roman forts, that of Gelligaer included, be compared, it will be found that while in no two do these buildings exactly agree, there is a general correspondence both in their forms and distribution.'

Essentially his observation remains true today. In spite of the considerable amount of evidence recovered since the beginning of the 20th century, in many ways it is still not possible to go further than Ward's statement. All too often latrines appear similar, and are arranged in familiar patterns, but, nevertheless, withhold their full meaning. While Ward's words remain true, few would now agree that latrines call for no comment. The very mass of latrine evidence, whose buildings, at least, are clearly all of the same family, challenges our understanding of its variety and shape. Furthermore, the variety we find in latrines is complicated by change and development through time, by location in different areas, by the vagaries of different architects and builders, and even by the impact of different building materials. This is the lasting testimony of the Roman achievement. Plenty of studies seek to determine patterns and similarities in the developments of structures within military establishments, such as barracks, granaries, *principia* and *praetoria* - yet why should one expect the Roman army to have reached a higher degree of organizational success? The purpose of most Roman military buildings is readily apparent, and it can be said with truth that 'there is no evidence, in either timber or stone forts, of a rigid plan or fixed set of dimensions for any type of building, and it is quite certain that there was no such thing as an unalterable blueprint which any fort builder had to follow.[57] Perhaps the real surprise is not that their plans went awry, but that they were ever built at all!

9.4 Domestic Toilets - Behaviors and Users
(Ann Olga Koloski-Ostrow)

The Latin word *publicus*, derived from *populus*, 'a people', 'the people', carried the meaning 'of or belonging to the people, State, or community'.[58] This is a significantly political word, as Riggsby has shown.[59] The word *privatus* is also a political word, meaning more than 'private'. It means 'apart from the State', 'peculiar to one's self', 'of or belonging to an individual', hence the sometimes applicable English adjective 'private'. Our English words 'public' and 'private' are rather differently structured from their Roman counterparts. In many respects, we consider what is defined as 'public' as less dignified, somewhat demeaning in stature, as opposed to our 'private' personal connections, which we place on a higher plane: primarily friends and family, our 'private' bank accounts, 'private' property, and 'private' affairs. A Roman would have viewed things quite differently and used the word *privatus* to describe anyone or anything not connected to the community as a whole.[60] This is to say that a *privatus* was not a magistrate, not in any public office, and therefore, not 'connected'. A *privatus* was a veritable 'nobody', a decidedly negative appellation. As we consider Roman domestic toilet use and custom, this rather reverse order of meanings for 'public' and 'private' should remain at the forefront of our thinking.

A few more words about the general Roman social context of toilet use, including the use of 'public' toilets are in order before turn to the domestic sphere, even at the risk of some overlap with Richard Neudecker's discussion in this same chapter (9.1). I am suggesting here that the privacy afforded by 'public' latrines to the Romans who used them, was not so much a right as a mandate - a mandate set by higher authorities within individual cities. The ruling classes eliminated from the 'public' sphere certain unseemly behaviors of the masses,[61] such as use of obscene language, raucous noisemaking, licentious dancing, frenzied drinking and eating, and its resultant vomiting, urinating, and defecating, by assigning them to a restricted place or time or occasion.[62] These behaviors were completely 'contained' or controlled by a subtle domination by the elite.

'Public' latrines provided a place where the nasty bodily evacuations of the *privati*, the dispossessed, could be controlled and hidden from sight. While it is certainly true that there were latrines used not only by the poor, such latrines gave to those same impoverished denizens the illusion of privacy, that sought-after intangible so envied of the wealthy, who could always escape to the peace and sanity of their villas and private gardens. Furthermore, latrines freed the urban poor from any sense of transgression associated with tending to their bodily functions. In the latrine, those with nothing could do what they wished and needed in a less humiliating circumstance.

When the Romans, such as Cicero, wrote about proper Roman behaviors, ancient customs, or necessary political and religious practices, the discourse was almost always directed to the elite, the social classes with political power. Everyone else could easily be dismissed as boorish, pathetic, and not worthy of attention.[63] We know that the Romans frequently assigned different activities to different areas, and they required that certain activities must, or must not, be carried out in public - certain rituals, for example. The Romans thereby understood a kind of unspoken code of behavior, particularly for their elite.[64] Observers - whether elites or people from other less privileged groups - could then compare actual behaviors of individuals to the unspoken codes, and thereby draw inferences regarding someone's character based on their behaviors. In other words, one had to act very judiciously in public.

Scholars have pointed out that the relative openness of the Roman elite house made it a stage for the theater that was Roman aristocratic public display.[65] Just as there were lines of 'public' and 'private' that could be drawn in different ways in all 'public' spaces and architecture in a Roman city, there were also such lines within the domestic house, and these were not always configured just as we might expect them to be. Such notions are important to keep in mind whether we are discussing toilets in houses or in public areas.[66]

An instructive passage from Vitruvius demonstrates the reverse thinking of the Romans in connection with the spaces in a so-called 'private' house, where rooms have public and private functions.[67] The passage makes it clear that there are rules about what areas of the house are open, or not, to outsiders, and which ones are exclusively for the family. One way to grasp how the levels of 'public' and 'private' in the Roman house[68] functioned is to realize that the moral scrutiny of the community penetrated the house. No Roman thought he could escape that moral scrutiny by running home. Whether he was *publicus* or *privatus*, the community always had an ethical primacy over the individual in ancient Rome.

When we move to the 'private' house and consider toilets constructed within it, it seems reasonable to think that Roman social rules were in force there too. As we have seen (chapter 8.1, p. 113, and see *fig. 11.2*, House of Apollo in Pompeii, VI 7, 23), one-seater house toilets can frequently be found in or near domestic kitchens.[69] This location would have made it possible for the kitchen slaves to dump dirty wash water and kitchen slop into the toilet - a convenient disposal system and a way regularly to drain the toilet's contents - and it also would give the slaves a specific and 'contained' area in the house for defecating and urinating out of the sight of guests and out of the sight of elite owners and their children. While it is impossible to know for sure if elites of the household (males and females) ever would have used these toilets, my hunch is that the richer the household the less likely it is that they did.

A slight digression into the world of Roman fiction can perhaps illuminate the situation of Roman codes of behavior even more. At the opening of the *Cena Trimalchionis* in Petronius' *Satyricon*,[70] we learn almost immediately that the main characters, Encolpius, Giton, Ascyltus, and Agamemnon, will be dining at the house of the millionaire freedman, Trimalchio, who is: *lautissimus homo, horologium in triclinio et bucinatorem habet subornatum, ut subinde sciat quantum de vita perdiderit*.[71] While Trimalchio himself seems very aware of time throughout the dinner - time to bathe, time to play ball, time to eat, time to urinate, and time to move his bowels - his dinner guests and we readers never know what time it is, or what is coming next.

Among the many things 'wrong' with this dinner party is the fact that the descriptions of many of the dishes served remind us of what food looks like when it exits the body more than food we would consider tempting to put into our mouths. We shall return to this point about the *Cena* and the literary trope that Petronius has employed here when we discuss the paintings in the Baths

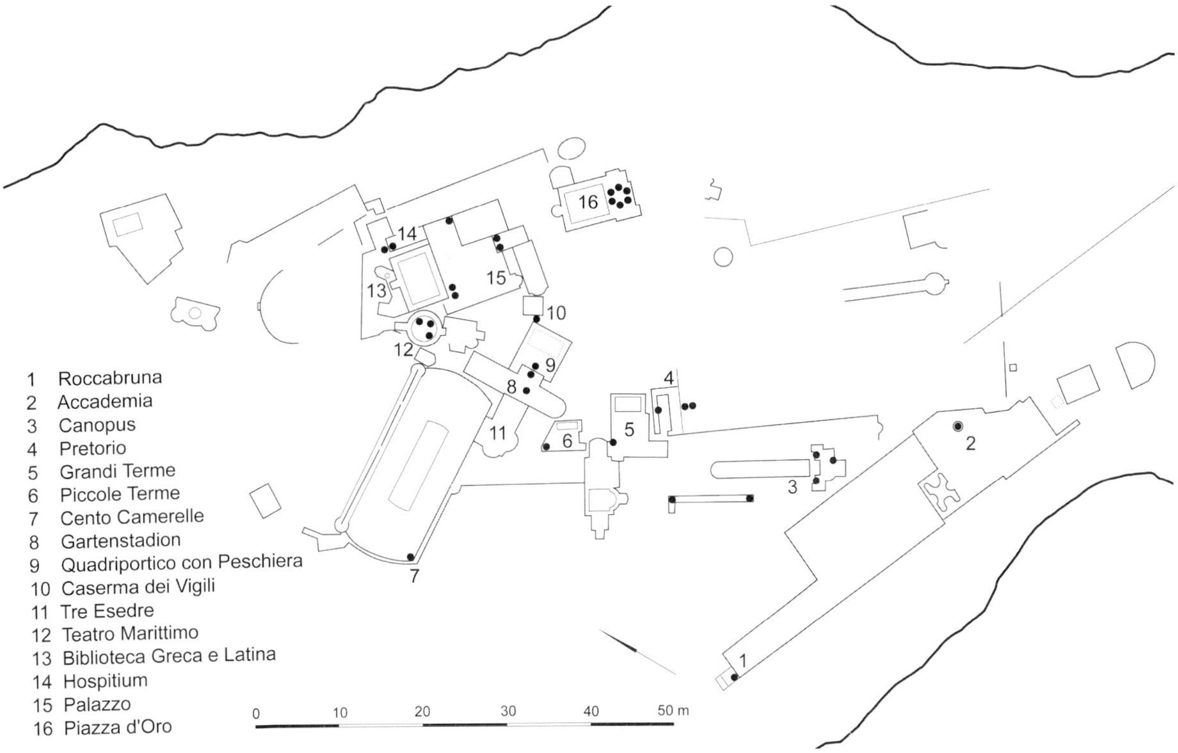

Fig. 9.5. Tivoli, Villa Hadriana, Punkte bezeichnen im Text genannte Toiletten (Zeichnung M. Schützenberger nach MacDonald/Pinto 1995).

of the Seven Sages in Ostia (see chapter 12, case study, pp. 178-181), but it is impossible not to notice that the *Cena* is so funny, in part, at least, because it is all so completely out of sync with expected elite behaviors and with expected 'public' and 'private' boundaries.

The Romans' belief in the moral superiority of their elite provided much ideological justification for the domination of the elite in the public arena. The very nature of the Roman social order itself, therefore, goes a long way toward explaining why latrines were increasingly apparent in the urban infrastructure during the late Republic, the time of Augustus, and most especially into the 2nd century AD, and may help us understand why the Romans increasingly built toilets within their domestic spheres in this same period as well. 'Private' house toilets were certainly sited within the house for functional reasons,[72] but they also were constructed with an apparent sense of social hierarchy for their use,[73] and they too, like 'public' toilets, provided a designated place for the 'containment' of undesirable behaviors, however necessary they were.

Case Study: Villa Hadriana *(Richard Neudecker)*

Eine kaiserliche Residenz setzt sich aus privaten Räumen und differenzierten Baukörpern mit erweiterter, öffentlicher Zugänglichkeit zusammen. Dementsprechend ist mit einem weiten sozialen Spektrum an Toilettenbenutzern zu rechnen. Die Toiletten der Villa Hadriana sind ein idealer Fall für eine solche Untersuchung, denn diese umfangreichste antike Residenz weist in ca. 30 Bauten mindestens 35 erhaltene Latrinen in mannigfachen Ausführungen auf, die zudem seit 1999 gründlich durch Gemma Jansen untersucht werden (*Abb. 9.5*).[74]

Die Villa Hadriana, errichtet zwischen den Jahren 118 und 138 n.Chr., bildet einen vielgestaltigen Baukomplex unterschiedlicher Bereiche wie etwa Canopus, Grandi Terme und Piccole Terme, Piazza d'Oro, Teatro Marittimo. Die meisten dieser Villenbereiche wurden für ein Gesellschaftsleben geschaffen, das sich bei *convivia* und Einladungen abspielte. Von diesen deutlich getrennt und zum größten Teil im Verborgenen befanden sich Arbeitsplätze und Quartiere der Bediensteten.

Baulichkeiten zu Empfang und Bewirtung großer Gästescharen sind auf kurzen Wegen zu erreichen, die keine exklusiveren Zonen tangieren. Die als Canopus bezeichnete Anlage diente derartigen Empfängen. Das Stibadium am Ende der Mittelachse, die davor angeordneten Pavillons und die Freiflächen für die Aufstellung von Klinen entlang der Wasserfläche dürfen auf Gäste unterschiedlichen sozialen Ranges bezogen werden, deren Zahl etwa 200 erreicht haben kann. Im Baukörper westlich entlang des Canopus befinden sich zwei Latrinen mit zehn beziehungsweise sechzehn Sitzplätzen. Durch Raumhöhe und Fenster garantierte Frischluft, Vestibül mit Brunnen und Mosaikböden entsprechen dem mittleren Niveau öffentlicher städtischer Latrinen. Ganz anders hingegen sind drei Einzeltoiletten in den seitlichen Pavillons und hinter dem Hauptsaal zu bewerten. Ihr Raumvolumen ist angesichts eines einzigen Benutzers gewaltig und reduziert Geruchsbelästigungen noch mehr, die Ausstattung mit Marmor hat höchste Qualität. Bemerkenswert ist aber auch die Position dieser Toiletten: Von den besten Plätzen am Stibadium und in den Pavillons aus waren sie ohne Zweifel schneller und leichter zu erreichen als von den Klinen entlang des Canopus aus die beiden Gemeinschaftslatrinen. Der kürzere und jedem sichtbare Weg dürfte klar gemacht haben, wer wohin zu gehen hatte. Der Latrinengang erfolgte im Verlauf einer solchen Veranstaltung nach individuellem Bedürfnis, wobei für die zahlreicheren Gäste auf den Klinen entlang des Canopus mehr Sitze erforderlich waren.

Piccole Terme und Grandi Terme befinden sich ebenfalls nahe dem Haupteingang in die Villa. Gemeinsamer Thermenbesuch in Verbindung mit einem nachfolgenden Gelage hatte einen festen Platz im Tagesablauf, so daß er auch hier zur Einladung gehört haben wird. Die luxuriösen Piccole Terme boten den Benutzern eine dreisitzige Latrine mit anspruchsvoller Marmorausstattung und Vestibül.[75] In den Grandi Terme hingegen verfügte die Gemeinschaftslatrine über mindestens zwanzig Sitze. Durch sechs Fenster wurde sie ausreichend belüftet. Der Dekor beschränkt sich auf einen Mosaikboden. Der bogenförmige Grundriss des Raumes und seine Lage im Außenbereich erinnern an die großen Latrinen der stadtrömischen Kaiserthermen. Wie üblich war ihre hygienische Grundfunktion erweitert um die Möglichkeit der Kommunikation einer gemeinsamen Körpersorge beim Badebesuch. Somit unterschieden sich Piccole Terme und Grandi Terme der Villa voneinander lediglich im Niveau der Ausstattung und in ihrer Größe, die einer einfachen Einteilung der Badegäste nach ihrem Status entsprechen könnte.[76]

Die Piazza d'Oro diente Gelagen mit hochrangigen Gästen und der Entourage des Kaisers. Dies ergibt sich unter anderem aus der Lage des Komplexes in einem exklusiveren Areal der Villa. In die Gewölbpfeiler des aufwendig gestalteten Saales an seinem Südende sind in raffinierter Weise sechs Einzeltoiletten eingebaut. Raumhöhe und Marmorausstattung entsprechen dem luxuriösen Niveau des Ambientes. Wesentlich war auch hier, sie bequem, das heißt schnell zu erreichen. Auch hier geschah der Gang zur Toilette im Rahmen eines längeren Abends individuell, motiviert einzig vom Drang der Natur und ohne schamhafte Sorge, dabei beobachtet zu werden.

Als innerer Bereich der Villa Hadriana darf das gesamte nordöstliche Areal vom Gartenstadion bis zum Palazzo gelten, das eine dichte Verteilung unterschiedlich großer Latrinen aufweist. Ein Kern mit unbestritten privaten Gemächern ist zwar kaum auszumachen, sicher war aber der Zugang von den Tre Esedre über das Gartenstadion zum Winterpalast am Quadriportico con Peschiera, von dort zum Sommerpalast, dem sog. Palazzo, zur Inselvilla und zu den Gesellschaftsräumen der sog. Biblioteca Greca e Latina auf den engsten und ranghöchsten Kreis um den Kaiser eingeschränkt. Am östlichen Garten und äußeren Peristyl des Sommerpalastes befindet sich ein runder Latrinenbau mit sieben Sitzplätzen. Seine Marmorausstattung ist von höchster Qualität, in seiner Mitte stand ein Brunnen. Die Sitze sind in einzelne Kompartimente installiert, so daß einerseits die Defäkation gleichsam im Schatten stattfand und zufällige Berührungen mit den Nachbarn ausgeschlossen waren. Die Distanzierung der entblößten Hintern galt ohne Zweifel als wünschenswert und darf als besonderes Qualitätsmerkmal einer Latrine gewertet werden. Andererseits beweist die kreisförmige Anordnung der Sitze, daß die Situation als solche nicht als peinlich empfunden wurde, ja sogar zur Kommunikation anregte. Man saß hier gemeinsam, weil im medizinisch geregelten Tagesplan der Stuhlgang seinen festen Zeitpunkt hatte.[77] Als Teil der Körpersorge wurde dieser Vorgang gemeinsam thematisiert, und zwar besonders in der höchsten Schicht.

Weithin verteilt finden sich in den inneren Villenbereichen zahlreiche Einzeltoiletten, zum Beispiel im selben Sommerpalast vier, im Winterpalast zwei, weitere im Gartenstadion, sowie im ebenfalls exklusiven westlichen Palast bei den Empfangs- und Gelagesälen von Roccabruna und an der

Accademia - insgesamt mindestens 24. Aufgrund der sehr hohen Qualität ihrer Ausstattung mit marmornen Wandinkrustationen und Böden in *opus sectile* waren sie zweifellos für Personen von höchstem Rang eingerichtet worden. Die in der Regel sehr hohen Räume mit großen Fenstern boten gute Luftqualität. Bemerkenswert ist, daß häufig die Fenster tief herabgezogen sind und dem Sitzenden zugleich eine inszenierte Aussicht boten. Auf diese Weise wird ein wesentliches Luxuskriterium der Villenarchitektur sogar auf den Latrinenbesuch angewendet. Freilich, eine besondere Intimität garantierten sie wegen der Fenster eben nicht.

Die Inselvilla gilt zu Recht als ein ausgesprochen privater Bereich des Kaisers. Aber auch sie muß auserlesenen Gästen zugänglich gewesen sein, die sich im Speiseraum und wohl auch im Bad versammelten. Dort galt das primäre Interesse sicher den Gesprächen und der Kontaktpflege. Die drei Einzeltoiletten auf der Insel hatten nichts weiterem als einem individuellen natürlichen Bedürfnis zu dienen. Der hohe Rang ihrer Benutzer zeigt sich an der prachtvollen Ausstattung mit Marmor. Auch hier sind die Fenster bis auf den Boden herabgezogen. Durch den Ringkanal nur wenige Meter von der Rundportikus entfernt, boten sie keinen besonderen Schutz vor Blicken von außen. Dies überrascht nicht, denn als beleidigend oder gefährdend galt stets der Anblick einer defäkierenden, insbesondere rangtieferen Person und nicht etwa, vom Personal gesehen zu werden.

Die erstaunlichste Toilette in der Villa Hadriana ist ein Zweisitzer östlich der Gesellschaftsräume der sog. Biblioteca Greca e Latina. Auch hier bieten die Geräumigkeit, ein großes Aussichtsfenster und eine kostbare Verkleidung selbst der Sitznischen mit Mosaik den höchsten Luxus. Dennoch wurde damit gerechnet, daß zwei Benutzer der Toiletten sich gegenüber saßen. Anders als bei einfachen Zweisitzern in Wohnhäusern, die stets eng nebeneinander angeordnet sind, wird durch die Positionierung in zwei gegenüberliegenden Nischen eine zu aufdringliche Nähe oder gar Körperkontakt verhindert. Aber daß der Benutzer beim Stuhlgang nicht allein war, verletzte offensichtlich nicht sein Schamgefühl. Wenngleich uns der Partner Hadrians in dieser Doppeltoilette unbekannt bleibt, kann hier aber auch der Blick auf das defäkierende Gegenüber nicht als beleidigend empfunden worden sein.

In allen diesen inneren Bereichen der Villa Hadriana ist mit selektierten Gästen und Mitbewohnern des Kaisers zu rechnen. Der hohe Rang der Latrinenberechtigten wird mit den architektonischen Mitteln angezeigt. Fast alle Einzeltoiletten befinden sich neben Gesellschaftsräumen. Die spezifischen Situationen von *convivium* und Empfang erforderten nicht mehr als eben eine Toilette, deren Raumvolumen um einen einzigen Sitz herum bereits als Luxus verstanden werden kann. Anders verhielt es sich in solchen Situationen innerhalb des Tagesprogramms, die an die Körpersorge gekoppelt waren und deshalb ein gemeinsames Sitzen sowohl zeitlich mit sich brachten als auch kommunikativ wünschenswert machten.

Die Zahl derer, die den Aufenthalt Hadrians in der Residenz begleiteten, und die Zahl der zu unterschiedlichen Anlässen Geladenen ist uns unbekannt. Sicher aber war die Zahl des Personals zu jeder Zeit entschieden höher. Unter den vielleicht 800 bis 1000 Sklaven, den Bediensteten, Handwerkern, Wirtschaftern, Wachen und Verwaltern herrschte eine soziale Hierarchie, die sich in unterschiedlicher Sorge um deren Lebensbedingungen ausdrückte. Einer gehobenen Stufe im Verwaltungsapparat ist das Hospitium mit Einzelräumen um einen zentralen Saal und Mosaikböden zuzuordnen. Die gleichförmigen Schlafräume lassen einen einheitlichen Status der Belegschaft vermuten. An den Bau ist eine Latrine mit elf Sitzen zur gemeinschaftlichen Benutzung angeschlossen. Ihre Ausstattung ist einfach und entspricht öffentlichen städtischen Latrinen der unteren Kategorie. Durch das Zusammenlegen wird Raum gespart und vom einzelnen Benutzer ein längerer Weg verlangt. Zugleich aber bot die Gemeinschaftslatrine einer sozial einheitlichen Gruppe auch eine Kommunikationsebene, auf welcher der elitäre Körperdiskurs in abgewandelter Form stattfinden konnte; man mag sich Gespräche vorstellen, wie sie in der bekannten Ostienser Latrine dokumentiert sind.[78] In analoger Weise kann man eine gleich große Gemeinschaftslatrine an der Caserma dei vigili sozial zuordnen, wobei die bessere Ausstattung auf höheren Rang ihrer Benutzer verweist, sowie drei weitere Latrinen im Personalgebäude des Pretorio. Auf unterstem Rang, nämlich ohne den geringsten Versuch einer Ausstattung, steht eine Latrine in den Substruktionen der Cento Camerelle. Mit einem Durchsickern der ursprünglich elitären Körpersorge und einer ihr entsprechenden Kommunikation ist hier nicht zu rechnen. Das gemeinsame Sitzen war von ökonomischer Raumplanung verursacht, bei der längere Wege in Kauf genommen werden mußten. Der Tagesablauf solcher Benutzergruppen wurde von Dienstpflichten bestimmt, der Gang zur Latrine erfolgte nach individuellen Notwendigkeiten und

Möglichkeiten. Freilich ist die Zahl der uns erhaltenen Latrinensitze dieser untersten Kategorie entschieden zu gering. Wir müssen damit rechnen, daß zum größten Teil die Bedürfnisbefriedigung in nicht nachweisbaren Winkeln und Küchenecken stattfand.

Es ist also möglich, die Latrinen der Villa Hadriana mit heute noch 135 gesicherten Sitzplätzen auf das soziale Gefüge ihrer Benutzer zu beziehen. Ein plausibles Kriterium dafür ist die Qualität ihrer Bauausstattung, die von Marmorinkrustation und *opus sectile* über Mosaikböden bis hinab zu *opus spicatum* und *opus signinum*, Wandputz und Holzbänken reicht. Eine architektonische Gestaltung mit luftigen Räumen, mit Nischen, Wasserspielen und Fensterausblicken vermittelt einer ranghöchsten Benutzergruppe die ihr geläufigen Konnotationen von Luxus. Die Verteilung solcher ranghöchsten Toiletten geschah nach dem Kriterium der bequemen Erreichbarkeit, weshalb viele von ihnen sogar mit zwei Türen versehen waren. Die hydraulische Grundausstattung ist bei sämtlichen erhaltenen Anlagen einheitlich zufriedenstellend; sie dürfte erst bei den uns nicht erhaltenen primitiven Abtritten unbefriedigend gewesen sein. Die Anzahl der Sitze in einer Latrine ist offensichtlich kein strikt anwendbares Kriterium. Denn Einzeltoiletten kamen dem individuellen spontanen Bedürfnis entgegen, weshalb die 24 erhaltenen mit guter Ausstattung sich weithin in verschiedenartige exklusive Villenbereiche verteilen, aber eine unbekannte Zahl einzelner Aborte auch im dunklen Abseits der verschiedensten Infrastrukturen zu erwarten ist. Gemeinschaftslatrinen mit gehobener bis höchster Ausstattungsqualität waren ebenso für ranghohe Benutzer vorgesehen, sobald die besondere Situation des Badeganges beziehungsweise des Tagesplans sie zu Kommunikationsorten prädestinierten. Mit dieser besonderen Funktion der Latrine ist bei den einfacheren Gemeinschaftslatrinen nach unten zu immer weniger zu rechnen. Bei diesen - und besonders bei den einfachsten Anlagen - geht es um die Ökonomie von Raum und Hydraulik. Ein Wunsch nach Intimität kommt insofern ins Spiel, als eine unmittelbare Belästigung beim dichten Sitzen nicht gewünscht wurde und damit zum Qualitätsmerkmal wird. Eine Scham, beim Defäkieren wahrgenommen zu werden, läßt sich keineswegs als sozial elitäres Kennzeichen feststellen. Denkbar ist hingegen ein Schamgefühl gegenüber oder von seiten weiblicher Latrinenbenutzer. Eine Unterscheidung von Männer- und Frauentoiletten ist zwar nicht nachzuweisen.[79] Doch immerhin befinden sich die luxuriösen Einzeltoiletten an solchen Stellen der Villa Hadriana, an denen die Präsenz von Frauen der gehobensten Schicht selbstverständlich war.

Notes

1 Dazu Wallace-Hadrill 1988, 43-97.

2 Neudecker 1994; Koloski-Ostrow 1996; Beiträge von A.O. Koloski-Ostrow, A. Merletto und A. Wilson in Jansen 2000b.

3 Dazu zählt eine kleine Latrine in den Substruktionen des Circus Maximus, s. Ciancio Rossetto 1985, 217. Im günstigsten Fall war eine Latrine in angrenzenden Thermen zugänglich wie in Bracara Augusta, s. Martins 2006, 218.

4 Mansel 1963, 99-101, 124.

5 Boeswillwald et al. 1905, 13-15.

6 Am Südostende des Theaters, s. Bellini 2002, 66.

7 Travlos 1971, 342-344.

8 Hallier et al. 1982, 55-71 Taf. 1.

9 Alarcão et al. 1977, 146-150.

10 Zwei unpublizierte an der Tetragonos-Agora, s. Scherrer et al. 2006, 52 Plan 4; so auch in Minturnae, unpubliziert, s. Bellini 2002, 36, 48.

11 Amici 1991, 116-136.

12 Zu den Traiansthermen s. Carettoni et al. 1960, Taf. 18; zu den Caracallathermen s. Piranomonte 1999, Abb. 27 an der Rückseite der Räume S; zu den Diokletiansthermen s. Candilio 1999, 54.

13 Für Frauenabteilungen plädiert Salza Prina Ricotti 1995 und 2001, 180-186.

14 An der Area Sacra des Largo Argentina, s. Coarelli 1981, 29 Taf. 27; an der Crypta Balbi, s. Manacorda 1993, 326-329.

15 Für Beispiele s. Neudecker 1994, 70 Anm. 241.

16 Bollmann 1998 und 2001.

17 Bollmann 1998, 323-327.

18 s. Abb. 2 bei Koloski-Ostrow 1996, 80.

19 Bollmann 1998, 291-295.

20 Bollmann 1998, 284-288.

21 Steuernagel 2005, 78-79, Abb. 3.

22 Keil 1929, 30-32; Börker et al. 1979, Nr. 454; Neudecker 1994, 65.

23 Broise et al. 1987, 33-38.

24 Crow 1995, 38

25 James 2000, 77.

26 Hodder 1982, 17

27 Collingwood 1926, 124ff. The 'standard' military latrines cited are Housesteads, Chesters, Caerleon, Piercebridge, 'and elsewhere' (p. 125) but not mentioned. Those further described are the latrines that do not drain into an outfall sewer, but drain into a cesspit or septic tank. There are timber lined examples at Hod Hill (Dorset) and Inchtuthil (Perthshire). Masonry built examples from Binchester (County Durham) and Ribchester (Lancashire) are covered.

28 Johnson 1983, 211-214. 'Less than twenty forts have yielded any evidence for soldier's latrines' (p. 211), yet only a few are mentioned; Castlecary, Vindolanda, and Neath can be added to the stone built latrines that Collingwood lists. Nanstallon and Gelligaer and Usk can be added to the list of timber-built latrines. Bar Hill is

mentioned for its latrine incorporated into the external military bath-house.

29 Jones/Mattingly 1990, 91, map 4.24.

30 Boon 1972.

31 Macdonald 1902-1903, 248.

32 Miket 1983, 159.

33 Birley 1977, 65.

34 Breeze 1984, 32-68.

35 Nash-Williams 1969, 98-101.

36 Richardson 1936, 235-266.

37 Philp 1981, 68.

38 Macdonald 1928, 339.

39 Birley/Blake 2007, 41.

340 Breeze 2006, 240.

41 Birley 1970, 97.

42 Breeze 2006, 440.

43 *Britannia* 17 (1986) 387.

44 McPeake/Bulmer/Rutter 1980, 19.

45 Gechter 1986, 155.

46 Wilkes 1961, 280-281.

47 Ward/Strickland 1978, 22.

48 Strickland 1982, 9.

49 Breeze 1972, 92.

50 Fink 1971, 110-11, papyrus no 9, 32g.

251 Wilson 2002, 493.

52 Wacher 1969, 19.

53 Ward/Strickland 1978, 23-24.

54 Fox/Ravenhill 1972, 81.

55 Bosanquet 1904, 193-200.

56 Ward 1903.

57 Wilson 1980, 45.

58 *OLD* 1513 s.v. *publicus*.

59 Riggsby 1997, 48-49.

60 Cf. Cicero, *De senectute* 7.22: *vita privata et quieta*, 'a "non-political" and quiet life', for example. See also *OLD* 1461 s.v. *privatus*.

61 Cf. Lendon 1997, 83-92 and see Lintott 1993.

62 Feeney 1992, 1-25. Further discussion in Riggsby 1997, 50-53.

63 Cicero, *De officiis*, 3.73.

64 Riggsby 1997, 53, lists, with ancient references, several particular examples of improper Roman behaviors, which, if executed, would bring the most severe reprimand upon the head of the perpetrator: not putting on one's shoes (*calcei*) before entering the atrium, not displaying too much affection towards one's wife in public, scratching one's head with one finger, wearing a tunic that was too long, and so on.

65 Wallace-Hadrill 1994 is the standard work on this topic. Cf. Koloski-Ostrow 1997.

66 Cf. Grahame 1997, 137-164. In his discussion of the private spaces in the Roman house (p. 146) Grahame says: 'Location within a space which permits the avoidance of scrutiny may allow privacy, but that privacy will be limited if there is no possibility of moving elsewhere without coming under surveillance. If the avoidance of surveillance requires remaining in a single location, we have *confinement*. It is through confinement that potential threats to the dominant structures of power are managed.'

67 Vitruvius, *De architectura* 6.5.1, and see further discussion in Riggsby 1997, 48-49.

68 See Wallace-Hadrill 1994, 5, and Cohen 1991, 71-83, for a complementary discussion of 'private' and 'public' in ancient Athens.

69 House of Apollo (VI 7, 23), House of the Silver Wedding (V 2, 1) in Pompeii and House of the Deer in Herculaneum (IV, 21) are good examples, but see Hobson in chapter 8.3, pp. 123-126 for many more examples.

70 Petronius, *Satyricon* 26, translation from Arrowsmith 1994, 38-84. Latin text used is Smith 1990.

71 Petronius, *Satyricon* 26, translation from Arrowsmith 1994, 38: 'Trimalchio's giving the meal. He is that real swank guy, who has a great big clock in his dining room and a uniformed bugler who blows a horn every hour so the old man won't forget how fast his time is slipping away.'

72 Hobson in chapter 8.3, p. 123 notes a number of toilets that were sited near front doors in order to locate their cesspits under the sidewalks at the front of the house, for example.

73 Jansen 2007, and see Neudecker (in this chaper 9.1 on *collegia*), and Goldwater (in this chapter 9.2 on Roman military latrines in Britain).

74 Gesamtdarstellung der Villa bei MacDonald/Pinto 1995 mit Rezension von Packer 1998; Salza Prina Ricotti 2001; zu den Latrinen Jansen 2002b, 2003, 2005 und 2007 mit neuestem Stand der Erforschung.

75 Neue Befunde bei Blanco 2007.

76 Salza Prina Ricotti 2001, 177-178 und Packer 1998, 588 halten sie für die Bäder der Bediensteten, angesichts der immer noch anspruchsvollen Ausstattung auch des marmorinkrustierten Zugangskorridors doch erstaunlich.

77 Dazu Neudecker 1994, 31-39; laut *M.Aur.* 6.30 mußte Antoninus Pius dank seiner guten Diät nur zu den festgelegten Zeiten aufs Klo.

78 Neudecker 1994, 35-37; Clarke 2003, 170-179.

79 Salza Prina Ricotti 2001, 180-186 erklärt so den verdoppelten Parcours der Grandi Terme, der sich freilich auch betriebsökonomisch erklären läßt.

10

The Economy of Ordure

10.1 INTRODUCTION *(Andrew Wilson)*

Human waste, like animal manure, has value in certain contexts - the solid waste, as a fertilizer or fuel, and liquid, as a chemical agent in some industrial processes. Despite the natural human disgust for our own excreta,[1] therefore, many societies make use of human excrement, and the ancient world was no different. This chapter examines the extent to which solid and liquid waste from latrines was collected and used, how this was organized, and how this activity functioned economically. A final section looks at the costs of building and the operation of public latrines.

10.2 THE USES AND VALUE OF EXCREMENT

The main use of human faeces in antiquity was as a fertilizer, like animal manure. There is no evidence, so far as we are aware, of the use of human (as opposed to animal) waste as a fuel in the Graeco-Roman world, although this does occur in some societies. Varro (*RR* 1.38.2-3) says that Cassius rated human excrement the second best (after pigeon dung) for manuring, ahead of the dung of goats, sheep and asses. As the Cassius concerned is evidently Cassius Dionysius of Utica, the translator into Greek of Mago the Carthaginian's treatise on agriculture, whom Varro lists as one of his sources (*RR* 1.1.10), this information presumably goes back to Mago and therefore also reflects Punic practice of the 2nd century BC. Columella confirms the use in horticulture of human excrement from latrines as well as animal manure as a fertilizer (*de Re Rustica* 10.80-85), but advises that human ordure, although generally thought to be excellent for the purpose of manuring, should not necessarily be used except for sandy or gravelly soils with little strength or nutrients of their own (*de Re Rustica* 11.3.12).

Human faeces are useful as fertilizer largely because they contain organic matter which acts as a soil modifier to increase the water-holding abilities of soils. Because urine and excreta are normally mixed, the fertilizer is also rich in nitrates, phosphorus and potassium. Human faeces, however, also contain billions of viruses and millions of bacteria as well as the eggs and cysts of many types of parasite such ascaris and hookworm. The removal of human faecal material from the living environment where it can come into contact with children, foods, flies, and fluids is thus a priority for public health. Wastes that are removed from households become a health problem for those who have contact with them, whether *stercorarii* (dung collectors) or farmers, and for those who consume products that have been fertilized with excreta, a practice which increases the risk of passing on intestinal parasites.[2]

Such fertilizer might be used for manuring private gardens, perhaps within a town house - this has been suggested at Pompeii for the waste from the baths and latrines in the *Praedia* of Iulia Felix,[3] and for a latrine drain leading to a cesspit in the garden in the House of the Silver Wedding.[4] In such cases, its use remains a part of the internal household economy and entails no financial transaction or complex organization. The same is true for the use of cesspit contents from a villa on that villa's estate; in discussing the construction of manure pits at a farm, Varro notes that some people site the latrines for the slaves over the manure pit (*RR* 1.13.4).

But many houses without extensive gardens will not have required this fertilizer all the time or even at all, and conversely, some farmers and market gardeners will have had a use for much larger quantities of fertilizer than their own households could provide. This imbalance of needs sets up the potential for a market exchange in human waste, which provided the business model for a group of professional cesspit emptiers and dung collectors, known as *koprologoi* in Greek, *stercorarii* in Latin. These provided a service to householders, whom they charged for emptying their cesspits, and then sold the excrement as fertilizer to farmers.[5] A graffito from Herculaneum records the emptying of a cesspit at a cost of 11 asses: *exemta / ste(r)cora / a(ssibus) XI* (*CIL* IV, 10606).

In classical Athens *koprologoi* seem to have been private entrepreneurs rather than public slaves or employees, though subject to the authority of the *astynomoi* or city magistrates, who enforced regulations stipulating that the *koprologoi* must deposit the *kopros* (manure) at least ten stades outside the city.[6] The same is likely to have been true for the Roman world; the relevant evidence refers chiefly to the economic transactions. In modern India cesspit-emptiers are so despised they fall outside the caste system;[7] in Africa the work is often done by outsiders to the community. We have no such evidence for comparable caste or social exclusion of *stercorarii* or *koprologoi* in the classical world, although it is likely that much of the foul work was done by slaves.

The necessity of the *stercorarii* to the life of major urban centers was recognized by legislation such as the *Lex Iulia municipalis*, which excepted their carts (*plostra stercoris exportandei causa*) from the general ban on wheeled traffic entering Rome during the day (*CIL* I^2 596.66-67).[8]

While the dumping of manure or refuse was prohibited in certain areas within towns or within a set distance of the city walls, there is nothing to suggest that these regulations were specifically or primarily aimed at *stercorarii* rather than casual polluters and defecators.[9] If such prohibitions were partly aimed at professional *stercorarii*, they might suggest that some could not find customers for their excrement within a cost-effective distance of the collection site, and that to some *stercorarii*, at least, the charges for emptying cesspits were a more important element of their revenues than the sale of excrement as fertilizer. Even the one text which does explicitly use the term *stercorarius* (rather than just *stercus*), however, is probably addressing casual foulers of the street: a graffito from Insula V 6 at Pompeii, only one block from the city walls, tells *stercorarii* to proceed to the wall, presumably to commit their nuisance there: *stercorari / ad murum / progredere si / pre(n)sus fueris poena(m) / patiare necesse / est cave* ('Dumper, proceed to the wall; if you are caught you'll have to pay the penalty. Beware!').[10] This is not an official inscription, however; it specifies no legal penalty, but rather a vague, generic retribution, and the second sentence is a hexameter, probably a common catchphrase. As such it falls into the general category of Pompeian graffiti telling would-be defecators to move on, and may have very little to do with professional *stercorarii* at all.

The market value of human excrement will have been determined by the factors of supply and demand. Supply was directly related to the size of cities, and whether or not their latrine arrangements were predominantly based around cesspits, from which material could be collected manually, or discharged into running sewers, in which case use as fertilizer seems to have been less common, although there are instances of sewage being deliberately run onto agricultural land (below). Demand was a function both of the land-use regime around a town, and of the perceived utility to the farmer of human excrement in comparison with animal manure, although both are equally useful in providing organic matter to improve soil quality. The natural fertility of local soils will also have affected demand - e.g. human excrement is not reused in the humid South of Vietnam today, but is on the poorer soils of the dryer North.[11] These factors in combination probably meant that the *stercorarii* found their greatest market among smallholders in the immediate surroundings of towns,[12] since the further the *stercorarii* had to transport the excrement from the city, the higher their costs; and the owners of large villa estates were more likely to have owned enough draft animals and other livestock to provide manure.

The main drain or sewer at Athens discharges into a tank from which ran terracotta pipes branching in several different directions to spread the liquid waste onto fields for irrigation; the tank was presumably emptied periodically of solid matter for use as fertilizer. The complete system in its present form dates from the Roman period, but many parts are much older.[13] Two sites in North Africa suggest comparable arrangements: at Sufasar (Dolfusville, Algeria) waste from a set of shower baths ran to a circular basin and seems then to have been used to irrigate an area below the town where the French colonists later established irrigated gardens.[14] At Zilil (Dchar Jdid, Morocco) the main drain from a set of public baths outside and below the town walls appears to discharge onto the hillside below the baths; as the baths included a set of latrines, the drain will have been a foul sewer carrying excreta. Although the area downslope has not been excavated, no remains are visible downhill, in contrast to the urban area uphill, and the ground is good agricultural land.[15] This site is a possible candidate for the use of sewage as fertilizer.

The frequency with which private cesspits were emptied was presumably a matter for the householders who summoned the *stercorarii* as necessary, but clearly there is a relationship between the size of container and frequency of collection - smaller cesspits would need to be emptied more frequently, given a similar level of usage, than larger ones. In houses with toilets the cesspits must have been emptied periodically; in any houses lacking toilets, chamberpots must have been emptied daily. In Strasbourg in the 10th century AD cesspits were emptied weekly.[16]

10.3 The Uses and Value of Urine *(Miko Flohr)*

Greek and Roman authors mention various applications of urine. This section discusses the practical aspects of such applications: in what way was the urine used and what was the intended effect? Are the medical or veterinary treatments mentioned likely to have been effective or are we to see the practice as some form of superstition? How was the urine collected and stored? Is there evidence for any trade in urine? The focus will be on practices where urine was used as some kind of agent in an economic context; other aspects, such as the role of urine in medical diagnosis, and its medicinal uses, of which there is ample evidence, will not be considered here.[17] The section will start with a short overview of the chemical qualities of urine and continue with an assessment of the uses of urine attested in Greco-Roman literature. Then follows a discussion of what we know about urine collection, including a reassessment of the written and archaeological evidence. The final section focuses on the famous urine tax introduced by Vespasian and its implications for the existence of a urine trade.

Chemical Qualities of Urine

Under normal circumstances, adult humans produce about 1-1.5 l. of urine each day, which contains a dry matter of 50-70 g. Urine contains a wide variety of substances, of which nitrates and phosphates are the most relevant here. An important element in urine is carbamide or urea ($(NH_2)_2CO$), not only because it makes up a large part of the dry matter of urine, but also because it is a very unstable compound. With the aid of urease, an enzyme produced by bacteria, it decomposes into ammonia and carbonic acid. This process is called urea decomposition, and its consequence is that urine, which on leaving the human body has a neutral pH value of about 6.5, transforms into a strongly alkaline substance with a pH that may rise to 9.2 or even higher. Recent tests have revealed that, without the addition of other agents, the process may take about 40 days.[18] While it must be stressed that the amount of nitrates and phosphates in urine varies according to diet, the basic properties of urine are not susceptible to change. The urine of other mammals shares the most important basic qualities with human urine.

In antiquity, there obviously was a very limited theoretical understanding of chemical processes and the details of urea decomposition, of course, were unknown, but there is evidence that people were aware of the gradual transformation of urine into something else: Roman authors like Columella and Pliny the Elder regularly advise using old instead of fresh urine for the treatment of land.[19] There also were ideas about the duration of the process: Columella recommends an aging period of six months.[20] It is hard to trace the origins of such ideas in terms of where and when. Probably, Columella and Pliny just wrote down what was common and successful practice in their own times. The practice of aging urine itself most likely was invented in prehistoric times.

Attested Applications of Urine in the Greco-Roman World

Agriculture and Horticulture

The most frequently mentioned application of urine was as a fertilizer in agriculture and horticulture, particularly for certain fruit trees and vines. Both human and animal urine could be used, either with or without faeces. For example, Cato advises adding the urine or dung of swine to the roots of pomegranates.[21] Columella gives a similar recommendation, though he prefers the use of stale human urine. He adds that the purpose of the treatment is to make the tree more fertile and to improve the taste of the fruit.[22] Urine is an excellent nutrient for plants as it contains two of the most important elements that plants need for growing. One of these is nitrogen, which is essential for the synthesis of proteins and is particularly necessary for the development of leaves and seeds. The other is phosphorus, which plays a central role in many biological processes. Of both elements, the quantities normally available in natural soil are not sufficient for agricultural production.[23] Compared to faeces, urine has the advantage that humans produce it in larger quantities, that it contains fewer enteric and potentially damaging microorganisms and that its application is technically very simple.[24]

Generally, it seems that aged urine was used: authors often add the adjective *vetus*.[25] The reason was not that aged urine was more fertile than fresh urine: the most important effect of ageing emphasized in modern studies about agricultural uses of urine is sterilization. Fresh urine is usually sterile, but may contain bacteria, if the urinator has a urinary tract infection. The increase in pH caused by urea decomposition makes it impossible for these microorganisms to survive and makes the urine safer to use. The fact that Romans preferred to use old urine may suggest that they appreciated the effects, even if they did not understand the cause.

Veterinary Uses

The chemical qualities of urine were also explored in stockbreeding. As the process of urea decomposition makes aged urine hostile to microorganisms, aged urine can be an efficacious antiseptic in the case of open wounds. Columella's handbook on Roman farming gives several examples of treatments that employed this quality of aged urine, especially for curing oxen and sheep. For oxen, Columella argues that aged bovine urine is useful for curing wounds caused by burns, whereas for cuts, pitch and oil are better suited.[26] If the animals suffer from suppuration (festering wounds) or scabies, the sores are to be cut away and the resulting wounds were to be washed thoroughly with aged bovine urine.[27] In the case of suppuration the use of tepid urine is recommended and the wounds afterwards are bound up with linen soaked in pitch and oil.[28] For sheep, similar applications of urine are discussed, but Columella also refers to some treatments in which urine was used internally.[29] The reader is told that problems with the bile are solved by having the animals drink aged human urine and, in the case of lung disease the shepherd is advised to administer a certain quantity of stale urine through the nose.[30] Here, Columella's emphatic advice to bring in the urine through the left nostril reminds the modern reader of the thin line between veterinary practice and ritual in the Roman world.

An interesting aspect is the provenance of the urine to be used for curing cattle. Whereas for oxen Columella explicitly tells his reader to use bovine urine, he advises aged human urine in the case of sheep. He does not explain why, but as there are no fundamental differences in the chemical qualities of human and bovine urine, the reasons for this distinction may be practical. One possibility is that Romans found it hard to collect ovine urine, as flocks often were on the move and only seldom stayed in permanent facilities that allowed for the collection of liquid excreta. It may also be imagined that most shepherds generally did not have large quantities of bovine urine at their disposal.

A remarkable use of urine was by bee-keepers. This is attested in the work of two authors. Varro has one of his characters say that, when bees are sick in early spring, they are cured by having them drink urine.[31] Columella mentions that some bee-keepers in case of illness follow the advice of Hyginus and bring urine, bovine or human, into the hives.[32] Urine was also used by poultry-keepers, in case their birds suffered from bird flu. According to Columella, the beaks of the birds had to be wetted with tepid human urine, the bitterness of which helped to drive out the parasites causing the disease.[33]

Industry

The chemical properties of old urine proved useful for some craftsmen too. The most important industrial applications of urine mentioned by ancient authors include those in leather production, in fulling and in dyeing.[34] For leather production, the evidence is limited to a single attestation. Pliny the Elder remarks that mulberry leaves soaked in urine were used to remove hair from animal hides.[35] Though no further information is given, it is generally assumed that Pliny refers to hides that were being prepared for tanning.[36] For the process of tanning itself other chemical agents were used.

Urine use by fullers is better attested. Fulling is the finishing or maintenance of woolen clothing by removing stains and animal fats by means of a detergent. Discussing the medical applications of animal and human urines, Pliny notes that the urine of camels could be very useful for fullers.[37] Further on, he also refers to medical possibilities of *urina fullonia* and explains that menstrual stains can only be removed from clothing by means of urine from the same woman.[38] Besides Pliny, there are three short references to fullers using urine in the vast medical corpus of Galen and one in Athenaeus' *Deipnosophistae*.[39] In the comic genres some allusions to urine use by fullers may be found. The *fructus fullonius* ('fuller's fruit juice'?) that the slave boy of the pimp Ballio fears to be obliged to drink in Plautus' *Pseudolus* must be interpreted as urine.[40] It may be imagined that the stinking old amphora of the avaricious fuller, to which the girl Thais is compared in one of the epigrams of Martial, stank so badly because, before breaking in the middle of the street, it had contained urine (see below).[41]

The importance of urine for fullers and tanners must not be overstated: we have no reliable information about the quantities that were needed or about its dominance in the production process. Urine was used by fullers in the first stage of the fulling process. In this phase, clothes were soaped in urine by trampling on them, scouring them, and wringing them out. This happened in tubs situated in small niches surrounded by low walls ('fulling stalls'), examples of which have been preserved at excavated fulling workshops at Delos, Pompeii, and Ostia. It is important to note that urine was used in combination with or as an alternative to several other chemical agents, including fullers' earth. In many fulleries, the surrounding walls of the fulling stalls contained built-in storage jars that sometimes contain a whitish deposit. The deposits found in a jar from a *fullonica* discovered at Barcelona were chemically analyzed by the excavators and turned out to contain not only traces of urine, but also of ash, which suggests that a mixture was used.[42] Remarkably, the only literary representation of this part of the fulling process makes no mention of urine at all, but only refers to water and fullers' earth:

> *Terra istaec est, non aqua, ubi tu solitu's argutarier Pedibus, cretam dum compescis, vestimenta qui laves*
> That is earth, not water, in which you usually slosh around with your feet,
> while you compact the clay, you, who wash clothes
> (Titinius, *Fullones*, fr. 10).

Similarly, Pliny's description of the fulling process does not make any reference to urine, but suggests that it began with clothes being washed with the aid of fullers' earth (*terra umbrica*).[43]

The fragment of Titinius also points to another issue: it seems to suggest that the usual amount of liquid under the feet of the fuller was rather limited. This is not contrary to logic. Fullers used urine and fullers' earth because their alkaline properties dissolved fats. Such agents work best without large quantities of added water. Some modern fulling machines employ a sprinkler to apply the fulling liquid to the textile, which is more moist than wet. In other cases, the cloth is soaked separately before being treated by the machine.[44] Moreover, the fullers' physical labor of trampling, kneading, and scrubbing the cloth did as much work as the chemical agents. Thus, even though there is evidence that Roman fullers used urine and were associated with it by several Roman authors, the image of a fuller standing all day long in a fulling tub filled with water and urine must be seen as a modern - and false - construct.[45]

The third craft in which urine was used as a chemical agent was the dyeing of wool. This application of urine is only explicitly attested in a rather obscure papyrus text from later antiquity. The Stockholm Papyrus describes a variety of chemical and alchemical procedures. Many of the recipes figuring urine are alchemical procedures for the production of silver or pearls.[46] Some, however, are seemingly realistic recipes for the dyeing of wool. In many of these recipes, urine was used as a mordant in the preparatory phases of the dyeing process.[47] This is likely to reflect common practice in late imperial Egypt, and it is not unlikely that similar procedures were common all over the Roman world. The use of mordants for such purposes is also known from early modern and industrial wool preparation.[48] Its use in wool preparation, however, is not the only application of urine by wool-dyers mentioned in the papyrus. Urine was also used to dissolve natural dyestuffs, so that they could be applied to the wool.[49] For example, alkanet is said to be dissolved by oil, water, and nuts, but it is emphasized that the best of all dissolving media is camel urine, because it would make the dye fast and durable.[50] The use of alkaline agents for the preparation of dyestuffs is also known from later periods.[51]

Urine Collection

The fact that farmers, shepherds and craftsmen used aged human and animal urine on a systematic basis meant that there must have been institutionalized systems of urine collection. The question is how and by whom this was organized. Unfortunately, Roman authors generally do not tell us from where comes the urine that they advise to use, so any account about urine collection necessarily will remain highly speculative.

Especially for users in rural contexts, it is hard to get an idea about their sources of urine. It may be imagined that urine used by farmers was collected on the farms where it was used and that it aged there, but it is completely unclear whether the urine produced annually by the humans and animals on one farm was enough to satisfy the needs there or whether it was necessary to have urine brought in from elsewhere. An important complication concerns the collection of bovine urine: it is not hard to make a man or a woman micturate into some receptacle, but oxen will urinate where and whenever they feel like it, so that it is either necessary to equip their stables with a system that automatically collects all urine or to observe the animals closely and wait for the right moment. In fact, all we know is that the Romans made systematic use of bovine urine, and that they, as a consequence, must have had some way of collecting it.

Our insight into the provenance of urine used in urban contexts, at first sight, seems to be a little bit better. There is a vociferous tradition claiming that fullers, who are the most prominent urban users of urine, had their stuff collected by means of jars that were positioned in front of their shops in the street. This idea can be traced back as far as the late 19th century, when it appears prominently in the dictionaries and handbooks that were produced in that period, and figures as an unquestioned fact in recent literature.[52] The generally accepted notion of urine collection by means of amphorae has made archaeologists identify the remains of amphorae in or near excavated fulling workshops as 'collection vessels'.[53] Apart from the fact that, without residue analysis (rarely performed), however, it is almost impossible for an archaeologist to determine whether one specific vessel was used for urine collection or not, there may be reason to have some doubts about the practice itself, as the evidence on which it is based seems to be very thin.

The standard body of references given as evidence for urine collection in vessels on the street consists of the same three texts: epigrams 6.93 and 12.48 of Martial and a passage in Macrobius (3.16.15). Epigram 6.93 of Martial is a not-so-subtle character assassination of a woman named Thais. With several metaphors, the poet explains to his public how badly the woman in question usually smells. The first metaphor compares her body odor with the smell coming from an old *testa* (crock) of a parsimonious fuller 'recently broken in the middle of the road'. While it may be argued that the broken vessel smells because it used to contain urine, it cannot be deduced from the text that it used to be at the disposal of male passers-by who needed to empty their bladders. Rather, the specific location referred to - 'in the middle of the road' - seems to suggest that the vessel fell on the ground during transportation and broke into pieces.

The second epigram, 12.48, is a critique of the absurd favors sometimes expected in return for a copious dinner. The argument is that no matter how fine the dinner is, as soon as the food is consumed, it is worthless,

> *quod sciat infelix damnatae spongea virgae*
> *vel quicumque canis iunctaque testa viae:*
> *mullorum leporumque et suminis exitus hic est, ...*
> ... a matter for a luckless sponge on a damned mop stick
> or some dog or other or a crock by the roadside to take care of.
> This is the end result of mullet and hares and sow's udder.

Here, Martial does not refer to fulling at all. Moreover, while the references to a sponge stick, a dog, and a crock may invoke an atmosphere of waste and excreta, it does not follow that the crock by the roadside is meant to be filled with urine. Given the consumed products mentioned in the following line, it is very possible that Martial refers to faeces or, possibly, to vomit (which is what dogs are notorious for eating).

The passage in Macrobius' *Saturnalia*, however, does refer to crocks in the street being filled with urine by passers-by:

> *Dum eunt, nulla est in angiporto amphora quam non inpleant, quippe qui vesicam plenam vini habeant*
> While they go (around the city), there is no amphora in an alley which they do not fill, those men who have a badder full of wine.

The text is part of a quote from the 2nd-century BC orator Caius Titius that is a long rant about the decadence of some judges who spend their day gambling and drinking before stumbling to the place of assembly only to avoid a charge of absence from duty. While Titius' account may be taken as an indication that amphorae were a regular element in Roman alleys, it does not follow that these functioned as intended urine collectors, nor that they belonged to fullers.

If there is no literary evidence for public urine collection, it may also be worthwhile reconsidering some of the archaeologically identified urine collectors. The best known of these is in the east part of the baths of Mithras at Ostia. According to Schiøler and Nielsen, the urine left by the visitors was transported by a lead pipe and collected in an amphora. It was to be used in the *fullonicae* in the basement of the baths. A significant problem with the theory of Schiøler and Nielsen, however, is that the establishments they claim are *fullonicae* do not satisfy any of the criteria used to identify workshops of this type. Moreover, there was no evidence for either a lead pipe or an amphora underneath the supposed urinal, and there is no underground through-route between the location of the amphora and the presumed workshops. It may even be questioned whether the so-called urinal actually was a urinal, as the only reason behind its identification is that there is a rectangular travertine plaque with a hole in it in the floor of the room parallel to the wall. There are no traces of wear and the room in question is much longer than the travertine plaque, which is in directly next to the entrance, an awkward position if it was meant as a urinal. Moreover, there are no parallel situations elsewhere in the Roman world suggesting that urinals of this type existed.

The urine collectors identified by Walter Moeller at Pompeii have recently been discussed by Mark

Bradley, who concludes that in all cases, there is no reason to assume that the vases in question were used for urine collection.[54] Laurence Brissaud's recent identification of a urine jar in Saint-Romain-en-Gal is equally doubtful.[55] The vase in question was at a distance of more than one house block from the nearest *fullonica* and was found between the street and the sidewalk with its highest remains 30 cm under the level of the present pavement. While this difference may be due to a hypothetical raising of the street level postdating the installation of the crock, the idea of a urine collector with a narrow neck fixed in the ground more than 100 meters away from the nearest fullery does not seem to make much sense. A series of jars in an alley at Berenice (Sidi Khrebish, Benghazi) have been identified as possible urinals, but have no necessary connection with a *fullonica*.[56]

Thus, on closer inspection, none of the material and written sources that have been presented as evidence turns out to give any substantial indication that fullers collected their urine through vessels in front of their workshops. This method of urine collection also seems contrary to logic. If urine is going to be used for cleaning clothes, it is important that it be collected in the purest form possible: any pollution would need to be removed afterwards as it might influence the process of urea decomposition or have other negative side-effects on the quality and color of the clothing. Obviously, this means that the usual seated latrines known from the archaeological record, where urine and faeces are collected in the same sewer, are unfit for urine collection. Public urinals, if they existed, are unfit as well, even if the liquids are collected in an accessible basin or trough: without someone watching over the space, a urinal can easily be abused for depositing waste-water, old wine, or even vomit. Further, once collected, it is necessary to keep the urine free from pollution and prevent it from being diluted by rainwater or from evaporation because of exposure to the sun. Both problems are likely to occur with urine collected in vessels along the street. For all these reasons, public collection without surveillance does not seem practical at all. In the absence of strong evidence, the theory must be seen as a scholarly fiction.

This, rather disappointingly, means that we do not know how Roman fullers got the urine they used. It is clear, however, that the urine must have been collected in some way or another. In early modern times, urine could be collected by the workers themselves in a vessel at home. This might have been a usual practice in antiquity too, even though there is no clear evidence for it.

Vespasian's Tax on Urine

An important problem with the above scepticism is that there is literary evidence that the imperial government drew taxes from some form of activity related to urine. According to several writers, Vespasian introduced a *vectigal* (tax) on urine. The classic reference is in the work of Suetonius and is part of a list of examples illustrating Vespasian's wit:

> *Vespasianus reprehendenti filio Tito, quod etiam urinae vectigal commentus esset, pecuniam ex prima pensione admovit ad nares, sciscitans num odore offenderetur, et illo negante, atqui, inquit, e lotio est.*
> When his son Titus displayed his disapproval that even for urine a tax was invented, Vespasian brought money from the first payment to his nose, asking whether the odor was offensive, and when Titus denied it, he said: 'Yet it comes from urine.'[57]

The same story, in similar words, can be found in the work of Cassius Dio, though here, the context is slightly different and the urine tax (τῷ τοῦ οὔρου τέλει) is mentioned to illustrate Vespasian's keen interest in gathering money.[58]

Unfortunately, neither Suetonius nor Cassius Dio reveals what kind of tax the *urinae vectigal* actually was. This has led to a certain variety in the interpretation of the nature of the regulation. There is a long tradition assuming it to be a tax paid by the users or owners of public latrines or urinals. This is based on a metonymical reading of the ancient sources that takes 'urine' to stand for 'urinal' or 'urinating'. Thus, when Claude-Philibert de Rambuteau, prefect of the Seine province from 1833 to 1848, had to invent a name for the public urinals he was locating in the streets of Paris (in order to prevent their being named after him), he chose to name them *colonnes vespasiennes* after the Roman emperor whom he thought to have made urinals part of his politics.[59] The term has also passed into Italian as a word for urinal: *vespasiano* (*fig. 10.1*). J.C. Rolfe, in the 1914 Loeb edition of Suetonius, translates *urinae vectigal* as 'a tax on public conveniences'.[60] Similarly, Cary's 1927 Loeb translation of Cassius Dio refers to a 'tax upon public latrines,' though the Greek text reads τῷ τοῦ οὔρου τέλει.[61] It must be emphasized that the origins of this metonymical reading of *urinae* and οὔρου are unclear.

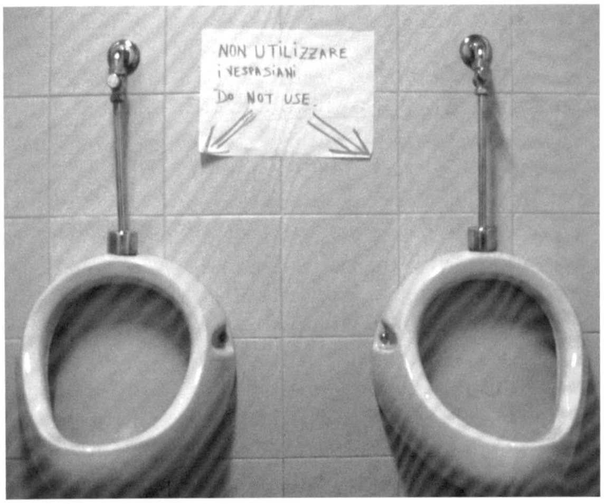

Fig. 10.1. Palazzo Massimo (Rome), Vespasian's legacy: urinals ('Vespasiani') (photo A. Wilson).

Moreover, there are no strong arguments why this interpretation should be preferred over a literal reading. It is not even specified in our sources whether the urine in question was of human or animal provenance. Hence, there also are commentators who take the text more literally and assume that the tax was related to urine. Some of these have come to believe that the urine referred to was used by fullers, so that, effectively, it was a 'fullers' tax'.[62] This also has been linked with the idea of fullers placing vessels for urine collection on the public sidewalks (see above): in his commentary on the work of Suetonius, Mooney argues that the tax was paid by fullers and tanners for the right to place these vessels and to empty them.[63] This seems overly determinative: none of the literary sources refers to any craftsmen or to the purposes for which the urine was used.

A key to a better understanding of the urine tax may lie in the fiscal terminology used in the sources. Though *vectigal* and τέλος were loosely defined terms that could be used for a variety of tax types, they both seem to belong to the realm of economy, trade, and commerce. *Vectigal* was the common term for almost every indirect tax related to the use of public space, including customs dues, auction taxes, and taxes on transactions in the slave market, but also the use of public land by farmers.[64] The Greek τέλος seems to have been the common way of translating the Latin *vectigal*.[65] In any case, it was used by Greek authors in similar ways.[66] In the case of the *urinae vectigal*, there seems to be room for two scenarios. One is that urine became subject to a *portorium* (a toll paid on goods imported, exported, or moved around between customs districts), so that anyone importing urine into a certain area had to pay a certain part of its value in money. The other is that commercial transactions involving urine within a certain area were taxed and that a certain part of the profit had to be transferred to the government. More important than ascertaining which of these scenarios is more likely (which is impossible), however, is the realization that the basic idea behind the measure must have been that collected urine was, more than 'waste', a commodity that could be transported and traded and that in this sense it was not fundamentally different from other commodities, such as oil, wine, animals and, indeed, slaves.

10.4 The Financing of Public Latrines
(Andrew Wilson)

Public latrines, or *foricae*, were a part of the repertoire of public buildings that any self-respecting city in the Roman empire needed to have, yet we have remarkably little evidence about who paid for their construction. In contrast to temples, theaters, markets, *basilicae*, baths, aqueducts, and fountains, and a whole range of other buildings for which there is abundant epigraphic evidence about who financed their construction and, often, how much it cost, there are very few inscriptions recording the building of latrines. Since public latrines were evidently common, we must surmise that they were seen by potential benefactors as a less desirable building type to be associated with, and the lack of inscriptions is therefore a function of particular features of the practice of euergetism and of the epigraphic habit that commemorated it. Furthermore, many public latrines formed part of larger complexes (e.g. the two sets of latrines in the market building at Puteoli and the numerous latrines forming part of public baths), and so may have been subsumed under their building dedications. Of the two surviving texts recording the construction of latrines, at Ephesus and Smyrna, one is ambiguous - the epigram in the Greek Anthology relating to latrines at Smyrna seems possibly to commemorate their conversion into something else, rather than their renovation as latrines:

> Χῶρος ἐγὼ τὸ πρὶν μὲν ἔην στυγερωπὸς ἰδέσθαι,
> πηλοδόμοις τοίχοις ἀμφιμεριζόμενος.
> ἐνθάδε δὲ ξείνων τε καὶ ἐνδαπίων καὶ ἀγροίκων
> νηδὺς ἐπεγδούπει λύματα χευομένη.
> ἀλλὰ πατὴρ με πόληος ἐναλλάξας Ἀγαθίας

θῆκεν ἀρίζηλον τὸν πρὶν ἀτιμότατον.
I am a place formerly hideous to behold,
divided by brick walls,
and here the bellies of strangers, natives, and countrymen
thunderously relieved themselves.
But Agathias, the father of the city, transformed me
and made me distinguished instead of most ignoble. (*Anth. Pal.* 9.662, tr. Paton)

The second text, from Ephesus, is reconstructed from fragments of an architrave found in the public toilets near the Baths of Scholastikia. The inscription, dated by letter forms to the late 1st or first half of the 2nd century AD, seems to refer to both a latrine and a brothel:

> τὸν θᾶκον σὺν τοῖς κατ' αὐτοῦ ἐπικειμένοις παιδισκήοις καὶ κοσμήσας πα[...].
> The latrine with the associated brothel and decoration [...]

The inscription was not found *in situ* in a primary context, and while it is simplest to assume an association between the latrine it mentions and the public latrine in which it was found, this is not wholly certain.[67] The mention of a brothel in a monumental inscription is as rare as the mention of a latrine, but, unfortunately, the fragmentary text does not preserve the name of the person(s) or body who paid for or erected these civic amenities.

Although it is an argument from silence, it seems plausible that public latrines were seen as ignoble, if necessary, and therefore less desirable targets for private benefaction; the costs of their provision, where this was separate from bath buildings, may therefore have been met from municipal funds, and such projects are less likely to have been commemorated epigraphically.

If we are poorly informed about their construction, we are almost as badly informed about their operation. There is one text, however, which certainly shows that public latrines (*foricae*) were rented out to contractors, and another that possibly alludes to the same practice. The first is from the *Digest* (22.1.17.5):[68]

> *Paulus l.S. de usura. Fiscus ex suis contractibus usuras non dat, sed ipse accipit: ut solet a foricariis, qui tardius pecuniam inferunt, item ex vectigalibus. cum autem in loco privati successit, etiam dare solet.*
> The Treasury does not give interest on its contracts, but it does accept it: as it is used to do from the latrine operators, who pay the money later, also from the vectigals. But when it happens in a private instance, it is used to pay interest.

Less informative is a passage in Juvenal, which mentions contracting for latrines in the context of other base activities, but is unclear whether the contracts meant are for constructing or managing latrines.[69]

This textual evidence shows two things: that the ongoing costs and trouble of operation were contracted out by civic authorities to individuals, and that such individuals must therefore have had reason to believe that they could obtain an income from the operation of latrines sufficient to cover their costs and to turn a profit. The services and costs of operation will have included the provision of water supply and payment of the charge for this; the provision of sponge sticks or other cleansing materials, including jugs, and presumably, the periodic cleaning of the facilities. Since the public *foricae* almost universally are multi-seater latrines set over a running sewer, the solid excrement was washed away immediately and so was not available for sale to *stercorarii*. There is no provision in *foricae* for urinals or collecting urine, so this could not have been a source of income either. The only remaining solution is to assume that the *foricae* operators charged users for the service they provided - in other words, that people had to pay to use public latrines. The evidence is indirect, but this conclusion appears inescapable - and there are, of course, abundant parallels in other societies, including much of the modern world. If this is accepted, at least one other observation follows - there must have been attendants to receive the payment. Such attendants could also have ensured the supply of sponge sticks and other consumables. Indeed, the widespread use of sponge sticks presupposes an extensive trade in sponges, to enable their use in inland cities.[70]

10.5 Conclusion

The direct evidence presented in this chapter for the economic uses of excrement and urine is limited, but there is enough to show that the use of cesspits generated a trade in the waste emptied from them and sold to farmers by *stercorarii*, and that urine was somehow collected, traded, and taxed for a variety of purposes related to dyeing, tanning, and other productive processes. Just as in the thriving economy of the Roman world there was a market for even the vilest of substances, so too the provision of public lavatories provided an opportunity to charge users for the service provided, not merely to cover the operating and maintenance costs, but to make a profit for private contractors.

NOTES

1 Curtis 2007.

2 Curtis et al. 2000. I am grateful to Valerie Curtis and Jeroen Van Vaerenbergh for the information in this paragraph.

3 Parslow 2001, 207-208. Cf. Van Vaerenbergh's use of this example in Ch. 6, p. 84.

4 Scobie 1986, 414 n. 116; Mygind 1921, 316.

5 Scobie 1986, 413-414.

6 Aristotle, *Athenaion Politeia* 50.2; Owens 1983.

7 Joshi/Ferron 2007.

8 The *plaustra quibus stercus evehatur* of Ulpian, *Digestae* 33.7.12.10, sometimes discussed in this context (Scobie 1986, 414 n. 115), are not relevant to the question of urban waste disposal. Ulpian is confirming that they are to be considered as part of the *instrumentum* of a villa or farm estate.

9 Rome: *CIL* VI.3823 (p. 3132, 4765, 4771) = *CIL* VI.31577 = *CIL* I.591 (p. 833, 915) = *ILS* 6082 = *AE* 1993, 111 = *AE* 1998, 24; *CIL* VI.31614 (p. 3799, 4772) = *CIL* I.838 (p. 957) = *ILLRP* 485a = *ILS* 8208a = *AE* 1993, 110; *CIL* VI.31615 (p. 3799, 4772) = *CIL* I.839 (p. 957) = *AE* 1993, 110 = *ILLRP* 485b = *ILS* 8208b; *CIL* VI.40885 = *CIL* I.2981 = *AE* 1993, 110. Herculaneum: *AE* 1960, 276 = *AE* 1962, 234; cf. *CIL* IV.10488. *Cingulum*: *AE* 1985, 358 = *AE* 1987, 344 = *AE* 1993, 611; *AE* 1988, 486. Verona: *ILS* II.2.8207b. Salona: *CIL* III.1966. Cf. Bodel 1986, esp. pp. 30-38.

10 *CIL* IV.7038.

11 Though this division probably originates in ecology, it is maintained by local cultural norms - so culture might well be a variable too, with potentially differing attitudes to the acceptability or desirability of reusing excrement (Valerie Curtis, personal comment).

12 On market-oriented horticulture, flower and fruit growing in the suburbium of Rome, see Wilson 2009.

13 Ziller 1877, 117-119; Guillaume 1887; Lang 1968, 22-26. For the collection of night soil for manure at Athens, see Owens 1983. In modern Hyderabad, city drainage waste is supposed to go to a settlement tank, but farmers like the run-off and often break the pipes further up to run untreated wastes onto their fields. Run-off from the settlement tanks is also prized by farmers (Valerie Curtis, personal comment).

14 Coste 1902, 35.

15 Personal observation in 1994.

16 Strasbourg: A. Hervé-Moretti, personal comment. Daily nightsoil collection continues in Indian cities such as Lucknow, although officially outlawed. Waste from bucket latrines is collected weekly in many Ghanaian towns. In China cesspits are emptied when full and waste transported to fields (Valerie Curtis, personal comment). For India, cf. Joshi/Ferron 2007.

17 For an overview of these aspects of urine use see R. Muth, s.v. Urin, *RE* S XI (1956) 1292-1303.

18 Gethke et al. 2006, fig. 1.

19 Cf. Columella, *De re rustica* 4.8, 5.9, 5.10, *De arboribus* 8.5, 23.1.

20 Columella, *De re rustica* 2.14.

21 Cato, *De agricultura* 7.3.

22 Columella, *De arboribus* 23.1.

23 Heinonen-Tanski/Van Wijk-Sijbesma 2005, 403.

24 Heinonen-Tanski/Van Wijk-Sijbesma 2005, 404.

25 Columella, *De re rustica* 4.8, 5.9, 5.10, *De arboribus* 8.5, 23.1.

26 Columella, *De re rustica* 6.7.

27 Columella, *De re rustica* 6.11: *calida bubula urina eluetur*; 6.32: *scabies ferro erasa perluatur urina*.

28 Columella, *De re rustica* 6.11; cf. 6.15 (discussing wounds caused by the plough): *calefacta bubula urina*.

29 Columella, *De re rustica* 7.5.9 discusses the treatment of *scabies*.

30 Columella, *De re rustica* 7.5.15 (bile); 7.5.18 (lung disease).

31 Varro, *De re rustica* 3.16.22.

32 Columella, *De re rustica* 9.13.6.

33 Columella, *De re rustica* 8.5.21.

34 Leather production: Blümner 1912, 266; Daremberg-Saglio I, 1505-1507; Forbes V (1957), 49; Fulling: Blümner 1912, 175; Daremberg-Saglio II, 1349-1352.

35 Pliny, *Naturalis Historia* 23.140.

36 Blümner 1912, 266.

37 Pliny, *Naturalis Historia* 28.91.

38 Pliny, *Naturalis Historia* 28.174, 28.84.

39 Galen. Kühn VI 228; XII 285; XVI 624; Athenaeus, *Deipnosophistae* 284a.

40 Plautus, *Pseudolus*. 779; cf. Kwintner 1992, 232.

41 Martial, 6.93.

42 Juan-Tresserras 2000, 249.

43 Pliny, *Naturalis Historia* 35.197.

44 See e.g. US Patent 4419871.

45 Cf. Bradley 2002, 37.

46 *Pap. Graec.* Holm. 9, 13, 22, 23, 29, 39, 43, 71, 75, 83.

47 E.g. *Pap. Graec.* Holm. 97, 102, 106, 108, 147, 151.

48 Nieto-Galan 2001, 3-8; Fairlie 1965, 493-497.

49 *Pap. Graec.* Holm. 88, 103, 105, 141.

50 *Pap. Graec.* Holm. 88.

51 For example, in the preparation of indigo; Schneider 1987, 428.

52 Smith 1875, 552; Blümner 1887, 175. More recently, Moeller 1976, 20; Scobie 1986, 414; Stambaugh 1988, 152; Bradley 2002, 30.

53 Brissaud 2003, 61-72.

54 Bradley 2002, 25.

55 Brissaud 2003, 61-72.

56 Lloyd 1977, 151-2 and Pl. XIa.

57 Suetonius, *Vespasianus* 23.3.

58 Cassius Dio 65.12.

59 Le Clère 1985, 536-539.

80 Rolfe 1914, 301.

61 Cary 1927, 289.

62 E.g. Geel 1828, 360; Ailloud 1957, 65; Bradley 2002, 30.

63 Mooney 1979, 459.

64 Rathbone in *CAH* X^{2}, 314; Fernández Uriel 1995, 168; Cf. *OLD*, s.v. *vectigal*.

65 Cf. *TGL*, VI 1998, s.v. τέλος.

66 E.g., Aristophanes, *Vespae* 658-659 (various taxes), *Acharniae* 896 (market tax); Plato, *Leges* 8.847B (toll), 850B (taxes on buying and selling), Politeia 4.425D (market and harbor taxes).

67 Jobst 1976-1977, 61-65. I am grateful to Gemma Jansen for this reference.

68 I thank Manfred Horstmanhoff and G. Thüry for this reference. See Thüry 2001.

69 *Satyra* 3.29-40, esp. 38 (*conducunt foricas*). I thank Barry Hobson for drawing my attention to this passage.

70 Cf. Buckland 1976, 14.

11

Toilets and Health

Gemma C.M. Jansen

The Roman world is generally regarded as highly civilized, an exemplary society from which many things can be learned: meticulous organization, building technologies, and artistic achievements.[1] For many centuries, aqueducts, large baths, communal toilets and even sewers have been cited as examples of sophisticated hygienic standards of cleanliness. Engineers and archaeologists constantly connect Roman provisions for discharging excreta and their water technology to cleanliness, and hence to hygiene. The connection, however, is too simplistic. We must not too casually label archaeological remains with our modern expectations clouding our perceptions.[2] Rather we must query whether our modern assumptions of a clean, Roman world are correct, and whether toilet and bathing facilities, nowadays installed to improve hygienic conditions, were laid out for the same reasons in Roman times.

To get to the root of these issues we first explore modern concepts of hygiene and understand how the Romans approached illness and health. We investigate some of the recent research on the topic of hygiene in antiquity and single out one case study: hygiene in baths. We consider hygiene in modern and Roman toilet rooms as well as the diseases present in these places, in order to arrive at some conclusion about whether Roman toilets were hygienic.

11.1 Modern Concepts of Hygiene and Roman Medical Thoughts

The concept of hygiene is fairly recent: after several cholera epidemics, John Snow discovered in 1854 that this disease was caused by water contaminated by faeces containing dangerous bacteria. This discovery, together with other insights into the appalling living conditions of the poor, led to the formulation of rules for public and private health, aiming to prevent disease and to maintain health. This set of rules is what we today refer to as hygiene.

Hygiene can be considered from other angles as well. The following two examples make clear that the concept of hygiene is not as solid as we are inclined to believe. Mary Douglas argued that our wish for a hygienic environment represents a longing for order. As an anthropologist she wrote: 'Dirt then, is never a unique, isolated event. Where there is dirt there is a system. Dirt is the by-product of a systematic ordering and classification of matter, insofar as ordering involves rejecting inappropriate elements.'[3] Recently, modern historians of science have proposed - along the lines of Douglas - seeing the germ theory of disease as having an ontological life of its own, as a social construction embedded within local social structures.[4]

Valerie Curtis, on the other hand, defines hygiene as the set of behaviors that animals, including humans, use to avoid infection.[5] She argues that hygiene has an ancient evolutionary history and that most animals exhibit such behaviors, because they are always striving to survive. Humans avoid infectious threats because they are motivated by the emotion of disgust. Both of these theories are interesting, but they are not among the mainstream ideas for understanding diseases, health, and hygiene that we follow in this chapter.

The Greek Word hygieia

That the word 'hygiene' is derived from the Greek word *hygieia* is confusing. The Greek word has nothing to do with our notion or definition of hygiene except that it gave our modern concept its name. The meaning of the Greek word is simply 'health'. Just as the goddess Hygieia, daughter, sister or wife of the god Asklepios, represents health in general (and not the battle against bacteria).[6] Together with Asklepios the goddess is among the favourite statues in Roman baths and in this way she illustrates the general concept of health.[7] No statues of this goddess have been found in toilets, though we will see in chapter 12 that a mosaic floor had the wish ΥΓΕΙ, 'stay healthy'.

Roman Medical Thoughts

Although the Romans had no word for our modern concept of hygiene, we might ask whether any rules for achieving hygienic conditions were developed or utilized in Roman times. Recent research has shown that in antiquity diseases were not regarded as contagious, but rather as the direct result of an individual's reaction to his or her surroundings and to climate.[8] No one tried to improve the situation; instead, people tried to adjust their personal way of life to the circumstances or tried to get away from the conditions that made them sick. We should also point out that health care was aimed more at the health of individuals and curing individual patients than at preventing diseases for larger groups. So the notion of 'infectious diseases' was absent, as was the concept of rules for public health care. Labisch and Kopitz stress this by stating: 'Die Menschen der Antike dachten nicht hygienisch (und schon gar nicht bakteriologisch).'[9]

One of the most important aims of ancient medicine was to teach people how to keep 'healthy'.[10] The most obvious way to do that was to study dietetics. The Roman physician Galen of Pergamon, who lived in Rome as court physician for the greater part of his long career, put down the rules in his *De victu* ('On dietetics').[11] Ancient doctors generally did not consider faeces and urine as health risks. On the contrary, uroscopy was practiced extensively and coproscopy (study of faeces) at least as much. Doctors even tasted urine and faeces and were called 'dungeaters'. Medicaments were often made of dung.

11.2 Recent Research

Recently, a few scholars have been bold enough to challenge the idea of the Roman world as clean and hygienic, stating that the mere existence of facilities such as aqueducts, toilets, and sewers does not necessarily indicate a high level of hygienic awareness. The first to question hygiene in Roman times was the classicist A. Scobie, who based his conclusions on ancient texts and available archaeological data (relatively scarce when he wrote his article).[12] Through his painstaking analysis, Scobie attacked the view of the Roman Empire as a pristine and glorious place. He argued that towns were over-crowded, streets appeared to be full of rubbish - a far cry from good public hygiene of today. Inspired by this more realistic version of antiquity, archaeological research into sewers and toilets has been increasing; new evidence has been presented at various international conferences devoted to dirt and waste as, for example, the *Sordes Urbis* conference in 1996.[13] In 2001, the classicist G.E. Thüry published the book *Müll und Marmorsäulen; Siedlungshygiene in der römischen Antike*, which is in fact an updated German version of Scobie's fifteen-year-old article. Thüry adds several significant issues, most importantly that of archeo-biology (research on insects, rat and mouse skeletons, food remains, etc.), a discipline which makes research into ancient waste finally possible. He frankly states that the notion of hygiene in the Roman world was not highly developed.[14] This causes current and popular 'dirt-free' reconstructions of Roman towns and villas in fact to be fallacious. Since archaeologists have become aware of this blind spot, more recent excavations have uncovered rubbish everywhere. Recently, moreover, two archaeologists studied what would have happened if the facilities supposedly created to improve hygiene failed to function properly: J. Van Vaerenbergh has studied toilets in Ostia and Hadrian's villa (near Tivoli) that did not flush well, and Camardo investigated a non-functioning sewer line in Herculaneum.[15] The academic repulsion towards investigating dirt is slowly diminishing, as the conference *Pollution and propriety: dirt, disease and hygiene in Rome from antiquity to modernity* held in 2007 in Rome has shown.

The research and conferences of the last decade have led to the conclusion that Roman society was far more polluted than has been recognized until now, and that - upon closer inspection - so-called hygienic facilities did not have the effects that modern researchers might expect. We will - as an example - first have a closer look at baths.

11.3 Hygiene in Roman Baths?

The many luxuriously decorated public baths of the Roman world, open for entire populations (rich and poor) of towns and cities, with their ample supplies of clear, running water are frequently referenced in discussions of hygiene. In his monograph on bathing G.G. Fagan concludes: 'it is not surprising that many modern commentators inspired by such evidence have presented the baths as palaces of hygiene, towering testaments to Roman appreciation of beauty, cleanliness and good order'.[16] He scales down this view in only a few steps, replacing the current idealistic reconstructions of baths with more realistic imagery, based on more close readings of the ancient texts, building inscriptions, and archaeological remains.[17]

Fagan looked at three things in particular: the state of bath buildings, the number of people using the baths, and the cleanliness of the bath rooms and the bath water. Not all baths displayed the great splendor we read about in the ancient sources, and we must not be misled by the actual remains of bits of marble and mosaics: most baths were small and had poor maintenance. Keeping up with maintenance was very important, because buildings not only suffered from large numbers of daily users, but also from the heat and the humid environment that destroyed decorations, plumbing fixtures, and even entire structures. Fagan discovered that baths could even remain in use right up until collapse threatened the bathers.[18]

The second item he discussed is the number of visitors sitting in the hot pools.[19] The fact that dozens of people (and in the baths of Caracalla thousands of people), including the sick, were soaking in these pools, gives no impression of hygiene. Ancient doctors actually advised the sick to go to the baths as a cure for their illness. Bath waters were thus both full of bacteria and also visibly polluted. Fagan illustrated this with an ancient text that tells us that the surface level of bath water could have a heavy layer of unguents from the cosmetics that Romans used floating together with bits of various plasters that were used to treat wounds. He also quoted a text about people washing their back sides in bath tubs. Knowing that the water in these pools was refreshed only once a day and that the Romans had no disinfectants, we can conclude that the quality of the water was extremely poor indeed.

The third subject Fagan investigated was Roman bathing habits. The bath floor was covered by a slippery substance called *gloios*, a combination of sweat, oil, and dirt that was scrapped off bodies with strigils. In addition, people ate snacks in the baths, and therefore we cannot be surprised that Pliny the Elder refers to baths as the breeding ground for cockroaches.[20]

To come from the glamorous picture of polished marble baths usually depicted in Roman archaeology texts to this loathsome view of filth and disease only requires a closer look at the evidence.

11.4 Were Roman Toilets Hygienic?

We need a similar approach for investigating the hygienic situation in Roman toilets.[21] As Roman toilets are as numerous and often as highly decorated as bath buildings, they too can give us the, perhaps false, impression that they were heavens of cleanliness. Although the ancient texts and inscriptions we have for baths are not available for toilets,[22] we can learn a great deal by studying the archaeological remains along the lines of Fagan's analysis. In addition to his research questions about the state of bath buildings, the number of users, and the overall cleanliness of each site, we also discuss what kind of illnesses might be lurking in toilets, in particular, and whether these were contagious diseases. In this section we have a closer look at the specific diseases that could be spread by toilet behavior, and we discover what were the critical points in public and private toilet rooms where caution should have been employed.

Toilet-Related Diseases

Illnesses caused by bad hygiene are faecal-oral diseases, and most of them are infectious. We become sick when swallowing bacteria present in human or animal faeces. These can be touched accidentally and then brought to the mouth by hand, or they can be in food or drinking water that is consumed. Diseases transmitted in this way are typhus, typhoid, cholera, diarrhoea, and amoebic dysentery, which, in fact are all intestinal infections. Also animals such as flees, lice, flies, cockroaches, mice and rats spread bacteria over a larger area by walking through faeces and spreading it around, or by biting humans.[23] Worms and parasites also derive from toilet behaviors.[24] These problems can also be transferred by swallowing faeces, but also by eating animals infected with worms or parasites. Some diseases are transferable simply by touching the toilet seat and the source of contamination: boils, for example. So, not all of these diseases require the faecal-oral route of transmission.

It seems save to assume that most of the diseases presently common in third-world countries were also common in antiquity. Whereas most diseases were fatal, some only effected the weak, such as children and the elderly, but spared people in their prime.

Hygiene Tests in Modern Public Toilets

In the Netherlands every year public toilets are tested and the results appear in November issue of the magazine *Service Management* as 'the national Dutch toilet research'. The conclusion is always the same: public toilets are not as clean as we wish or imagine they are. Every fifth public toilet is not up to the hygienic standards of the investigators. In these tests, contact points for the spread of bacteria are listed: toilet seats, flush buttons, toilet paper holders, door handles, water tap, soap (or soap dispenser) and linen towels. The contact point that contains the most bacteria changes a little through the years, but the seats are usually found to be the most dirty, followed by water taps, door handles

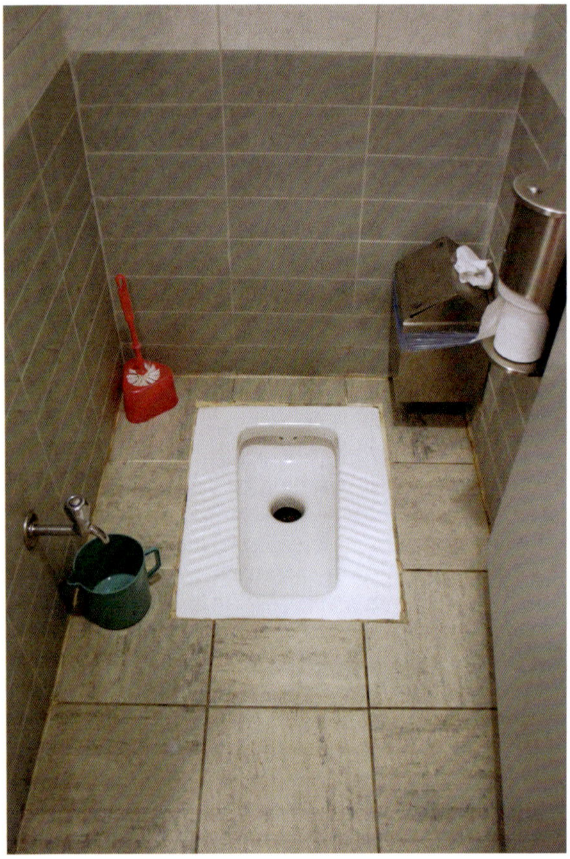

Fig. 11.1. Airport Izmir, Turkish toilet with juglet at left under water tap (photo G.C.M. Jansen).

and then flush buttons. We can easily conclude from this list that every contact with faeces is potentially dangerous, especially in the act of cleaning the backside, or in the case of befouling the toilet room because of a sudden attack of diarrhea.

Hygiene in Roman Public Toilets

What parts of a Roman public toilet would score high on the modern inspection list? The areas with the most striking amount of bacteria would be the cleaning device, the sponge on a wooden stick, the water in which these are rinsed, and the toilet seat. Wooden toilet seats are difficult to keep bacteria-free, since even a good scrub does not remove these germs completely. Therefore, stone seats are much better from a hygienic point of view.[25] The sponge and the stick would have been full of faecal traces and thus full of bacteria. The water in which they were washed could not free the cleaning device from bacteria, as much stronger disinfectant would be needed for that. By 'cleaning' the sponge in the gutter full of water, both the hands of the toilet user and the water got infected. As the water was flowing in the gutter with fresh water continuously added, this was not a mayor problem, although the best seat - from a hygienic point of view - was, in most cases, the one closest to where the fresh water was coming in, that is, the one directly next to the entrance.

The use of water juglets to clean oneself was a much more hygienic alternative. These juglets were found in drains of a private toilet in Ephesus and in a public toilet in Ordona.[26] The juglets were probably used in the way they operate in present day Turkey and in modern Arab countries (*fig. 11.1*). One hand is used to pour out water at the back and the other hand is used from the front to wash off the faeces. In this way the juglets themselves remains clean, only one hand would need to be washed off afterwards in the gutter at the feet of the toilet. Clearly, with this method the gutter would be just as dirty, the cleaning device would not become a container of bacteria, and cross contamination would be substantially limited. When this method of cleaning was combined with discipline in hand use (one hand for washing and the other for eating), the result would be a higher degree of hygiene. Washing hands after toilet use would have helped to improve the situation considerably. Several researchers think the Romans did, and refer to the many ancient toilet rooms with water basins, apparently used for hand washing. We have, however, no texts referring directly to such a habit and the basins might be for storing sponges or for water to be drawn with juglets.[27]

Hygiene in Private Toilets

The toilets in private houses were not open for the general public and were, therefore, used by fewer people, and mostly by the same people: these conditions would have reduced the risk of cross-infection considerably. On the other hand, private toilets also harbored serious health risks. The sponge sticks were just as full of bacteria in house toilets as they were in public toilets, and perhaps even more so, as virtually no private toilet had a gutter with running water to wash the sponges. In private toilets there was a basin, or a *dolium* with standing water, for this purpose, and it was not connected to the tap water supply. This standing water was a good breeding place for bacteria. The other factor that makes a dramatic statement about poor hygiene in the private house was the presence of kitchens in or very close to toilets. In

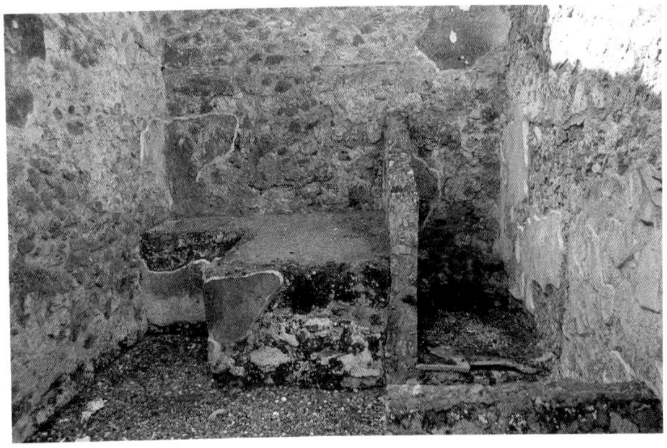

Fig. 11.2. Pompeii, House of Apollo (VI 7, 23), toilet next to kitchen hearth (photo G.C.M. Jansen).

many houses the toilet is situated next to the kitchen hearth (*fig. 11.2*).[28] The locus of infectious disease was therefore very near the food supply. Not only were people carrying bacteria through the kitchen when they finished in the toilet, but surely animals and insects were coming up from the open sewer and looking for the food in the kitchen, which greatly contributed to the spread of faecal-oral diseases.

These observations put the use of chamber pots into a different perspective. While it is probably true that the *dominus* and his guests used chamberpots, this might be a more hygienic alternative than the use of the private toilet near the kitchen.[29] At least the chamberpots were more hygenic for the *dominus*, if not for the slave/servant who had to empty the pot and clean it (in the kitchen?).

Cleaning the Toilet Rooms

The next question is how often were toilets cleaned and how dirty were they anyway. When we see remains of marble seats, immediately modern shining white toilets spring to mind, and it is hard to imagine these Roman toilets being dirty. In reality, however, Roman toilets must have been dirty most of the time. Besides unseen bacteria befouling their surfaces, all kinds of visible dirt must have been apparent. The floors of the toilets were always wet from the splashing of sponges or juglets. People walked into public toilet rooms from the dirty streets, which were covered with dust, mud, house waste and animal dung. The floors of public toilets, therefore, must have been - despite marble and mosaics - horribly soiled. Also faecal remains must have been everywhere in the environment, as it is most likely that many people suffered from some kind of diarrhea. The large numbers of people using public toilets made the situation much worse. As we discuss in chapter 12, we have inscriptions on the outside of toilets that indicate waiting lines, and suggest that the toilet seats were occupied during a large part of the day. For us in the modern world, this is a horrifying picture of a hygienic nightmare. So cleaning was needed, and indeed toilets floors were paved with easily cleanable surfaces such as tiles, marble slabs, whereas the walls had water resistant coatings or marble veneer. The floors were slightly declining towards a drain, which facilitated the cleaning process. Plautus (*Curculio* 580) refers to a lady who cleaned a toilet.[30] The only conclusion we can draw from this, is that toilets were cleanable and that cleaning personnel existed, but we do not know whether the toilets actually were cleaned, or when they were cleaned, so we do not know with what intervals: once an hour, once a day, once a week, or once a month.

Cleaning Sewers and Emptying Cesspits

Excreta in toilets, whether public or private, were directed either to sewers or to cesspits, which had to be emptied and cleaned on a regular basis. Roman sewers were not self-cleaning and their shape was not designed so that fluids and more solid materials flowed away easily. Now and then men had to go down into the sewers to clear away debris. The sewers were small and dark, and workers cleaning them must have slipped often and suffered many serious injuries.

Dampness might bring about hernias and arthritis. The fauna of the sewer could be dangerous, too: spiders and poisonous centipedes caused nasty bites that turned easily into infections, as the sewer environment was full of bacteria. The rotting material in the sewers attracted swarms of flies. Rats were dangerous when cornered: they could jump from the small ledges on the walls and bite the hands and faces of the workers. In the worst cases, they infected workers with fatal viruses. Dangers also included poisonous gases and the risk of drowning, especially when a sewer filled up quickly from a downpour.[31] The Romans were well aware of these dangers, and as the sources suggest, working in the sewers was not an attractive option, so the work fell to slaves, captives of wars, or convicted prisoners.[32] When the health of the sewer workers of Paris in about 1900 was studied, the research showed that the work was so unhealthy that one third of the working crews died within ten years of the start of such underground work. Most died of tuberculosis.[33]

Emptying cesspits and cesspools was also dangerous. Apart from falling in and drowning and inhaling deadly gases, this work could cause many bodily discomforts such as premature aging, blindness, paralysis and all the known faecal-oral infections.[34] Although the openings of cesspits in Pompeii were often in the sidewalk outside the houses, which was an effective precaution preventing huge messes inside the house, for the men who emptied the cesspits, the health risks remained the same (*fig. 11.3*).

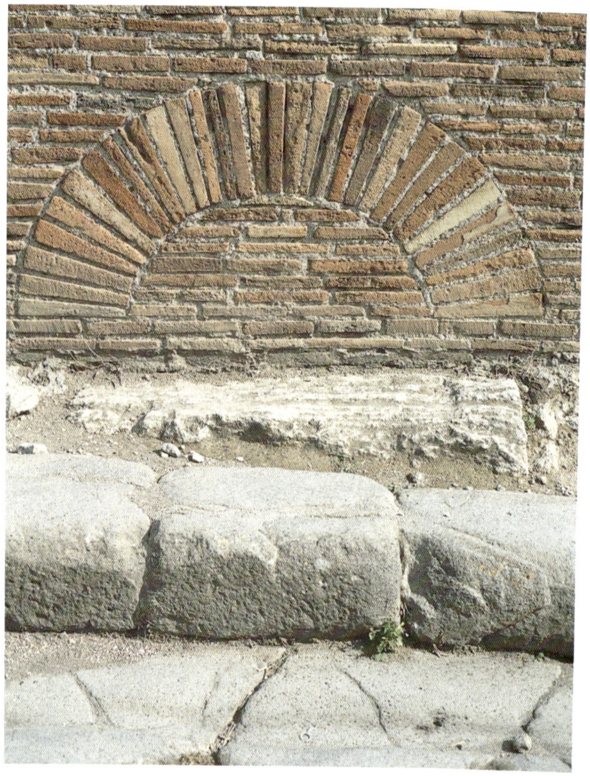

Fig. 11.3. Pompeii, cesspit cover in side walk of street (photo G.C.M. Jansen).

11.5 Conclusion

Roman toilets were clearly far from hygienic. Romans must have contracted many (for them deadly) diseases from using these toilets, resulting in a high mortality rate. As they did not know the relation between these illnesses and these death causes, it was hard to improve this situation. We will see in chapter 12 that Romans regarded a toilet as an unsafe place where demons roamed around, demons that could make you sick, or in the worst case, could cause your death. We will discuss the goddess Fortuna as a protector of the toilet users and carved apotrophaic symbols on toilet seats and walls. Clarke might be right in stating that we, modern people, fear bacteria on toilets as the Romans feared demons.[35]

Everywhere in Roman toilets and sewers there was a very high risk of contamination through direct or indirect contact with human or animal faecal matter. The time has come to review the notion that the Roman promoted advanced hygienic standards and cleanliness. Rather than using the Romans as a role model for modern hygiene, we can understand their sanitary facilities and hygienic customs best if we compare them to the conditions found in third-world countries, not to conditions in the industrialized west.

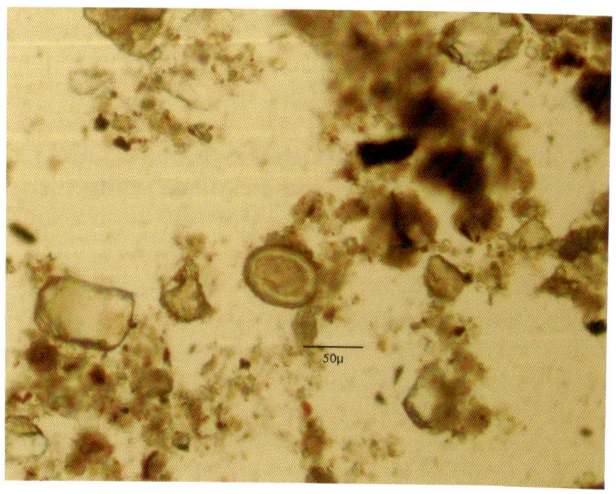

Case Study: Detection of Eggs of the Intestinal Parasite *Ascaris Lumbricoides* in Samples from the Roman Sewers of *Carnuntum* (*Horst Aspöck, Ingrid Feuereis and Silvia Radbauer*)

The excavations in the civil town of Roman *Carnuntum* yielded large amounts of backfill from the sanitation system. Due to the archaeological interpretation of these structures as sewers, parasitological investigations were undertaken. Samples were drawn from the 2nd-century AD sewer K5, deliberately backfilled with urban rubbish, and from the 3rd-century AD sewer K14, filled up with latrine deposits, and also solid waste in the course of its abandonment (see case study chapter 2, pp. 18-20).

Two methods were applied: suspension in 0.3% trisodium phosphate and the SAF (Sodium acetate+Acetic acid+Formalin) method respectively. The first method showed considerable disadvantages as the suspension hardly adhered to the microscope slides; the SAF method proved, however, very suitable. The samples were suspended in the stock solution (1.5 g sodium acetate, 2 ml glacial acetic acid, 4 ml 40% formalin, 92 ml aqua dest.) and left therein for several hours, then shaken intensively, filtered through gauze and finally centrifuged. The supernatants were decanted, the sediments were resuspended in some drops of 0.9% NaCl and examined microscopically. Altogether twelve vials of each sample were processed in the described manner, and twenty-four slides from each of the vials were examined for parasites. In all samples from the main sewer K14 eggs of the roundworm *Ascaris lumbricoides* (*fig. 11.4*) were found, in the material from the sewer K5, however, only two *Ascaris* eggs could be detected in only one of the samples. With respect to the fact that the materials from the sewers have an age of about 1,800 years, the eggs are in surprisingly good condition and can be identified as *Ascaris* without doubt.[36]

The occurrence of *Ascaris lumbricoides* among the civil Roman population of *Carnuntum* is not surprising. This parasite has been detected in various prehistoric samples in Central Europe, e.g. rather frequently in preserved excrements of the salt miners of Hallstatt and Hallein of the Late Iron Age (450-15 BC),[37] and also in Roman pit latrines.[38] Today this parasite is the most frequent helminth (intestinal worm) of *Homo sapiens*, and it is estimated that at least 1,6 billion people are infested by *Ascaris*. One person may harbor up to several hundred roundworms. Each female of *Ascaris* may produce up to more than 200,000 eggs per day, which are excreted with the faeces and need (depending on the temperature) several days up to several weeks to become infective. Humans become infested by ingestion of these embryonated eggs, e.g. from contaminated vegetables. The parasite (which can reach and even exceed the length of 30 to 40 cm) lives in the small intestine and has two calamitous behavioral properties, which may lead to serious and life threatening complications: on the one hand, worms, when irritated by certain substances (food, drugs), may form a ball and lead to an intestinal obstruction (*ileus verminosus*); on the other hand, they like to crawl into small openings and ducts, thus e.g. blocking the biliary duct or the pancreatic duct. The latter condition may cause a necrotizing haemorrhagic pancreatitis, which is usually lethal. Today possibly 60,000 up to 100,000 people die of ascariosis every year.

There is no doubt that also the population of *Carnuntum* suffered from abdominal pains, from loss of appetite, reduction of productivity, and sometimes even death due to *Ascaris* infestations. As these people did not know anything about the life cycle of the parasite, they could not perform any prophylactic measures in order to avoid parasitic infestations. *Ascaris* worms do not live long - about twelve to eighteen months - and are then excreted with the faeces. Due to their large size, they are very conspicuous when found in the excrement. It is very likely that people were thinking of a causal connection between the abdominal disorders and these worms, and possibly they tried certain remedies, particularly certain plants against the parasites.[39] In summary, *Ascaris* and ascariosis were certainly of considerable significance in the every day life of the Roman population and may even have influenced the course of history, simply due to the fact that throughout the ages numerous humans - rich and poor people of all professions - have suffered from this parasite and have been impaired in their activities and that many thousands may have died from ascariosis.

Fig. 11.4. Eggs of the roundworm Ascaris lumbricoides (photo I. Feuereis).

NOTES

[1] I am most grateful to Manfred Horstmanshoff, Jens Köhler, Ann O. Koloski-Ostrow and Eric M. Moormann for their useful comments on the first drafts of this chapter.
[2] Winkelmann 1988, especially p. 159 and 168-169.
[3] Douglas 1966.
[4] See Curtis 2007, 660 for more about these arguments.
[5] Curtis 2007.
[6] Schnalke 2005, 443.
[7] Manderscheid 1988, 120; Fagan 1991, 88-90.
[8] See among others, Nutton 2000 and Labisch/Kopitz 2005.
[9] Labisch/Kopitz 2005, 446.
[10] This paragraph is by Manfred Horstmanshoff.
[11] Wöhrle 1990.
[12] Scobie 1986.
[13] Dupré y Raventos/Remolà 2000.
[14] Thüry 2001, 59-61.
[15] Van Vaerenbergh (chapter 6) has studied toilets in Ostia and Hadrian's villa (near Tivoli) that did not flush well. For Camardo see case study at chapter 6.
[16] Fagan 1999, 179.
[17] Fagan 1999, 177-188; 2000.
[18] Fagan 2000, 281.
[19] The following examples are from Fagan 1999, 181-186; 2000, 282-284.
[20] Pliny, *NH* 11.99.
[21] For this paragraph I am most grateful to Carol de Bell, bacteriologist, who discussed this subject with me and provided several starting points for this chapter.
[22] For texts about toilets see Thüry and Hoss chapter 4, for building inscriptions see Wilson chapter 10 and for graffiti inside toilet rooms, see Jansen chapter 12.1.
[23] See Thüry 2001, 52-53 for a first analysis of the presence of rats in the Roman Empire and for photographs of Roman fleas on fig 62a and b.
[24] For Roman worms and parasites see Hoeppli 1959 and the case study of Aspöck/Feuereis/Radbauer at the end of this chapter.
[25] In fact most Roman toilets had wooden seats. Marble seats are in the minority, although these are the ones always shown in photographs.
[26] See in this book chapter 7 with references. The juglets of Ordona can be found in Mertens 1995, 219, 220: they date from the 2nd and 3rd century. For the ones of Ephesus see Outschar/Thür, 1997; Wiplinger forthcoming has an extended discussion of this method of cleaning. The Ephesian juglets date from the second part of the 2nd century and the first part of the 3rd.
[27] In Petronius' *Satyricon* (2.27) the principle person Trimalchio washes his hands after using a chamber pot. As this is a comic situation, it cannot be taken for granted that this was a common practice. I thank Jens Koehler for this reference. Cfr. Koloski-Ostrow, here p. 140.
[28] See Hobson, chapter 8.3.
[29] Scobie (1986, 410) states that high status Romans did not use the toilet in their own house, but used a chamber pot. One wonders how people cleaned themselves after use of the chamber pot.
[30] See Thüry, chapter 4.1.
[31] These are the dangers of working in the Parisian sewers in the 19th century, described by Reid 1991, 149.
[32] Scobie 1986, 412, n.105, especially gases and the potential danger of chocking to death are mentioned. See also Thüry chapter 4.1 (in particular Pliny, *Ep.* 10.32.2).
[33] Reid 1991, 153-155.
[34] Reid 1991, 88-95.
[35] Clarke 2005-2006, 294: 'Just as we believe, (on basis of modern science) that the world is filled with bacteria and viruses, so the Romans believed that demons surrounded them.'
[36] Theoretically, they could also represent *Ascaris suum*, a closely related parasite of swine, with eggs morphologically indistinguishable from those of *Ascaris lumbricoides*, but this is very unlikely, and it is a more than reasonable assumption that *Ascaris* eggs from sewers which had contained human faeces represent *Ascaris lumbricoides*.
[37] Aspöck et al. 1973, 1974, 1999.
[38] Goppelsröder/Sommer 1996, Gonçalves et al. 2003.
[39] The prehistoric salt miners may have used butterbur, *Petasites*, against their abdominal pains due to helminthoses (Aspöck et al. 1974).

12

Cultural Attitudes

12.1 Interpreting Images and Epigraphic Testimony *(Gemma C.M. Jansen)*

In the previous chapters we have seen where Roman toilets were located, what they looked like, how they functioned, whether they flushed properly, and other facts about them. We must now insert into this rather technical framework the experiences of the users. Images of urinating and defecating figures are presented together with images and graffiti that can be found inside toilet rooms. With the help of this new information we attempt to reconstruct the feelings Romans had regarding their toilet visits.

The Iconography of Defecating and Urinating

Quite a few defecating and urinating figures from Roman antiquity have survived in wall paintings, mosaics, graffiti and also as statues. In this section, I present them and attempt to find meaning for them.

Pygmies

Most of the defecating figures are so-called pygmies who are defined by Clarke as the opposite of the dominant power and as the typical non-Roman.[1] They are all but the ideal Roman body type. When pygmies are mentioned in classical literature, the designation is, in fact, aimed at a larger group of people: 'the normally-proportioned but black-skinned Aethiops, Pygmies afflicted with dwarfism, and humans with physical deformities, including dwarfs and hunchbacks'. Many of them are represented with large, ithyphallic penises. These are, according to Clarke, constructions of the Other rather than accurate records of the ethnic Aethiops or actual Pygmies. In addition to having a non-Roman appearance, pygmies do non-Roman activities. In visual presentations they occur in exotic Nile landscapes and are caught up in burlesque adventures and lascivious behavior.[2] They overestimate their own strength and try to fight crocodiles, hippopotami and large water birds, much bigger and stronger than themselves. From the many presentations it is obvious that their *hybris* will be fatal.[3] Their 'weapons' are somewhat strange: sometimes, for example, they use the neck of an amphora as a shield. Moreover, they are not able to control their physical desires, as Romans were supposed to do. They have sex in the open wherever they please, even in dangerous situations as, for example, in little unstable boats among hungry crocodiles.[4] These actions are comic and provoke laughter.

Apotropaic Forces

The pygmy in his Nilotic landscape occurs in several kinds of rooms or buildings, though mainly in gardens, baths, and tombs. Why is that? To the Romans these places were regarded as extremely unsafe: the graves obviously because of the bad demons roaming around, and the baths because the moisture supposedly attracted the demons. The Romans believed that the evil eye or demons lingering in baths and tombs could be expelled by laughter and the unbecoming behavior of 'ugly' pygmies made Romans laugh.[5] Clarke shows four examples in graves, and Dunbabin lists six pygmy or blacks on mosaics in baths, who had an apotropaic function.[6] For us, people of the 21st century, fear of demons is a less common phenomenon, but for the Romans it was second nature to watch for them everywhere and try to avoid them. To protect themselves, they used amulets, they performed what we call superstitious practices, and they paid attention to prophetic omens. They had to do so, because, if a demon possessed you, he could make you sick or kill you. This also holds true for the evil eye that some one could cast on you.

Clarke has also found three toilets with pygmy decorations, all with the intention to protect the toilet user.[7] The fact that, in the eyes of the Romans, there was apparently a frightening aspect to toilets, is also clear from small magic symbols, like graffiti depicting letters of the alphabet (the so-called *abecedarius*) and *phalli*, which were there to divert evil.[8] Furthermore, one also finds snakes painted on the outside of toilets, meant to protect the people inside.[9] The most important proof, however, of the belief that demons lurked in toilets is a late antique text that is part of the 5th century *Life of Saint Thecla* (*Miracle* 7):

> 'In the middle of the night, (the priest) Dexianos was sitting on the privy, when a demon raised itself in front of him, a demoniacal creature, savage and enraged. As soon as Dexianos perceived the demon's presence, because of the

deep and hellish obscurity and also because the demon was breathing, throwing crazy looks and proffering insanities, Dexianos was stunned, seized by fear and trembling, filled with terror and covered with sweat.'[10]

To understand this fear of demons in toilets, we have to keep in mind that the Roman toilet experience is different from ours in having no gooseneck or stench trap. This implies that one was sitting over an open connection to either a sewer or cesspit. Underneath the toilet user was a deep dark hole from which all kinds of animals could climb up, and perhaps even a demon.

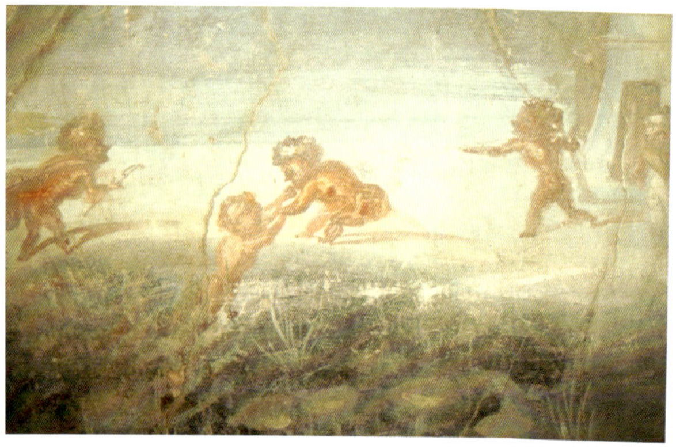

Fig. 12.1. Pompeii, Sarno Baths (VIII 2, 17-21), frigidarium, *defecating pygmee (photo S.T.A.M. Mols).*

Defecating and Urinating Pygmies

Many paintings or mosaics of pygmies or black men are shown in the act of defecating or urinating, which enlarges their comic effect (*fig. 12.1*).[11] As Neudecker shows that body control is a virtue deeply entrenched in Roman culture, Romans were not supposed to relieve themselves whenever they felt the need, and this is exactly what the pygmies are doing in these decorations.[12] It seems that they do this out of fear,[13] and in some instances, their stream of faeces or urine seems to be a weapon against the crocodiles and other animals (*fig. 12.2*).[14] The act of defecating also enlarges the effect the images have on demons and the evil eye. The defecator can blind the evil eye, which can be seen clearly on a famous bas-relief (*fig. 12.3*) on which an evil eye is under attack from a gladiator with a trident, a raven, a long-beaked bird, a scorpion, a snake, a lion and a defecator.[15] We see a squatting man with his back and naked bottom turned towards us, carrying a Phrygian hat, and he looks over his right shoulder. He sits right on top of the eye to ensure that the blinding will be most effective. This image puts the attacks of the pygmies in another light too; they might be aiming to blind the eyes of the large animals with their excreta. This implies that the evil eye will not feel comfortable in the presence of a defecating person.

Apart from the comic context of the pygmy presentations and the evil eye protection, there are several illustrations of defecating people. The row of defecators at the bottom of the famous painting in the Baths of the Seven Sages at Ostia (III x, 2) seems set in a humorous context. For a discussion of these men, see below pp. 178-181. The two other defecating men, the one next to Fortuna on a painting found at Pompeii (*fig. 12.5*) and the one struck by Jupiter's lightning, appear in a much more serious, even religious, context. They are discussed below.

Urinating Men

Understanding the many small statues of urinating men is perhaps more difficult. Researchers have discussed them for their chronology and typology, but they have not tried to reconstruct their original context. The statues, called *mingentes*, represent two groups: urinating children and drunken men who urinate. The most famous

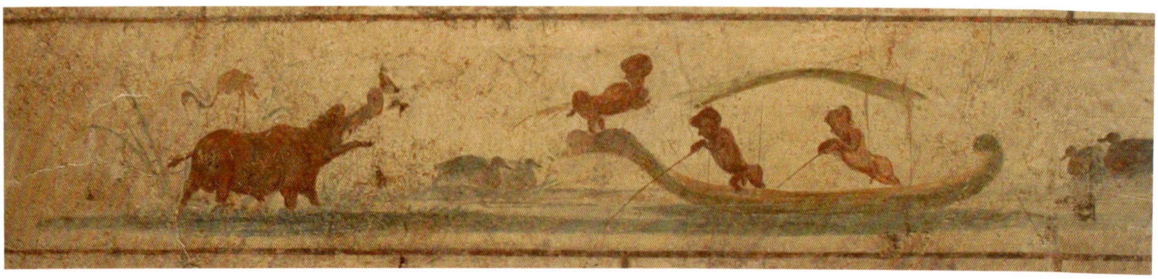

Fig. 12.2. Rome, Columbarium of the villa Pamphilj (wall E, IV), now in Palazzo Massimo, pygmy defecating towards a hippopotamus (photo S.T.A.M. Mols).

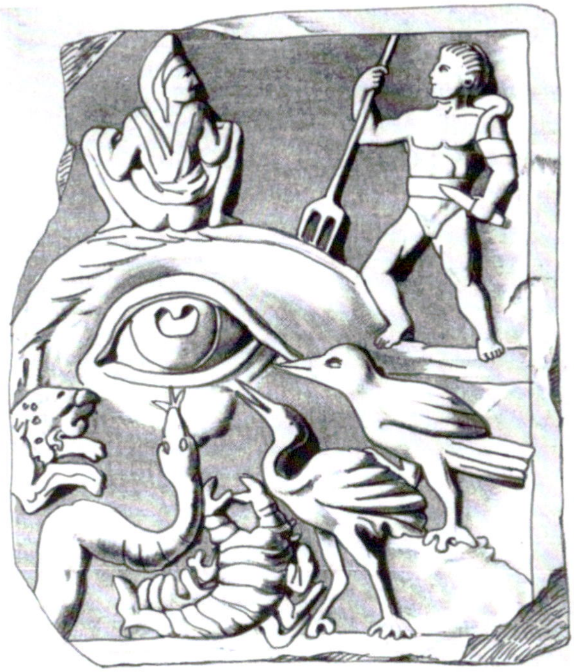

Fig. 12.3. Bas-relief from unknown location with the evil eye under attack (from Millingen 1821).

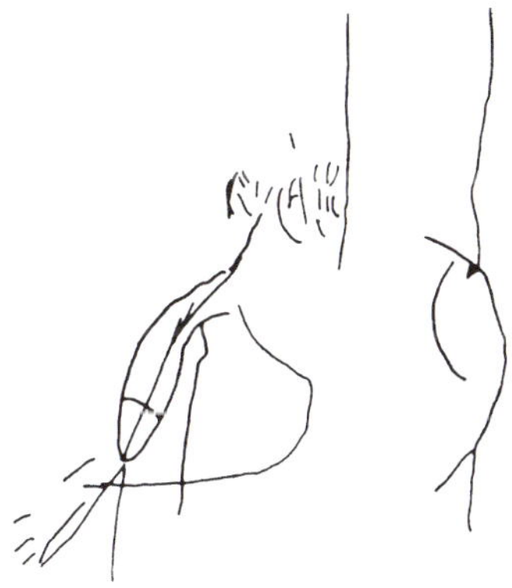

Fig. 12.4. Rome, Paedagogium, *graffito of urinating man (printed with permission from Langner 2001, number 1258).*

statue is perhaps the inebriated Hercules *mingens*, found in the garden of the House of the Stags (IV 21) at Herculaneum.[16] The immediate impression is even more powerful when the statue is a fountain and a stream of water splashes down from the statue's penis.[17] At Ephesus there is a fountain statue of a komast returning home from a symposium, lifting up his shirt to urinate.[18]

Langner lists four graffiti found in Rome representing urinating men (*fig. 12.4*). According to

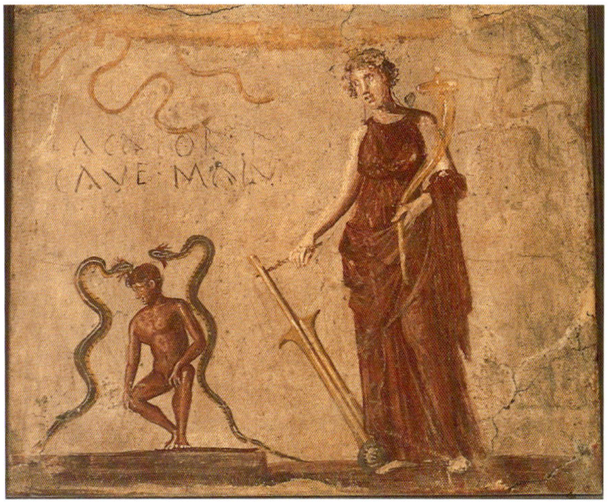

Fig. 12.5. Naples museum, Fortuna painting from Pompeian taberna *IX 7, 22 (photo G.C.M. Jansen).*

him, they might have a provocative character. He is wisely cautious, however, to acknowledge that without context this is hard to determine.[19]

Without the context both of the graffiti and the statues we are not yet able to reflect on the function of these urinating men.

With Help of Fortuna

Some people used other protections in the toilet room and brought in a real goddess, namely Fortuna, to help. Several paintings of her have been found in or near toilets at Pompeii, the most famous image - now in the Naples museum - is the one excavated in a narrow corridor that led to a single-seat toilet of *taberna* IX 7, 22.[20] The painting shows a woman, two snakes and a naked man (*fig. 12.5*). Underneath the painting, the excavator discovered a small terracotta altar. The woman in the painting is dressed in a red chiton; her shoulders are covered with a red shawl. In her left hand she holds a yellow horn of plenty, with her right hand she leans on a yellow rudder, and there is a dark green globe at her feet. On her head she has a corn-measure and two ribbons hang next to her ears. All these attributes indicate that this is the goddess Fortuna, and the corn-measure on her head specifies her as Fortuna-Isis, a very common figure at Pompeii. She looks at a naked, sun-tanned man, squatting on a small platform. The man is smaller than the goddess, and most researchers agree that he is defecating.[21] Two brightly colored snakes rush towards him. Above this scene a flower garland with more ribbons has been painted.[22]

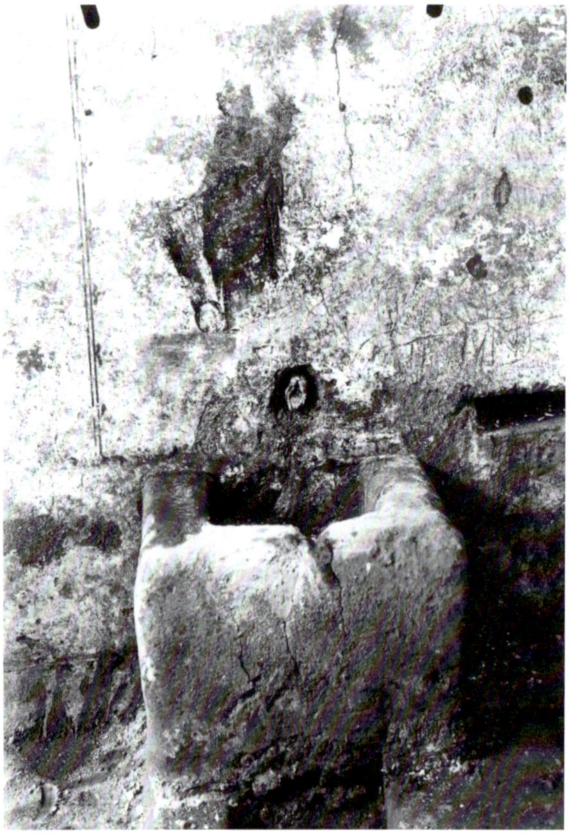

Fig. 12.6. Pompeii, Praedia *of Iulia Felix (II 4), painting in toilet room (printed with permission of the Soprintendenza Archaeologica di Pompei. Neg A/1404).*

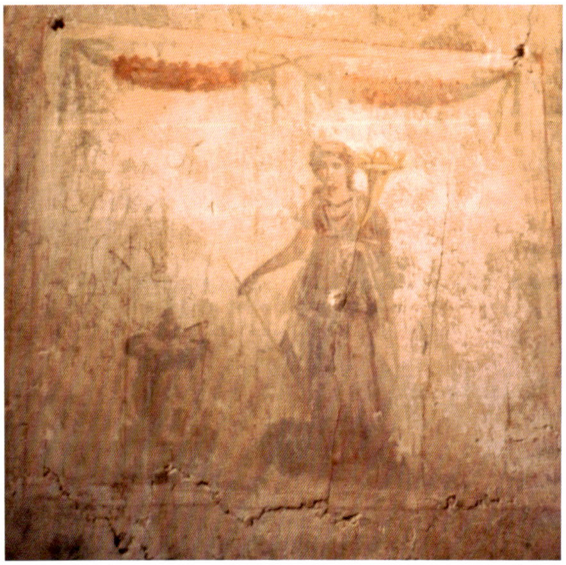

Fig. 12.7. Pompeii, Suburban Baths (VII 16, a), Fortuna painting in toilet room (photo G.C.M. Jansen).

Four other paintings of Fortuna inside toilets in Pompeii are known. Two paintings have been found in toilets belonging to private households: Fortuna was present in the two-person toilet of the rather large and wealthy house of the Greek Epigrams (V 1, 18) and in a single-seat toilet in the much more humble house V 4, 9.[23] Today, not much of either one survives. Two other Fortunae were painted in multi-seaters belonging to the most luxurious baths of Pompeii, where the richer clientele went. One was found in the ten-seater toilet belonging to the bath complex of the *Praedia* of Iulia Felix (II 4) (*fig. 12.6*). This one has fallen off the wall, but a rather clear picture taken just after excavation shows us the position of the painting: above the water basin in which the sponges could be rinsed so that all the toilet users could see Fortuna.

The only surviving painting still *in situ* has been discovered in the six-seater toilet of the Suburban Baths (VII 16, a) (*fig. 12.7*).[24] Fortuna is just in front of the toilet users and above the spot where water once filled a *labrum*. The painter has drawn a small altar with flame burning on it next to Fortuna and, above her head, a flower garland. In fact, remaining parts of nails lead one to believe that fresh garlands were also hung here.[25]

The discovery of a 2nd-century Fortuna painting in a one-person toilet in the so-called house of Domitia Lucilla in Rome illustrates that this was not a local Pompeian phenomenon.[26] This Fortuna has, just as the Pompeian ones, a garland painted above her head. In addition, she is bringing an offering with a *patera* to an altar with a burning flame.

A twenty-seater toilet in the Barracks of the Firemen (II v, 1) at Ostia (*fig. 12.8*)[27] is furnished with an *aedicula* (small, temple-like niche) for a statuette of Fortuna. Since this toilet had no entrance from the street side, it could only be used by the people inside the building, the men of the fire brigade or the night watchmen. The *tympanon* bears the inscription *Fortunae sanct(um)* (*fig. 12.9*). The *aedicula* was placed rather high above the floor level. From this position Fortuna could watch over all the users of the toilet, whatever seat they would have taken. In the middle of the room was an altar dedicated to Fortuna; the inscription reads *C(aius) Valerius / Myron b(ene) f(iciarius) pr(aefecti) / coh(ortis)IIII vig(ilum) / Fortunae / sanctae / v(otum) s(olvit) l(ibens) a(nimo)*. 'Gaius Valerius Myron, beneficiary of the prefect of the fifth cohort of the night watch has gladly paid his vow to holy (or sacred) Fortuna' (*fig. 12.10*).

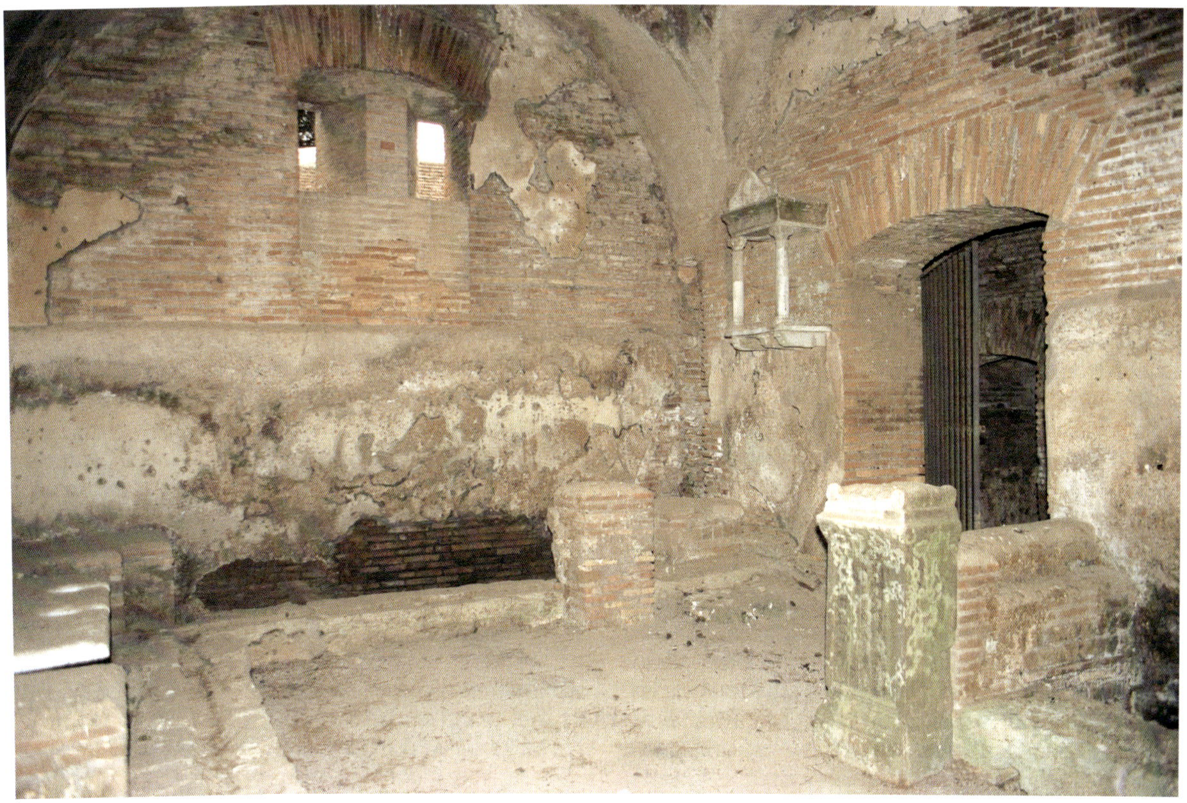

Fig. 12.8. Ostia, Barracks of the Firemen (II v, 1), Fortuna shrine and altar in toilet (photo G.C.M. Jansen).

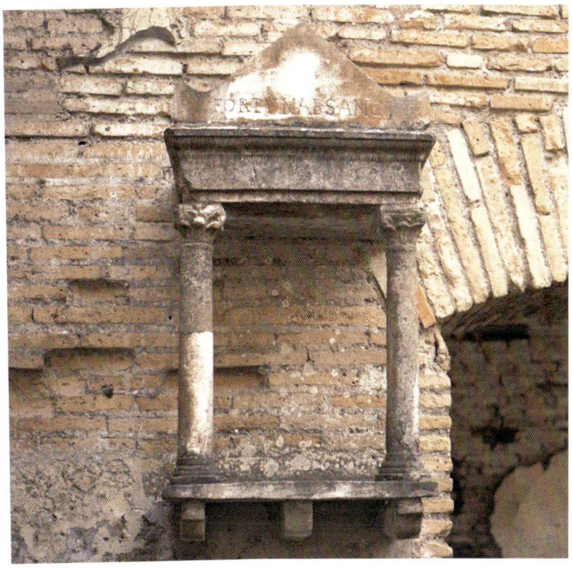

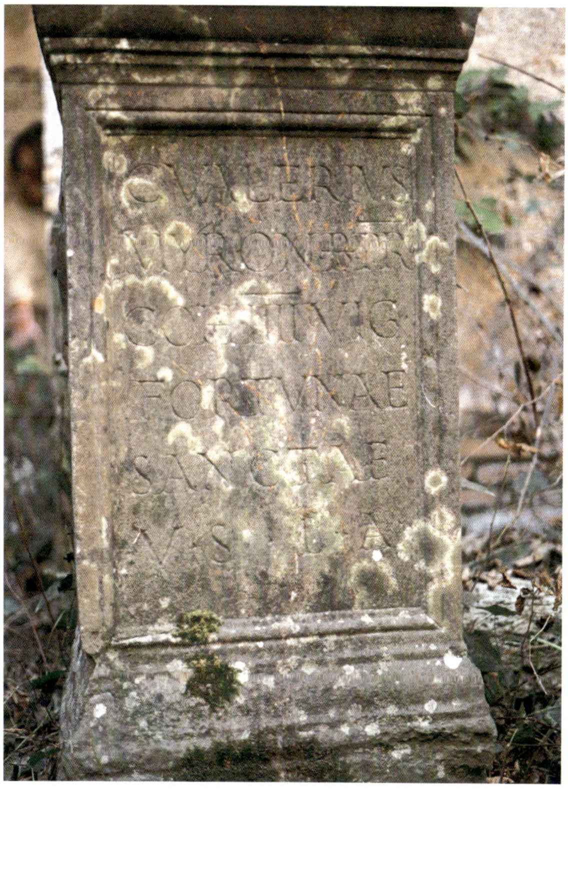

Fig. 12.9. Ostia, Barracks of the Firemen (II v, 1), Fortuna shrine in toilet (photo G.C.M. Jansen).
Fig. 12.10. Ostia, Barracks of the Firemen (II v, 1), altar in toilet devoted to Fortuna (photo G.C.M. Jansen).

A reference by the Christian philosopher Clemens who lived at the end of the 2nd and beginning of the 3rd century AD at Alexandria indicates that most Romans were probably familiar with the presence of Fortuna in toilet rooms. In a discussion about the strange 'religion' of the pagan Romans, Clemens comments that, in his opinion, Fortuna in the toilet was the height of ridiculous superstition: 'The Romans, although they ascribe their greatest successes to Fortuna, and believe her to be the greatest deity, carry her statue to the privy and erect it there, thus assigning her a fit temple.'[28]

Fortuna has been found in both private and public toilets, with a seating capacity varying from one to twenty. In three of the toilets discussed here the interaction between Fortuna and the toilet users can still be reconstructed: Fortuna was in a central position in the room and all people on the seats could see her, apart from the toilet of the Barracks of the Firemen in Ostia, where the view from some seats was not ideal. Fortuna herself, however, could keep an eye on all toilet users from her high position and this might be the intention. It is remarkable that all these toilets were well lit, thus assuring a clear view of the painting.[29] What is also striking is that Fortuna is not just present in these rooms in a passive sense, but that she is also worshipped and asked for favors. The presence of an altar or the nails for fresh garlands above the paintings clearly indicate this. It is a pity that we do not know what favors Fortuna granted that inspired the *beneficiarus* to erect the altar.

Though the evidence in itself is scarce - seven depictions of Fortuna inside toilets and one reference in a text are not much - from it we can conclude that Fortuna helping in a toilet was a well-established phenomenon both across time and in different regions: she can be detected in the 1st century in Pompeii and in the 2nd century in Rome, Ostia, and Alexandria. We can also conclude that all social classes called upon her, from the rich elite (house of the Greek Epigrams and the two baths in Pompeii for more selective clientele) to the workmen (in the tavern and the humble house in Pompeii, and the Barracks of the Firemen at Ostia). The question, 'With what is Fortuna helping here, and against what is she offering protection?' has puzzled many scholars and some possibilities are discussed here. Fröhlich thinks that the goddess protects the toilet user against the evil eye (*Böser Blick*) in form of the '*übler Geruch*'.[30] What the '*übler Geruch*' means is not completely clear from his text. Neudecker argues that the goddess protects against problematic bowel movements and the health problems that they might cause. Koloski-Ostrow[31] combines both solutions in stating that the goddess helps with bowel movements and at the same time turns away the effects of the evil eye.

Following the conclusions of the previous section on the apotropaic function of the images of burlesque pygmies in general and in toilet rooms in particular, the goddess as protector against the evil eye and demons seems a fit interpretation to me. This is also underlined by the image of the defecator and two snakes on the Fortuna painting of tavern IX 7, 22 at Pompeii (*fig. 12.5*). This naked man, with whom the toilet user could identify, is not only guarded by Fortuna, who is bending protectively towards him, but by the two snakes that shelter him, too. Snakes are known to guard specific places against all evil, as we can see in decorations on *lararia*.[32] The Pompeians who used this specific toilet would have felt very safe. This aspect of protection and safety is also well expressed by the title of Clarke's article *Forica security*.[33] And just as demons can bring good and bad luck, Fortuna is an ambivalent goddess who brings good and bad luck. What goddess could better neutralize a change of fortune?

'Shitter, beware of evil' (*cacator cave malum*)[34]

In the previous section we saw that the goddess Fortuna was used to protect toilet users. Here we consider how gods and curses were used to threaten unwanted defecators in places other than toilets. We are talking about the well-known *dipinti* (texts painted on walls) from Pompeii expressing variations of the expression *cacator cave malum*, 'Shitter, beware of the evil'. Philologists have interpreted the word *malum* as 'evil' in the sense of evil eye, the evil eye that can bring you bad luck, disease, and even death.[35] 'Shitter, beware of the evil', then, would than mean 'When you defecate here, the evil eye will get you'.[36]

Examples from Pompeii

Five such *dipinti* have been found as well as two variations on facades at Pompeii. *Cacator cave malum* is written three times (*CIL* IV. 5438, 7714, 7715), once *cacator / cave malu* (*CIL* IV. 3782), and once *cavu malum cacator* (*CIL* IV. 4586). There is a sixth *dipinto* with an additional phrase, *cacator cave malum / aut si contempseris habeas / iove(m) iratum* (*CIL* IV. 7716), 'Shitter, beware of the evil, or if you neglect this, Jupiter will be angry with you'. While another says *cacator, sic valeas / ut tu hoc locum*

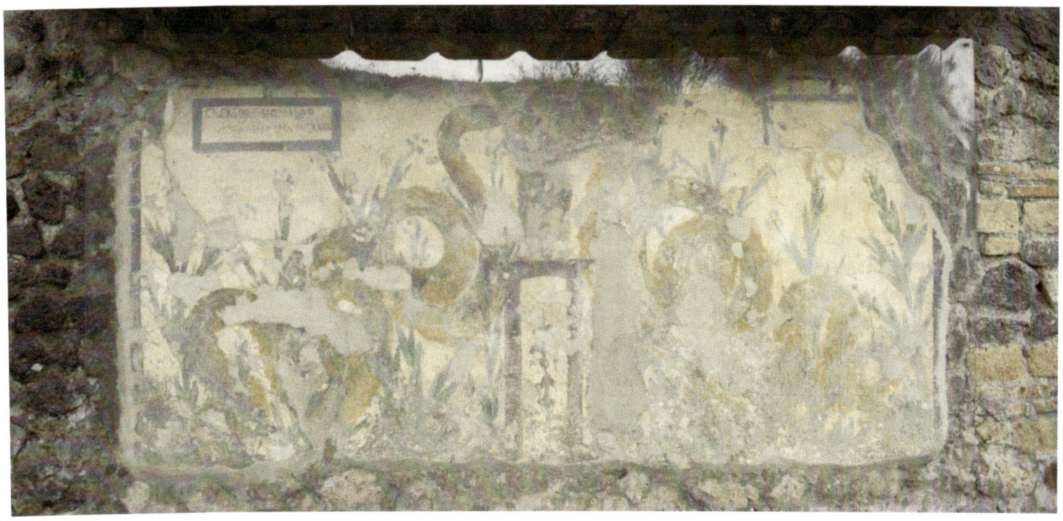

Fig. 12.11. Pompeii, near Vesuvian gate (CIL IV. 6641),
dipinto*:* cacator sic valeas ut tu hoc locum traseas *with snakes (photo G.C.M. Jansen).*

tra(n)sea(s) (*CIL* IV. 6641; *figs 12.11-12*), 'Shitter, may you feel well, if you go past this place'.[37]

This only *dipinto* that has survived (*CIL* IV. 6641) adds some contextual information: the warning is painted in a so-called *tabula* to give it a semi-legal status and the statement is underlined by two large snakes, as protectors of the place. It is hard to reconstruct the context of the other *dipinti*, as they cannot be seen in situ any more, and no photographs or drawings exist. Some conclusions, however, can be drawn from the find spot alone. All *dipinti* occur far away from the town center; to be more precise, on walls of small back-alleys diverging from the main roads. Here, there was little traffic and no entrances to houses. When the excavators mention the height of the letters of the *dipinto*, we can draw some additional conclusions. For example, Spinazzola describes the find of the three *dipinti* clustered in a small alley of the Via dell'Abbondanza, in the neighborhood of the amphitheater.[38] He saw the *cacator cave malu* paintings on each side of the street, with letters that were about one meter high with the whole threat covering over ten meters of wall. The third one, with 'Iupiter will be angry' added, is smaller, but even so seven meters long! The neighbors must have often taken offence at people defecating in this street.

We modern people assume implicitly that human excreta troubled the Pompeians because of stench and the unpleasant sight of it. We also imagine that removing excreta would have been an endlessly unpleasant task. These things probably did not bother most Pompeians, since cleaning away dirt was not a job for citizens, but for slaves. Smell and the constant unpleasant presence of excreta cannot have been much of a problem either, since human excreta would have blended well with the extensive amounts of street dung: in addition to all other rubbish, animal and human excreta were a part of the street pavement. If we think the Pompeians took offence at defecating in the streets, there must have been another motive. Here we must return to the pygmies, the Others, who did everything inappropriately, including defecating in public. It seems safe to conclude that public defecation was not considered civilized. In other words, 'We educated Romans should not act like animals.' If we can accept this argument as valid, then the *cacator* message that one reads immediately after entering Pompeii at the Vesuvian gate is a very powerful one (*figs. 12.11-12*): It might be interpreted to mean: 'Watch out, you enter a city in which defecating in public is not considered civilized.'

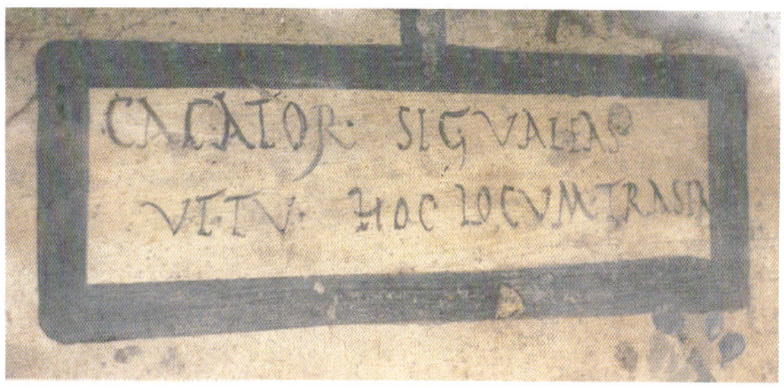

Fig. 12.12. Pompeii, near Vesuvian gate (CIL IV. 6641), detail of dipinto*:* cacator sic valeas ut tu hoc locum traseas *(photo G. Jansen).*

Examples from the Rest of the Roman Empire[39]

Petronius (*Satyricon* 71.8) makes his character Trimalchio say that he wants to place a guard at his grave monument: *Praeponam enim unum ex libertis sepulcro meo custodiae causa, ne in monumentum meum populus cacatum currat*, 'I will put one of my freedmen in front of my grave to guard it and to prevent people from rushing to my monument to defecate'. While Trimalchio's proclamation may be said to evoke laughter more than to reflect reality, it is not hard to imagine abandoned tombs used as toilets. When there was no living guard available to protect a tomb, however, a written threat would be a good alternative. This situation can be seen in a grave inscription found in Rome (*CIL* VI. 13740): *C(aius) Caecilius C(ai) / et (mulieris) L(ibertus) Florus / vixit annos XVI / et me(n)sibus VII. Qui / hic mixerit aut / cacarit, habeat / deos superos et / inferos iratos*, 'Caius Caecilius Florus, freedman of Gaius and his wife lived sixteen years and seven months. Whoever will have urinated or defecated here, let him incur the anger of the gods above and below'.[40]

The poet Persius (*Satyrae* 1.11.2-4) makes a reference to snakes guarding a place against befoulers: *hic inquis veto quisquam faxit oletum / pinge duos anguis. Pueri, sacer est locus, extra / meite*, 'Here, you say, I forbid anyone to defecate; paint two snakes. Boys, the place is holy, urinate outside (of it)'. Snakes are also part of a large dipinto in cryptoporticus 19 of the Domus Aurea (*fig. 12.13*).[41] In fact, the complete ensemble resembles very much the painting near the Vesuvian gate at Pompeii. The threat itself, however, is different: *duodeci(m) deos et Deana(m) et Iovem / optumu(m) maximum habeat iratos / quisquis hic mixerit aut cacarit*, 'Anyone who urinates or defecates here, may he incur the wrath of the twelve gods and also both Diana and Jupiter the Best and Greatest'. Mars is used in Thigibba for such a curse, and Jupiter in Aquileia.[42] In Ephesus it is the goddess of the place herself, Hecate, who tries to protect a gateway from urinators at a T-forked road. She appears on a relief in the west passageway, and on the opposite (east) side, she appears again with an ominous stance with raised arms. Below her is written: 'Whoever urinates at this place, Hecate will punish.' (*fig. 12.14*).[43] Hecate also speaks to potential befoulers on a relief found at Split.[44]

One can confidently conclude from these *dipinti* that urinating and defecating in public was not considered civilized in the Roman world. Those who had intentions to do so in Pompeii were threatened with the powerful words, *cacator cave malum*, painted on the facades of the houses. In one of those threats, the god Jupiter himself comes to help. He and his fellow gods occur in many other threats of the same type all over the Roman Empire. Painted snakes underline the message.

Inscriptions, tituli picti *and Graffiti in Toilet Rooms*

There are three kinds of texts and drawings to be found in Roman toilets: official inscriptions, *tituli picti* put upon the toilet walls as an intended decoration, and occasional inscriptions scribbled by the toilet users.

Official Inscriptions and *tituli picti*

It is not surprising that in toilet rooms there are hardly any inscriptions carved in stone. I was able to discover only four and, as we shall see they either do not provide much information, or they are not part of the toilet room. We have already discussed the inscription *Fortunae sanct(ae)* on a marble slab in a shrine for the goddess Fortuna in the Ostian toilet of the Firemen's Barracks (II v, 1; *fig. 12.9*). From Ephesus, another inscription in marble is known, this time a building inscription

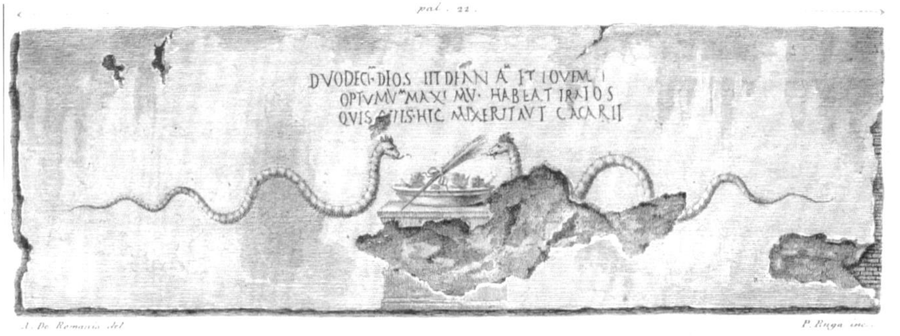

Fig. 12.13. Rome, Domus Aurea, dipinto *with two snakes (from De Romanis 1822, 7).*

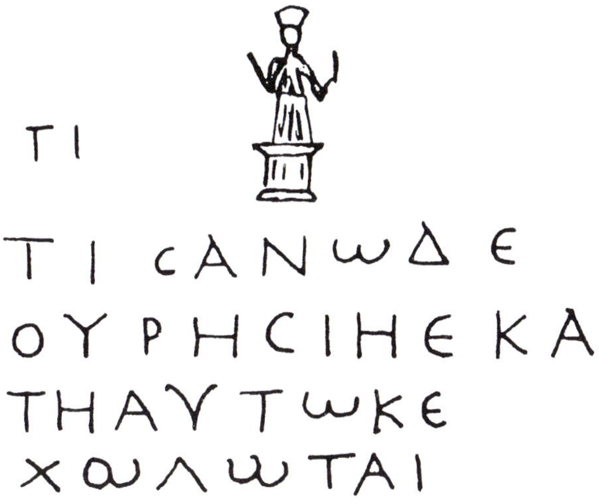

Fig. 12.14. Ephesus, Hecate grafitto (from IvE, *567).*

mentioning both a toilet and a brothel. As the inscription is now in the so-called Scholastikia toilet, people have thought for a long time that it was the building inscription of this specific toilet. The present toilet, however, is much later in date, and it is possible that further up hill there was another toilet (and brothel), and that the architrave came down the hill in the course of centuries.[45] Ephesus is also famous for the seat reservations found in the toilet of the Vedius baths. This toilet is of the so-called peristyle type and in the columns names of several different professions are cut. Recently, however, after a close study of the building and the toilet, La Torre has come to the conclusion that the toilet was composed of many *spolia* and that the columns together with inscriptions might come from a nearby stoa or market.[46] Therefore, it is very likely that the inscriptions have nothing to do with the toilet and seat reservations.

The last 'inscription' I have come across is a word laid out in a mosaic floor in Sepphoris (Israel). It reads ΥΓΕΙ meaning 'stay healthy'.[47] The lettering is positioned in such a way that those sitting on the toilet seats could read it well. The word seems to indicate a wish 'to stay healthy' in the sense of the *bene lava* wishes, also in mosaics, and found on the floors of baths.[48]

The archaeological evidence suggests that Roman toilets could contain *tituli picti* with poems and other texts. A line from Martial (12.61.8-10) advises someone, who wants a poem to glorify himself, to look for a drunken poet who writes verses in toilets. He is not referring to graffiti, but to official *tituli picti*, since he says: *carbone rudi putrique creta*, 'with raw charcoal and smelly clay'.[49]

The evidence is meager. Not many toilets have decorations and even fewer have *tituli picti*. The kind of poem that Martial is writing about might resemble the one from a toilet of Smyrna or the one excavated in a toilet in Ephesus.[50] From Ephesus other *tituli picti* in toilets are known: in Hanghaus 2.2 on a nine-person toilet three philosophers were depicted in caricature. Two are easily recognizable and have a riddle painted above their heads. These riddles are rather absurd and have not yet been solved. Maybe they were not meant to be solved and instead illustrated the strangeness of those philosophers thus creating the apotropaic laughter that was needed in the toilet.[51]

Graffiti on Toilet Walls[52]

> '[...] i muri delle latrine non meno di oggi erano anche nell'antichità coperti di iscrizioni, che ci dànno spesso utili e interessanti indicazioni.'[53]

The Romans are (in)famous for their fanatical writing on walls. If no charcoal was available for writing or a *stilus* for scratching, some sharp device was always near, for example, a *fibula* that held clothes together. With this in mind and given the fact that modern toilets often are covered with graffiti, we would expect a lot of graffiti in Roman toilets, and several researchers underline this point.[54] The same view is expressed in many popular reconstructions of Roman toilets (*fig. 12.15*). Langner on the other hand, suggests that there are only a few wall inscriptions in Roman toilets.[55] By way of explanation, he argues that normally Roman wall inscriptions occur in rooms where people stay for a long time, like the *atrium*, peristyle or *triclinium* in a Roman house. The graffiti are scratched at eye level (1.5 m) and evoke the

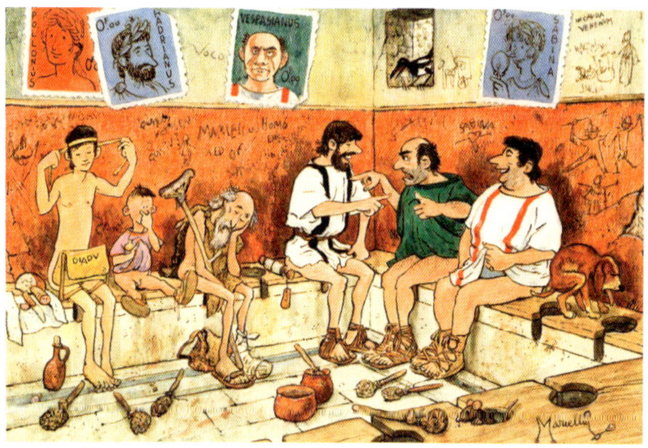

Fig. 12.15. Vaison la Romaine, reconstruction of the latrines (ill. J. Marcellin).

viewer to interaction with the message.

The fact that so few inscriptions have been found in Roman toilets seems to indicate that this interaction between the message on the wall and the reader of the message did not take place in toilet rooms.[56] The best example that underlines Langner's conclusion is the toilet in the large *palaestra* (II 7) at Pompeii. The walls of this building, and especially the columns of the peristyle, are completely covered with graffiti, but in the twenty-person toilet connected to it, not a single graffito has been found.[57] In addition, Langner points to another modern assumption about Roman graffiti with which we must deal.[58] Is the meaning of a Roman graffito's message (when there is one) different from the kind of unfulfilled wishes we find in modern graffiti? A modern toilet user usually sits alone on a toilet and can write in anonymity. This was usually not possible in a Roman toilet. Let us test whether Langner's conclusions that a) there are few graffiti in Roman toilets and b) that the graffiti that do exist differ in meaning from ours, are valid notions. We do this by looking at the evidence of toilet graffiti from the Roman world that are available at the moment.

First of all, Langner is right in saying that the evidence is thin. Many toilets have been found without wall plaster, or the plaster has fallen off at a later time, so that we will never know whether graffiti were scratched there or not. Several toilets have been published, but there is no word about writing on the walls.[59] Sometimes researchers find toilets with graffiti, but do not publish them, hence we remain in the dark about what the writings might mean.[60]

Most evidence is known from the cities around Vesuvius where many toilets with plastered walls have survived. Nevertheless, of the more than 200 toilets that are excavated in Pompeii, only thirteen toilets have graffiti;[61] of the more than 60 toilets discovered in Herculaneum, only four have graffiti (*fig. 12.16*).[62] In these seventeen toilets 48 wall inscriptions and drawings occur. What are these wall inscriptions about? They contain mostly statements such as 'Mister so and so was here', 'We were here on such and such day', and 'Mister so and so salutes Miss so and so'. Some have a sexual significance and state 'Penis for rent for five sestertii', or a person boasts about his success with women. Other graffiti are related to the action in the room, as someone mentions having diarrhea, another tells us 'I am a midwife', and several graffiti mention having a good shit (*hic cacavi bene*). Furthermore, the alphabets (*abecedarii*)

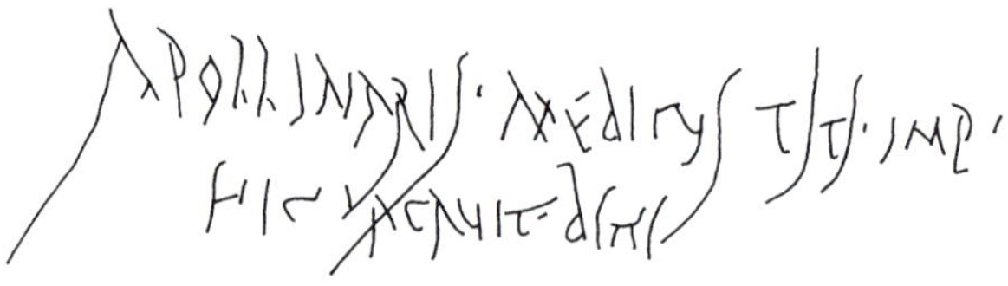

Fig. 12.16. Herculaneum, House of the Gem (Ins. Or. I, 1), CIL *IV. 10619 (drawing G.C.M. Jansen).*

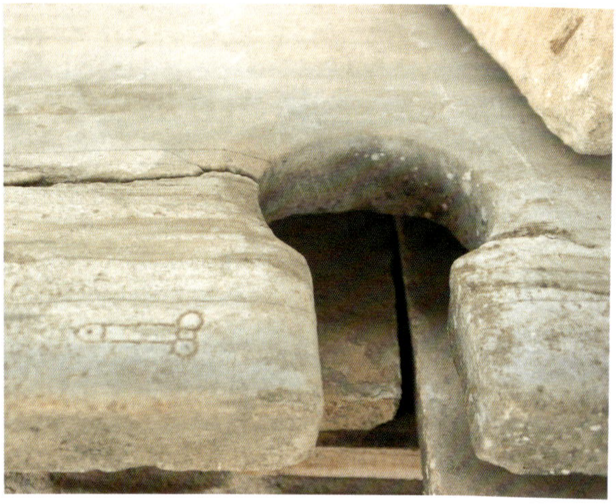

Fig. 12.17. Ephesus, 'Steindepot' behind the lower agora, marble toilet seat with carved phallus *(photo G.C.M. Jansen).*

(six) and the drawings of the *phalli* (three) are worth mentioning, as they indicate protection against the evil eye or demons.

How do wall inscriptions from elsewhere in the Roman Empire inform about this issue? We can compare the inscriptions of Pompeii and Herculaneum with only six other toilets in the Roman empire: three in Ephesus,[63] two in Rome[64] and one in Hadrian's villa (see case study Molle pp. 176-178). The inscriptions in these toilets contain some apotropaic symbols, such as concentric circles, *phalli*, and alphabets (*fig. 12.17*). Wall inscriptions can also offer good wishes. They differ, however, from the ones in Pompeii, because they represent human faces, animals, birds (*fig. 12.18*) and ships.

What can we conclude from the location of graffiti in toilet rooms? It is clear that most graffiti occur next to seats (50%) and must have been written by someone seated on the toilet. This pertains, for example, to the birds in the Ephesian toilet, and to the phrase 'I am a midwife' from a Pompeian toilet, which has been written vertically down from seat level to the toilet floor. 30% of the graffiti occur in front of the toilet user on

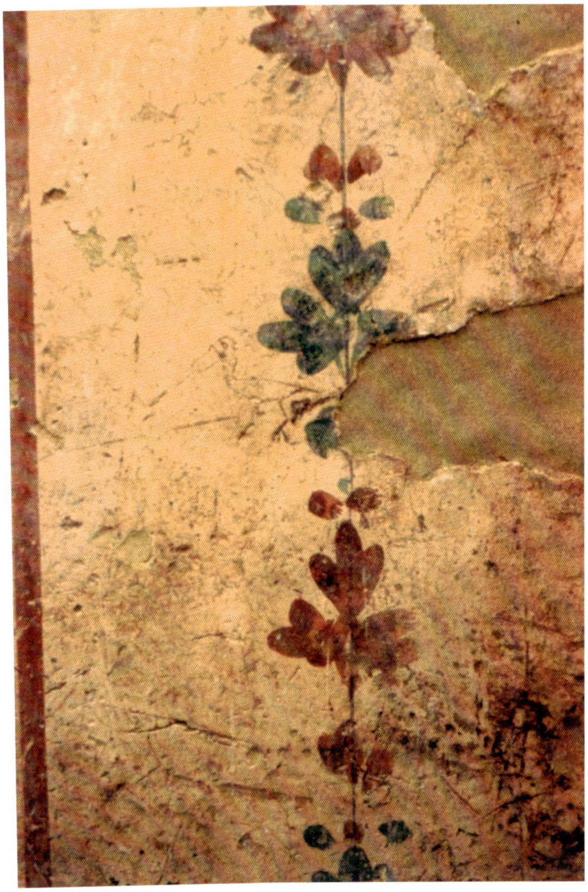

Fig. 12.18. Ephesus, Terrace House 2, 2, so-called Philosophers toilet SR 29, two incised birds next to the toilet seat (photo G.C.M. Jansen).

the blank wall and only 20% are written behind the user, above the seats.[65] We only have a few notations by the excavators at which level the graffiti were written, but the evidence we have shows that the average height is 1.2 m above ground level (in contrast to the normal Roman height of 1.5 m). It is important to realize that most of the graffiti have very small letters of about 3 to 4 cm in height and are scratched in the white plaster of the toilet room. The words and drawings are not very visible; and the darkness of the toilet rooms would not help the situation either. These graffiti, therefore, have a different effect from the ones scratched in the much brighter rooms of the Roman house, such as triclinia and peristyles where darker surfaces (red and black, for example) would offer better contrast. The interaction between the graffitist and the reader, as discussed by Langner, indeed would be much more difficult in a toilet.

The other interesting thing is that the names that occur on these toilet walls are nearly all male and that messages are written from the male perspective, like 'I had sex with many women' or 'Male x had sex with female y'. In the latter phrase, the man is the subject and the woman the object. The two women appearing as subject are Mystice and Martha. Are these inscriptions helpful in solving the question that keeps popping up in this book: 'Did women frequent public toilets?'. After a closer look at the inscriptions, it appears that we have most evidence from private single seaters, and here this issue is not relevant. A possible explanation might be that the women were not as literate as the men, or that they did not feel the need to make their presence known.

Two toilets have been found with no graffiti in the toilet room itself (at least not recorded), but just outside, for example, on the walls of the staircase leading down to the 60-persons toilet underneath the Domus Flavia on the Palatine that was intended for the palace staff. Here many graffiti have been discovered, one scribbled on top of another, and among the words are sketches of birds, ships, circles and lozenges.[66] Other examples are the graffiti on the walls of a corridor leading to a toilet at Ordona (in South of Italy), where the walls are covered with drawings of ships.[67] These very much resemble the ones scribbled and drawn by persons that had to wait before entering the large theater in Pompeii.[68] Is it possible to conclude that these toilets were very crowded, and that one had to wait outside a long time, evidently long enough to draw these huge ships? And are there no graffiti inside, because one had no time for drawing as people from outside were pushing to get in?

What about the statements of Langner (that there are only few graffiti in Roman toilets and that the graffiti that do exist differ in meaning from ours) discussed at the beginning of this section? The evidence of graffiti in toilets is indeed meager, more meager than one would expect. And indeed the effect of the graffiti is different from the architecture of the room alone: the relative darkness inside and the light-colored walls would make it more difficult to communicate through graffiti. The assumption that the nature of the graffiti differs from ours, since the users of these toilets were usually not alone, seems invalid. Besides the apotropaic wall inscriptions, which we, of course, do not have in our toilets, we find cries from the heart, humor, nonsense, names, and greetings - just the kind of things one can find in a modern toilet. Although the inscriptions themselves are not that

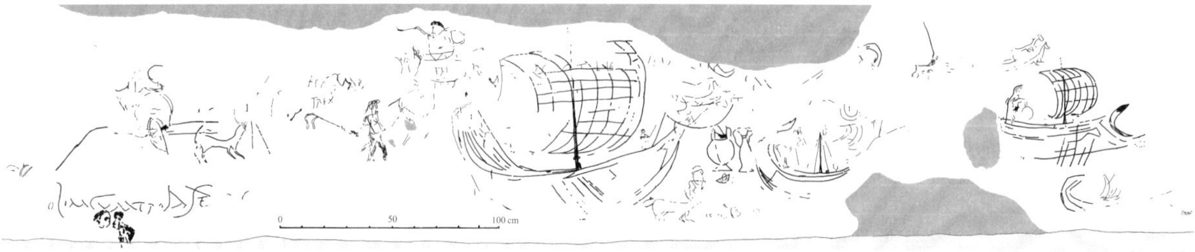

Fig. 12.19. Hadrian's Villa, Canopus *toilet, southern wall, charcoal graffiti in their actual condition of visibility (drawing C. Molle).*

revealing, and do not say much, their place in the room and the person who wrote them gives us some insight about what was going on in a Roman toilet. We can imagine someone sitting in this room and scribbling on the wall his thoughts of that very moment. We must not forget that we draw these conclusions from 22 toilets only.

Conclusions

The images of defecation, the paintings for protection in the toilet rooms, and the epigraphic testimonies reveal sanitation habits completely different from our own. Although Romans did not worry about the presence of fellow toilet users, they were afraid of something else: the evil eye or demons. The Roman went to great length to protect himself with *phalli, abecedarii*, laughter-provoking pygmies, and the goddess Fortuna. The things they feared inside toilet rooms, like the evil eye or the *malum*, they used to threaten potential defecators near their houses. Also gods, among others Jupiter and Hecate, were used to scare off those who would defecate in public places. Whereas we are afraid of germs and bacteria, and feel the need to protect our privacy, these were apparently of no concern to the Romans. They had their gods and superstitious beliefs that played a considerable role in their sanitary behavior, and this shows us a unique part of Roman society, a part that deserves more exploration.

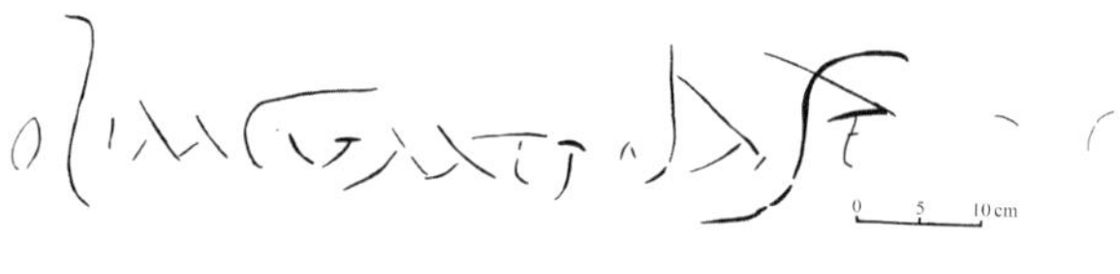

Fig. 12.20. Hadrian's Villa, Canopus *toilet, southern wall, detail of fig. 12.19: the inscription of Trojan subject, detail drawing (drawing C. Molle).*

Case Study: Graffiti in a Toilet of Hadrian's Villa *(Carlo Molle)*

In the multi-seater toilet south of the western substructures of the *Canopus* of Hadrian's Villa (Tibur),[69] there are Roman drawings and inscriptions made in charcoal or by scratching the plaster.[70] They are disposed both on the thick hydraulic plaster of the lower part of the walls and on the thinner white plaster of the upper part, the latter surely and clearly preferred for the charcoal graffiti. Since the plasters are not restored and the graffiti are partially invisible, this note is to be considered as a brief preliminary study.

On the eastern wall, to the right of the door, we see at least a scratched inscription, whose visibility is at the moment compromised by concretions.[71] On the southern wall we find many charcoal drawings, made by one or more persons who stood on the plain of the perforated seats of the toilet (now lost) and drew almost exclusively on the upper white plaster (*fig. 12.19*). We can distinguish, on the left, an interesting inscription, probably part of an unknown verse (spondaic metrum) and possibly the first line of a poem (*fig. 12.20*):[72]

Olim cum Trọia se[---].

On the same wall, we can see a quadruped[73] and a fighter with a crested helmet, apparently shaking what seems to be a pole with two floating objects on its end. One can think of a warrior or a gladiator, maybe in connection with the nearby inscription which could concern a *Thrax*, but the presence of an unusual 'breast' suggests more probably an Amazon or an armed woman (*fig. 12.21*).[74] Further

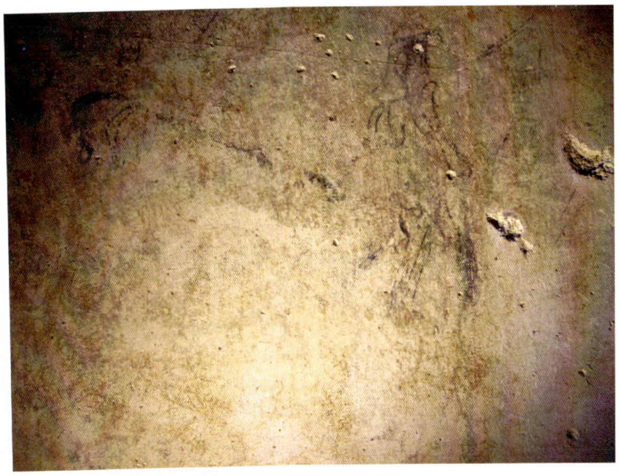

Fig. 12.21. Hadrian's Villa, Canopus *toilet, southern wall, the 'Amazon' (photo C. Molle).*

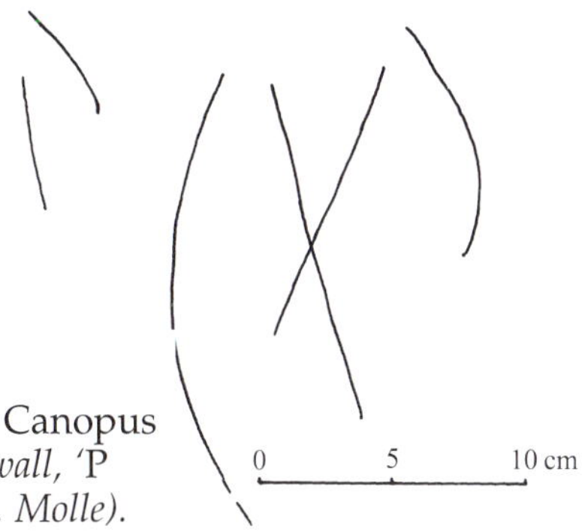

Fig. 12.22. Hadrian's Villa, Canopus *toilet, southern wall, 'P (X)' (drawing C. Molle).*

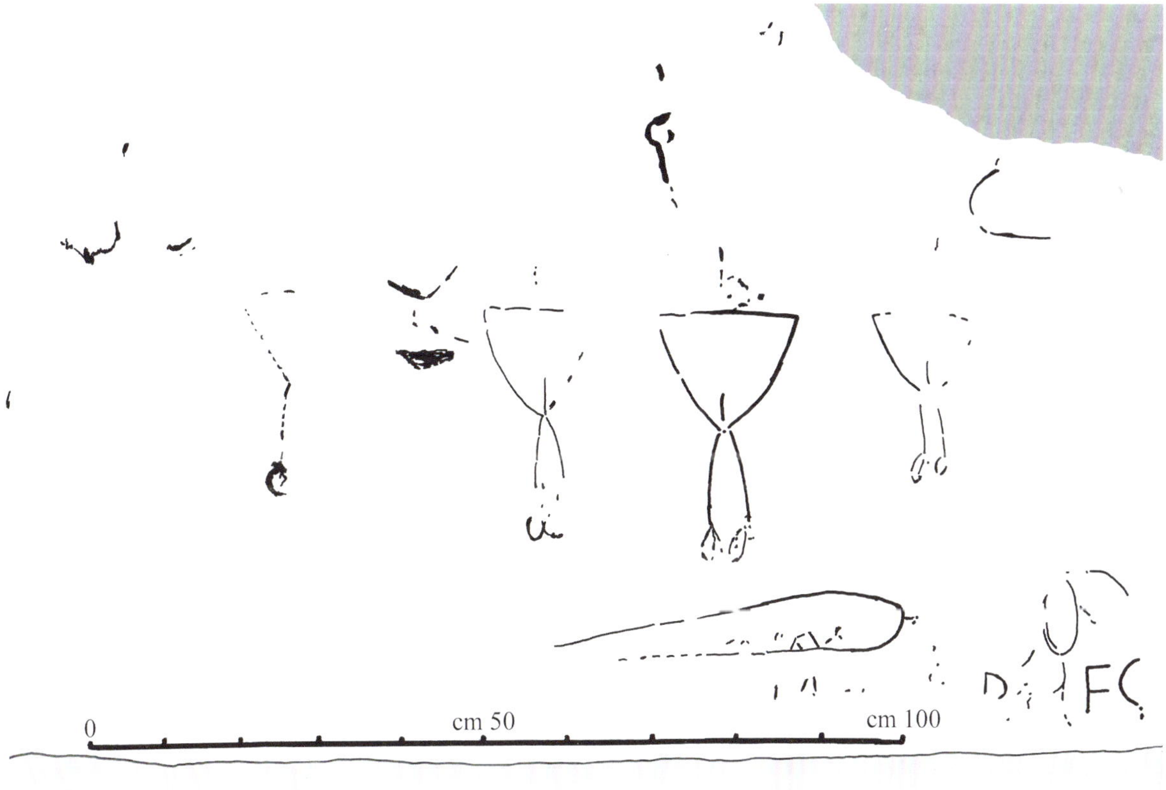

Fig. 12.23. Hadrian's Villa, Canopus *toilet, western wall, traces of charcoal graffiti (drawing C. Molle).*

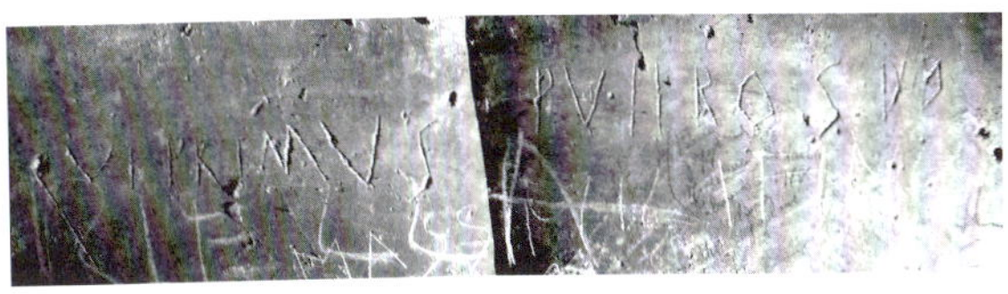

Fig. 12.24. Hadrian's Villa, Canopus *toilet, northern wall, the inscription concerning the* pueri*, photo composition (photos C. Molle).*

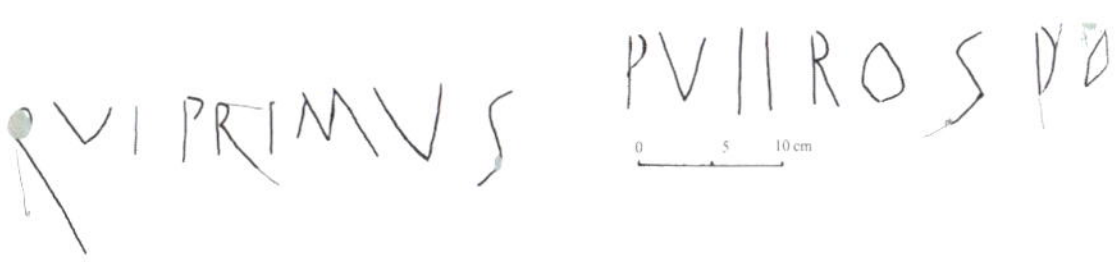

Fig. 12.25. Hadrian's Villa, Canopus *toilet, northern wall, the inscription concerning the* pueri *(drawing C. Molle).*

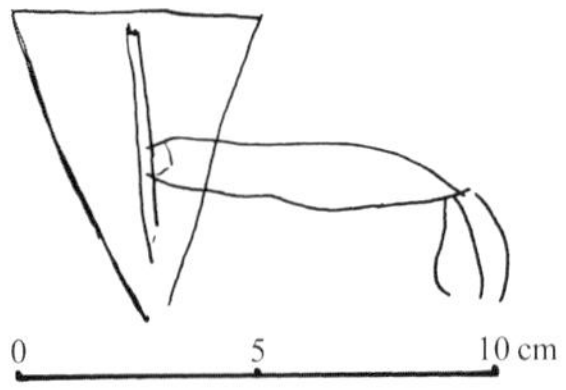

Fig. 12.26. Hadrian's Villa, Canopus *toilet, northern wall, scratched representation of a* coitus, *(drawing C. Molle).*

on to the right, there are at least four ships, with sails bloated. Before the first ship, above, there may be a man holding out a twig in his hand.[75] The first ship, more than one meter long, is probably a *navis oneraria* ('merchant vessel'): we can distinguish the mast, the big square sail, some oars, and a little man on the boat deck.[76] Further on there is another quadruped and at least three pots (amphoras) of different shape (harbor scene?). We can see also a second ship,[77] and a third, in this case showing a beaked prow, with a *gubernator* ('helmsman') wearing a sort of hood and having something round in front of him.[78] Above there are at least two animals with long necks.[79] Under the third ship, we see the rest of a fourth ship (the stern and a part of the sails). A scratched graffito is clearly visible on the hydraulic plaster underneath (*fig. 12.22*).[80]

On the western wall, and always on the white plaster, we can again observe traces of charcoal. Here I see at least three or four very curious triangular shapes with 'legs', possibly personified female genitalia (*vulvae*), a long horizontal shape (*phallus*?), and the remains of an inscription (*fig. 12.23*).[81]

On the hydraulic plaster of the northern wall, there are some scratched graffiti. The most evident one was already published by Aurigemma,[82] but I am proposing to read it differently, as part of an unknown verse (hexameter or pentameter), probably of an erotic nature (*figs 12.24-25*):

Qui primus pueros do(---?). [perhaps *do(cuit)*]. 'Who first [taught] the boys.'

The same wall has a singular representation of a *coitus* (*fig. 12.26*)[83] and a very disarticulated inscription of about six lines, maybe beginning with *hic* and mentioning a *puella*.[84]

The chronology of these documents is not before the 120s AD and probably not later than Severan times.[85] We can observe that almost all the graffiti are of an extemporary sort: the poetic (and erotic) subjects are of no surprise on the walls and the big charcoal scenes represent themes very loved by the Romans: naval subjects, fighters, and animals.[86] What is remarkable is the size and the visibility of the scenes[87] that dominated the surface of the walls. That is unusual for graffiti in private contexts, but I think more comprehensible in a less controlled place, such as a public, multi-seater toilet.[88]

Case Study: The Paintings of Philosophers in the Baths of the Seven Sages in Ostia
(Ann Olga Koloski-Ostrow and Eric M. Moormann)

The painted decoration in the Baths of the Seven Sages (III x, 2-3, room no 6) at Ostia deserves attention in the context of Roman messages concerned with 'toilet talk'.[89] Heavily robed Greek philosophers,[90] (*fig. 12.27-30*) seated not on latrines, but on *bisellia*, converse with each other (or with us viewers) in a hand-lettered, cartoon-like dialogue about ways to effect good digestion and defecation. Their 'advice', written in street Latin above their heads, and their names and cities of origin are inscribed beside them in Greek.

Not much was written about them for many years after the first publication by the excavator Guido Calza,[91] but in recent decades some fascinating interpretations have been made. As they concern acts that are performed in a toilet, we find it appropriate to include them in this book. Three of these Sages are still visible: Solon (*fig. 12.28*), Thales (*fig. 12.29*), and Chilon (*fig. 12.30*), and part of the name of Bias. While we might expect philosophers to expound about the soul or meaning of life, much to everyone's surprise, these messages concern the functions of the body and hence are rather non-philosophical. In a lower register the heads of some seated men are preserved (*fig. 12.30*), originally numbering about twenty. Their bodies were probably destroyed when the room was renovated and received a new dado for decoration. Apparently, these men were sitting on a multi-seater toilet and chatting to each other.

The texts from the mouths of the philosophers are written in iambic *senarii* which belong to a form of poem appropriate for Roman mimes. Next to Thales (*fig. 12.29*) we read: (1) *durum cacantes monuit ut nitant Thales* ('Thales advised those having a difficult shit to strain (or push hard)'); (2) *verbose tibi / nemo / dicit dum Priscianus / [u]taris xylospongio nos / [a?]quas* ('No one speaks to you with many words

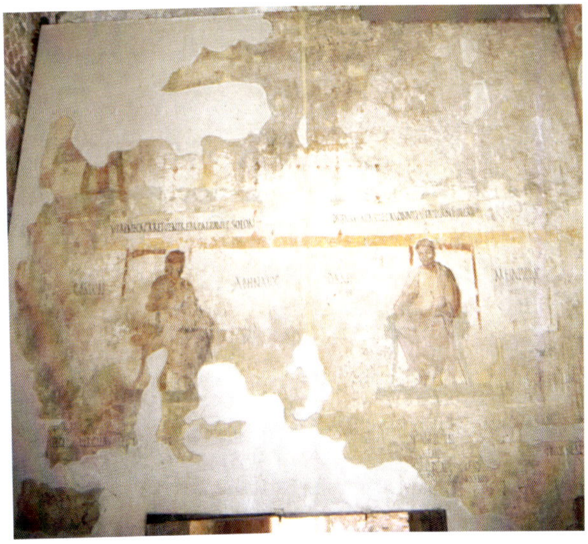

Fig. 12.27. Ostia, Baths of the Seven Sages, Solon and Thales (left to right) (photo S.T.A.M. Mols).

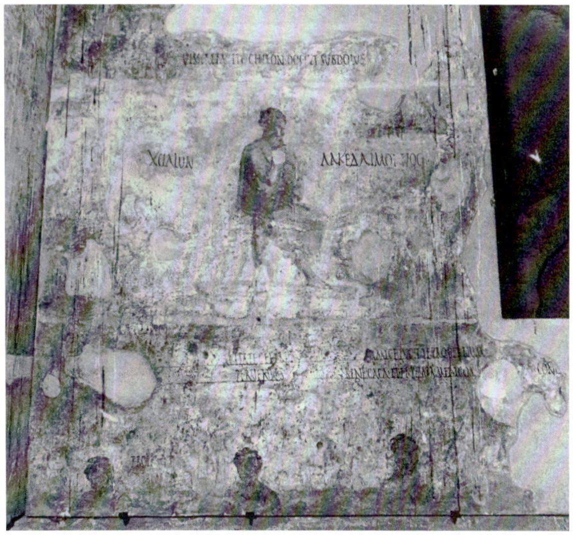

Fig. 12.30. Chilon with heads of toilet users below (from Neudecker 1994, 37 Abb. 8).

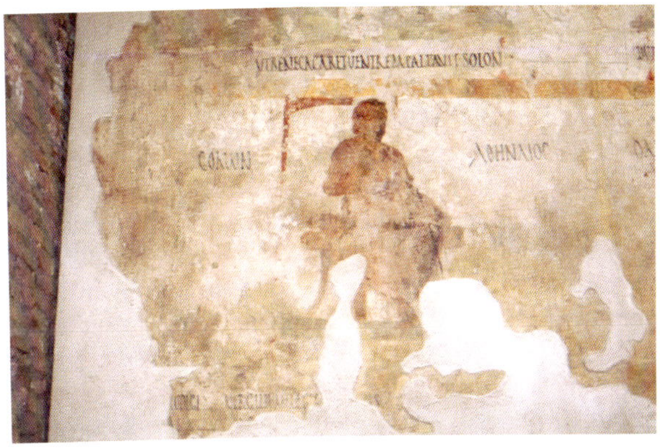

Fig. 12.28. Ostia, Baths of the Seven Sages, Solon (photo S.T.A.M. Mols).

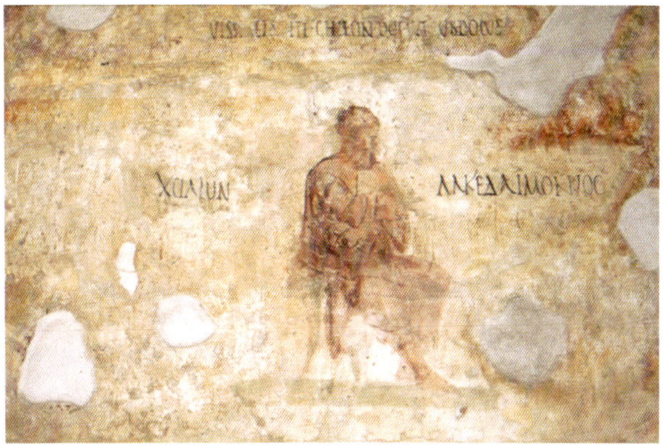

Fig. 12.31. Ostia, Baths of the Seven Sages, Chilon (photo S. Mols).

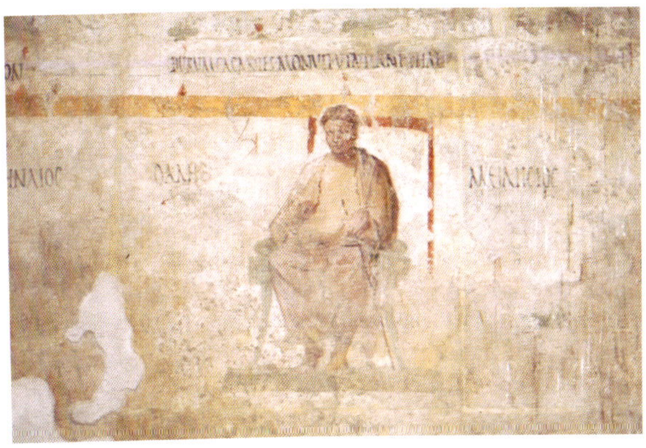

Fig. 12.29. Ostia, Baths of the Seven Sages, Thales (photo S.T.A.M. Mols).

while you, Priscianus, use a sponge on a rod. [...] we... water...'). Perhaps the biggest joke of all suggested by the painter of the room is that the small rods wielded by the notable philosophers during their 'lectures' may just as effectively be used for cleaning sticks in the toilet (cf. above A. Wilson, p. 103).

Above Solon (*fig. 12.28*) we see: (1) *ut bene cacaret ventrem palpauit Solon* ('In order to shit well Solon rubbed his belly'); (2) *iudici (?) / or(di)na (?)* ('Order to the judge/to be judged'); (3) ... *Vergilium legis(se) pueris* (?) ('... that Virgil read to the boys' or '[a text of] Virgil read to the boys'). Chilon (*fig. 12.31*) declares: *mulione sedes / uissire tacite Chilon docuit subdolus* ('You sit on a muleteer.' (or, if we read *mulio ne sedes/* 'Don't sit down, muleteer.' Then,

'Sly Chilon taught (how) to fart silently').

Figures, presumably of more regular, run-of-the-mill 'contemporary' Roman visitors to the room, are in a band beneath the Seven Sages (see again *fig. 12.30*, bottom). They too converse together in comic strip manner, and their discourse is even more colloquial and basic. Unfortunately, many of the words and portraits are poorly preserved, but enough survives to be certain that all the walls were covered in such a manner. In this lower section, above the heads of these men, we read texts: (1) *...]enis Bias*; (2) *agita te celerius /pervenies* ('Move yourself and you will arrive faster.'); (3) - as an answer to this - *propero* ('I am hurrying'); (4) *amice fugit te proverbium / bene caca et irrima medicos* ('Friend, the saying escaped you: shit well and let the doctors suck you.'). The best doctors of the day could not possibly have delivered more pointed or honest advice about emptying the bowel. Fortuna would have gladly stood by any of these gentlemen to assist them in their hard labors of evacuation and breaking wind, or to protect them from the dangers of the open sewers under the seats.

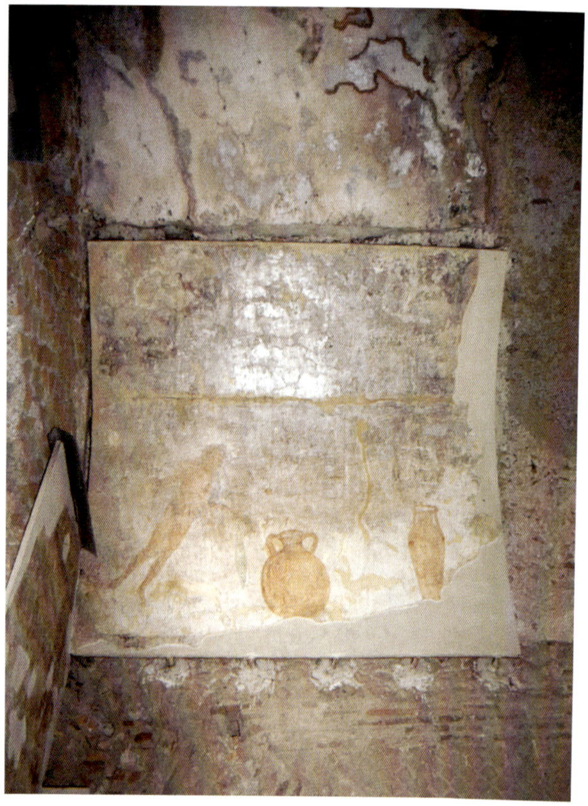

Fig. 12.32. Ostia, Baths of the Seven Sages, ceiling (photo S.T.A.M. Mols).

Several fundamental problems must be tackled first: the building history of this part of the complex, the date of the decorations, and the function of the room. Clarke called it a tavern, pointing to the amphorae painted near the ceiling (*fig. 12.32*). Others have seen it as a latrine, but in this dark and gloomy space we find none of the necessary constructions to suggest such a function, so that, at present, no definitive interpretation can be given.[92] As to dating, most authors agree that the murals belong to the early 2nd century AD.

Secondly, we should ask to whom these messages were 'sent': were they for 'lower-class' people, as Clarke argues *expressis verbis*, or could they be for a more sophisticated clientele, such as the visitors to the baths? The fact that precious wine (*falernum*, see note 95 below and *fig. 12.30*, where the word is visible) is depicted on the upper register of the south wall, and that the Greek Sages speak in street Latin suggests the notion of bilingual literacy for those who wanted to understand the overall message. The images of the Sages were probably easily recognizable, thanks to their standard iconography, but their humor was only fully grasped if their words could be understood.

Richard Neudecker suggests that the decorations endorse the philosophical ideas described by Plutarch in his *Convivium septem sapientium* 159B, whereas Clarke analyzes the images as an example of heteroglossy, philosophers using language that they are not normally known to use.[93] For Clarke, the scenes are lowbrow, instead of highbrow, as Neudecker posits, and they rather show an example of what the Romans really found funny: overturning power. Stephan Mols, contra Neudecker, denies the connection with Plutarch and other literary texts, and sees the humor in the fact of the combination of such serious persons as the Greek Sages - depicted in the standard fashion of Greco-Roman art - and the humble, and sometimes embarrassing, matters of defecation that they discuss. Therefore, he thinks the humor is even more subtle than we find in the philosopher paintings at Ephesus. We agree with Mols that the decorations are probably not just caricatures of famous philosophers, but '...a parody of the customary behavior of the wealthy, in showing off their own *humanitas*, their own humane sensibility, by means of portrait galleries, a parody that is inspired by the Roman genre of mime.'[94]

But to push even further the notion at the heart of Mols' argument - that insult to authority was what stimulated the most laughter for the Romans - we propose another, similar way to understand the paintings in the room. To do so, we must consider relationship of the Seven Sages paintings to a type of Roman literary trope, not just to the influence of mime. The toilet-talk pun expressed in these painted walls is indeed exceptionally clever, but perhaps it can only be fully appreciated if the whole wall is considered together, including the decorations in the uppermost band of the room - the band near and on the ceiling. Not quite symmetrically placed above the heads of each of the surviving Sages are different types of amphorae, containers for beverages like expensive wine or foodstuffs (*fig. 12.30* with the word *falernum*).[95] Such amphorae can be seen on the ceiling as well, along with a big fish and a man who seems to be floating beside them. There is no question that Falernian wine brings luxury to mind. The fish on the ceiling, although very poorly preserved today, might also be another type of comestible meant to signal more wealthy tastes. We believe that these Trajanic paintings may be a visual representation of the kind of literary trope we can find in Petronius' *Cena Trimalchionis*. The 'authority' figure, Trimalchio, is the real laughing stock from beginning to end, despite his display of erudition, which at every turn is faulty, his wealth, which is continuously excessive, and his gluttonous generosity, which itself becomes an agony for all his dinner guests, who will need toilet facilities for relief, and who most of all will themselves need to evacuate from his house in the end. The 'authority figures' in the paintings, of course, are the philosophers, and they bear the brunt of our laughter in the painted scenario.

Petronius deliberately (and ingeniously) employs descriptive language that reminds us of bodily evacuation in a whole parade of overwhelmingly lavish, greasy, and rich foods mentioned in the course of his dinner party. In reading the satirical novel, we come to visualize those foods almost as excrement itself (soft, brown, wet, creative culinary lumps), and ultimately to imagine the whole overstuffed dinner party as a preparation for a massive bowel movement.

The painter of the Ostian room also plays upon the relationship between luxury and excess (at the top of the room, manifested in expensive wine like Falernian, and perhaps in the fat fish near the amphorae) and the dregs (*faex*), the ordinary toilet users and their production, at the bottom. The upper register mainly represents costly drinks. These savory pleasures are 'digested' into excremental advice from the mouths of famous philosophical authorities in the middle register. Finally, in the lowest register, itself at the very bottom of the room, the heads of contemporary Roman *cacatores*, babbling their 'silly' conversation seat to seat in the *forica*, will themselves create the ultimate end-product of the whole sequence, fresh urine and excrement. It all boils down to that! The paintings allow the humor of a sophisticated literary trope, like the one in Petronius, to become easily accessible to clientele of these handsome baths, even to those clientele who might not know all the words or who might themselves be illiterate.

12.2 Interpreting the Archaeological Evidence: Latrines and the Senses *(Zena Kamash)*

The aim of this section is to approach an understanding of the experience of using a Roman-style communal, public latrine. In recent years, an increasing body of inter-disciplinary work has looked at the role of the senses in human experiences of the material world.[96] The sensuous interrelationship of body-mind-environment ('emplacement') is our way of finding out about the material world around us. A sensual archaeology of latrines in the Roman world must, therefore, be considered in any attempt to understand the complexities of latrine use across the Roman world.

There is a tendency in the western world to prioritize vision over the other four senses. In experience, however, our senses are knitted together; that is, we do not necessarily experience them simultaneously, but rather they are woven together sequentially.[97] In what follows, I hope to bring out some of the ways in which four of the fives senses, vision, smell, touch and sound, might have been knitted together in the experience of a Roman public latrine.[98] In order to make as secure a sensory interpretation as possible, this analysis draws on the well-researched data presented by Wilson in chapter 7. I focus on public latrines because many of the issues discussed here, particularly those related to the social gaze, seem to be a greater threat in public, rather than private latrines.

Most latrines were screened from exterior view, which would have afforded a degree of privacy to the people inside the latrine. Once inside the latrine, two factors suggest that there may also have been visual privacy of the body. It has been argued convincingly in chapter 7 that the wearing of voluminous clothing would have prevented in practice very little of the body from being seen. There is also textual evidence referring to bathhouse practices that has a bearing on this question. Carlin Barton has demonstrated that in the face of visual temptations and inhibitions in the bathhouse there should be *oculorum verecundia*,[99] i.e. according to Seneca,[100] the restraint and modesty of one's gaze. It seems plausible that this concept of averting one's gaze may also have a bearing on the question of the view inside a latrine, as the implication is that if one's gaze is withdrawn, others' private parts would not have been on display (as no-one should have been looking).

The nature of lighting inside a latrine is also key here. The extent to which good lighting was desirable inside a latrine was probably governed by whether the overriding concern was with bodily privacy or ease of movement. Several different light sources have been recognized in chapter 7, including from lamps, from windows, and from above in unroofed examples, such as 'peristyle' latrines. This variety of different levels of lighting is likely to be due to the fact that uses of light can be culturally constructed.[101] Tanizaki, for example, expressed disappointment for the growing trend towards tiling bathrooms in Japan.[102] He felt that it made the space shiny and bright, whereas he preferred the seclusion provided by the shadows. Interestingly, this concern was expressed over private bathrooms, so the problem was one of aesthetics, rather than bodily privacy. Tanizaki seems to have been reacting against the western trend for tiled, white surfaces in bathrooms, which we deem to indicate cleanliness. These examples show, then, that a variety of complex, cultural sensibilities may have lain behind lighting options, which makes it difficult to offer a single interpretation of the archaeological evidence.

The unroofed latrines would not only have been bright, but would also have provided good ventilation from the various smells that would be wafting around a latrine. The evidence from public latrines indicates that there were no stench traps and that the users were sitting directly above the sewer or cesspit. This suggests that latrines were smelly places, though it is recognized that it is difficult to provide any quantitative assessment of how much public latrines may have smelt in comparison to other parts of a Roman town, for example, *fullonicae* and other industrial areas. Given the potential for visual privacy of the body discussed above, it is still possible that in the unroofed examples, ventilation may have been one of the key motivations behind the design. This seems likely when one considers that smell is well-documented as having strong and complex, cross-cultural cognitive effects.[103] It has, for example, been regularly associated with theories of contagion and has often been used as moral indicator to exclude and stigmatize others.[104] Smell, then, may have played a strong social role in latrines that would have been difficult to ignore.

As discussed in chapter 7, p. 101, the choice of sitting over squatting on a toilet is cultural, not biological. In a Roman latrine, it is more than likely that the user had to sit, which would involve touching the seat. It is conceivable that it may have been problematic for some users to sit in the same place as an unknown, previous user. It is also possible that proximity to another user may also have been a concern. Again, this probably links in to conceptions of personal privacy (see below). In addition, the user would have been sitting above a deep, dark hole, which may have been unsettling, not only because of the smells emanating from it, but also due to the potential for contact with, for example, flies and rats in the sewer or cesspit or sewer demons.[105]

Some of the potential sources of sound in a toilet include passing wind, the sound of running water in the gutter and from fountains, and the sound of chatter between users. The running water may have to some extent masked some of the human sounds made when going to the toilet, but this would have varied depending on proximity to other users. The likelihood of chatter between users is probably dependent once again on how notions of privacy have been constructed. The wall-paintings and *dipinti* in the Baths of the Seven Sages are one potential source of information on this subject.[106] Below the heads of the seven philosophers are the heads of people who are commonly assumed to be sitting on a communal latrine. These heads seem to be having conversations about going to the toilet, which might point to an open and chatty atmosphere inside a Roman toilet in Italy, but the painting was clearly meant to be humorous, so it needs to be used cautiously as evidence for everyday activities. As well as these regular users, the seven sages themselves are also depicted as conversing about digestion and going to the toilet. One of these snippets of conversation says: *vissire tacite Chilon docuit subdolus* ('The cunning Chilon taught how to fart quietly'). This suggests that hearing and possibly smelling of farts were something of a social taboo.[107]

Therefore, it seems that latrines must have elicited a variety of sensory responses in past users through a complex intermingling of smells, sights, sounds and tactile sensations. The effect of these sensory experiences seems to have been closely tied to social taboos, notions of privacy and aesthetics. Interestingly, several of these experiences bring to mind potential elicitors of disgust noted in cross-cultural psychological and anthropological studies of the emotion. Disgust elicitors include bodily excretions (with faeces always occurring as a disgust elicitor), certain categories of 'the other' who are perceived as bringing in poor health, of lower social status, contaminated by contact with something disgusting (including toilets), or immoral in their behavior and things that are thought to be damp, slimy or stinky.[108] Furthermore, disgust can be triggered by concerns about what something is or where it has been.[109] An overarching element of disgusting events is that they remind us of our animal nature. Humans often seem to feel the need to distinguish themselves from animals, but our bodies do things that are animalistic, such as excreting, bleeding when our outer skin is cut, or having sex. In a Roman latrine, in spite of the lack of vision of your private parts, there was still plenty of potential for other people to be aware of your animalistic behavior, such as the smells, and sounds made, and the act of going to the toilet in the presence of others. In addition, sitting on the same seat might have meant coming into contact with other people's body products, urine, and excrement. These areas of social engagement were and are, of course, culturally variable, which suggests that there may have been a high degree of regional diversity in responses to Roman latrines.

12.3 Regional Diversity in Latrine Use

North-Western Provinces (Adam Goldwater)

Buildings are often seen by archaeologists and historians as manifestations of a material culture, with an emphasis on architectural appearance, socio-political impact, dating, and historical associations. There is a bias towards the grander, public buildings and those built of substantial and archaeologically durable materials. When more mundane buildings are considered, the emphasis is often on appearance. One of the major themes of future research should be to see Roman military latrines as not simply cultural objects, but also the remnants of a process; design, supply, construction, and maintenance, and the planning and organization of this process. An understanding of these processes can tell us a great deal about the abilities, resources, socio-political conditions, and values of the culture that produced them.

The evidence for latrines in military establishments covered in chapter 8 highlighted that the most outstanding examples of latrine architecture in Britain come from the military bases and fortifications. This raises important questions about the nature and degree of Romanization, particularly within the frontier zones, and it is worth considering this for a moment. The high degree of regional diversity in the evidence is encapsulated in the extreme cultural variance evident within Britain. Here especially the social, moral, and religious concerns discussed by Zena Kamash (below pp. 186-187) combine, and in particular along Hadrian's Wall, where we find a unique microcosm of amalgamated cultural traditions. Here cultural attitudes, particularly among the native populations, were tied to the environment.

The population of Roman Britain can be recognized as an amalgamation of indigenous culture along with the Roman military culture - which was itself a mixture of different traditions from across the Empire and beyond its boundaries. The adoption of Roman customs, including that of latrine facilities was an intensely variable phenomenon - depending much upon the momentum of the military. To the existing local population, the army brought a completely new social, moral, and religious ways of perceiving the world - not exclusive to the army, but the army was the main force driving these new cultural traditions. Colonies and towns in Britain are prominent installations of Roman society, devised as models of civilized Mediterranean life. But they were initially occupied largely by veteran soldiers - inhabited by people with military experience and thus a model of Roman society in military form. This is in stark contrast to the Mediterranean, North Africa, and the East where sophisticated urban cultures were already well established.

Consider this for a moment against a background of existing native populations venerating wet places as *foci* for religious activity, and the ritual deposition of metal objects in lakes and rivers as a tradition stretching back into the pre-Roman Iron Age.[110] It is plausible that the native populations found it abhorrent to pollute water courses with their waste. Little can be said on the basis of available evidence, but with native religion firmly rooted in the local environment, springs and wet places certainly retained sacred significance into the period of Roman occupation, of course. We have no written or archaeological evidence at present to confirm this, which is why we can make a plea for future researchers in this area. The bias towards the study of Roman military sites has been at the detriment of the study of everyday life in rural areas - particularly in the vicinity of Hadrian's Wall. The Romans did not arrive in a barren land occupied by primitive savages - but in one that was already a complex environment developed over millennia and ripe with significance for its people. Conventional views which contrast the civilized Romans with ignorant barbarians are themselves ignorant - the native way of life (including the disposal of human waste) was very different from that of Rome, but not necessarily any less complex or significant.

Studies have tended to distinguish between 'military' and 'civilian' in Roman Britain. It is now recognized, however, that such divisions are not so straightforward.[111] This military-civilian 'dichotomy' is particularly relevant to the topic of sanitation - the Roman military machine was distinct spatially inside the walls of its bases and installations and seen as an encapsulated presence bounded territorially in its 'military' zone, and the Romanizing civilian population in the demilitarized 'civil zone,' constituting the Romanized heart of the province. The imperial military presence in Britain was fundamentally different from the common image of a monolithic 'war machine,' and the boundaries between the military and civilian were nowhere as simple or sharp as usually assumed. Our modern construct of the 'Roman army' as a monolithic machine bears no relation to the way in which the Romans saw their armed forces.[112] 'There was no such thing as the Roman army because there was no such concept.'[113] Thus what should be seen instead is a community of soldiers - an awareness of a common interest and identity stretching across the empire, and the soldiers themselves developing their own powerful sense of an 'imagined community' of fellow soldiers. Effectively, the soldiery in Britain represented a distinctly provincial experience of becoming Roman, a view (it is suggested) that is fundamentally different from that seen in the demilitarized 'civil' communities.

Seeing each fort as representing a different 'community' may go some way to explaining the differences in sanitary provisions between forts, particularly on Hadrian's Wall - all planned generally along the same lines, but interpreted and used in different ways by the different units stationed there.

When it comes to the sanitary provisions in the *vici*, small towns, information about drainage is scarce. Lancaster, for example, has a rather haphazard *vicus* developed on all four sides of the fort. There appears to have been no planned street network, and presumably no planned drainage.[114] At Housesteads the *vicus* developed south and west of the fort, but there is no indication of whether it had an effective drainage system. The vicus outside Vindolanda had some street plan to it, but it is unlikely that it had a system of street drainage. Excavation reports for Corbridge[115] say nothing about the extensive drainage system of the various phases of the forts and later town. The need for sanitation would certainly remain, but economics of construction, maintenance, and technical ability favored smaller or separate systems - simple latrines with wooden supports constructed over a cesspit.

The population of settlements (*vici* or larger urban centers), as opposed to the native rural communities, was very cosmopolitan (including people from all corners of the empire, as well as large numbers of native peoples). The nature of this population must have meant a great exchange in the variety in cultural practices, attitudes, and interactions - there is, however, no escaping the fact that the most predominant examples of communal latrine facilities still come from military sites, or sites with strong military associations, and this continues to raise important questions about the nature of Romanization among civilians in Roman Britain. It is the relationship between the diversity of communities and populations that provide the greatest challenge to future archaeologists studying this subject. If we are to progress in this area the barriers between 'Roman' and 'native', military and civilian need to be broken down and an integrated study of human activity surrounding sanitation in Roman Britain addressed.

Palestine (Stefanie Hoss)

The Jewish people considered defecation ritually impure, resulting in the fact that a toilet was considered to be an impure place. In addition to this, communal nakedness was also considered dangerous and as something to be avoided (see chapter 4.2, pp. 47-48).

Considering these facts, it is not surprising that only five public toilets are known from Palestine, all of them located in the vicinity of public baths.[116] According to the various excavators' preliminary reports, the latrines all date to the 3rd or 4th centuries AD. With the exception of one latrine - which was situated near a fort in the Negev - they are located in larger cities with ample financial means, a strong urban tradition, and a large non-Jewish population. The number of seats can be extrapolated from the plans to have been in excess of four in two cases and at least 25 in another. The latrine in the Eastern Bathhouse of Beth-She'an - the largest and most luxurious in Palestine - had

75 seats and was accessible from both the bathhouse and the street. It was built as a peristyle courtyard, with mosaic flooring in the open part and limestone slabs in the covered part. The architectural elements of the portico and the marble slabs forming the seats were a collection of reused materials. Both this latrine and the latrine of the Western Bathhouse in the same city had a gutter running in front of the seats.

The position of the latrines inside or near bathhouses seems to indicate that they were perceived as belonging to a 'proper' Roman bathhouse and thus may be considered an appendage to them rather than an individual phenomenon. Like other forms of Roman amusement, Roman bathhouses were accepted rather reluctantly in Palestine. It took at least until the mid-2nd century for the habit of bathing in the Roman way to become established among the Jewish populace, and even then it was only accepted with certain adjustments that allowed religious Jews to use the facilities.[117] While passages on bathing in Roman bathhouses are numerous in the Palestinian Talmud, public latrines are mentioned only twice (see pp. 47-48). This also seems to indicate that this convenience was not frequented by religious Jews.

One latrine with sluicing channels and an uncertain amount of seats is also known from a private bath belonging to a Byzantine *villa suburbana* in the vicinity of Caesarea Maritima.[118] Private toilets with single seats can be found in wealthy houses from Hellenistic times onwards.[119] They are usually located in a small building on the inner courtyard and seem to be connected to cesspits. A house in Kurnub also had a latrine on an upper storey.[120] Less wealthy people might have had a wooden construction above a cesspit in their courtyards, but traces of wooden structures in the earth keep less well in the climate of the region and no bio-archaeological tests were done on most of the 'storage pits' found in courtyards or near houses. As single-seat toilets do not pose a problem with exposing oneself before others, they may have been the favored sort of installation in Palestine.

Syria (Zena Kamash)

Until recently comparatively little research had been carried out on latrines in Syria, reflecting in part a bias towards research in Italy.[121] Only two were included in Neudecker's work on Roman public latrines (the 2nd-century latrine in Apameia and the latrine in Bath F3 at Dura Europos),[122] yet at least fourteen other latrines have been located in Syria.[123] Ten of these latrines were located in or close to public bathhouses, three were independent structures, and the urban contexts of three are unknown. This pattern reveals that across the empire as a whole latrines were located in areas with easy access to water supply.

Eight of the latrines had evidence for the gutter running in front of the seats, which was a common aspect of latrine design. This small gutter was 0.10 m wide in all examples where the width was recorded. A stone basin (ca 0.5 m x 0.4 m) on the floor in the south-eastern corner of the Zeugma latrine may have been used as a water basin, but it was not on a pedestal, so may have been too low for such use. If it were a water basin, it would be the only example from the East, which is in marked contrast to North Africa, Asia Minor, and Italy where water basins were common features in latrines. The number of seats has been estimated for five of these installations and varies from four to eighteen. The notable exception is the 2nd-century latrine at Apameia that could have seated between 80 and 90 people.[124]

The chronological patterning of latrines in Syria allows some insights into the attitudes towards latrines in the region. In other parts of the empire latrines were introduced commonly in the 2nd and 3rd centuries.[125] While five of the latrines in Syria may belong to this bracket, the majority of the latrines (eight) in Syria date to the 4th century or later. This late introduction of latrines can be paralleled with the late introduction of latrines in Palestine (see above). In the latter case the low numbers of public latrines and their late date has been attributed firmly to religious taboos that would have made it problematic for latrine use to be incorporated into Jewish society. Evidence for similar explicitly religious concerns in Syria is lacking, but the similarities in date and distribution between the two areas are striking. This implies that the inhabitants of Syria may also have found Roman-style latrines culturally problematic. A comparison with the spread of public bathing in these eastern provinces further enhances this picture. Public, communal bathing presented similar problems for the Jewish population, as did public latrines.[126] Yet baths, while slow to develop, did become frequent features in the urban landscapes of Palestine from a significantly earlier date than latrines. A similar developmental trajectory can be seen in Syria.[127] This easier acceptance, as shown by a faster spread of baths, suggests that there were broader, more deeply embedded, concerns specific to latrine use that need to be explored (see below).

12.4. Perceptions of Latrines: Socio-Cultural, Moral and Religious Issues *(Zena Kamash)*

The aim of this section is to explore some of the social and cultural forces at work in latrines using the epigraphic, art historical, and archaeological evidence presented above. I bring together here several key strands drawn out in this chapter: the protective imagery and epigraphy associated with latrines or defecation and urination more generally, the sensory experience of latrines, and the disparities in the geographical and chronological spread of latrines across the Roman world. I begin by looking at the evidence for toilet sensibilities in the areas of the empire with widespread latrine use, in particular Italy and North Africa. I will then consider the areas of the empire, such as Britain, Syria, and Judaea, that saw lower numbers of latrines.

From the 2nd century AD onwards comparatively high numbers of latrines were in use in Italy and North Africa. Initially, it may seem that a simple correlation might be drawn between widespread latrines and a lack of socio-cultural and moral concerns with latrine use. The majority of the known protective imagery and epigraphy also, however, comes from these same areas, which suggests that such a simple interpretation might be misleading. Protective devices, such as Fortuna, the pygmies, the *phalli* and the alphabets, are similar to those found in bathhouses.[128] In both cases they seem to have been used in response to a non-specific threat from disease or pollution, i.e. they function as a hazard-precaution system.[129] Recent research in clinical and evolutionary psychology and anthropology has shown that humans have a hazard-precaution system that responds to potential (as distinct from actual) contaminants.[130] This system, which malfunctions in obsessive-compulsive disorder, produces ritualistic responses to potential hazards, which may seem to threaten fitness. These responses have cross-cultural similarities and include having lucky or unlucky numbers, taking measures to prevent harm, or saying special prayers and incantations.[131] Furthermore, they do not necessarily require a scientific understanding of disease, but are commonly identified with broad categories of danger from our evolutionary past, including contamination from pathogens.[132]

The epigraphic evidence from Italy and North Africa also strongly indicates that there are social rules governing where it is appropriate to defecate or urinate. This preoccupation seems to be mirrored by the archaeological evidence for visibility. The distinction here seems not so much to be between what is considered a public or a non-public space (as a public latrine is by its nature public), but rather where one is considered to be under the social gaze or not under it.[133] It is this distinction that seems to set up the boundaries of being in place and being out of place. William James' definition of dirt as 'matter out of place' (made famous by Mary Douglas) is a helpful concept here.[134] In the case of defecating or urinating under the social gaze not only is the matter polluting, but also the behavior. The act of defecating or urinating in public is animalistic, as shown by the images of the pygmies, and so does not conform to human, social rules. Therefore, it needs to be controlled and protected against, hence the religious curses. The need to control the potential pollution (both actual and behavioral) can also be seen in the construction of the latrines themselves, i.e. in the designation of a particular place for these animalistic activities to be performed, from where the social gaze can be temporarily diverted.

In the discussion of regional diversity in latrine provision, several striking patterns were brought out. Firstly, in Britain latrines have been found predominantly on military sites or sites with strong military associations (such as Wroxeter). Secondly, the spread of latrines in Judaea and Syria was significantly later than elsewhere in the empire and particularly restricted in Judaea. Discussions of Judaea tend to explain this pattern solely in terms of the religious taboos concerning impurity and nudity, which undoubtedly presented severe problems for a Jewish population. A full explanation, however, requires us to look behind such cultural and religious taboos to find out what motivates them. There appear to be at least two main areas where motivations may be found: the use of water for the disposal of excrement and the communality of latrines.

The water problem is seen explicitly in Jewish religious texts and can maybe be implied from negative evidence from, e.g. Britain and the early period in Syria. One obvious problem is that putting excrement in your water creates a potential source of disease. The associations that water has with life and death are intricate and multifaceted. Attitudes towards water in both the past and present seem to be caught up in a complex network of negotiations of its life-giving and potential death-bringing aspects.[135] It seems possible that the depositing of excrement in water might have been a step too far in this negotiation. The deliberate contamination of water may also be viewed as the contravention of basic order.[136] It is conceivable, then, that the person who pollutes could come to be a pollutant himself, i.e. that an evolutionary concern could become a moral problem, hence framed in terms of ritual purity and impurity.

The problems associated with the communality of latrines need not equate just with nudity, but may also incorporate issues of proximity and the perception of the social gaze. The problems with proximity, as discussed above, include potentially coming into contact with the bodily products of other people, especially faeces, and being made aware of one's own animalistic behavior in the company of others. Both of these things have been noted to produce the disgust emotion cross-culturally.

Shame must have been an important factor here too, as it governs what is deemed appropriate behavior. In other words to do something that is deemed shameful is to behave animalistically and show no awareness of human social rules. For Romans to have a sense of honor was also to have a sense of shame, of *pudor* or *verecundia* or shyness. A Roman was expected to withdraw his gaze from a person (see above) or a god so as to augment that person or god.[137] The Jewish strictures on graven images, however, suggest that they may have conceived of the gaze separately, i.e. that there was no option for withdrawing one's gaze out of sense of shame or to confer honor. This could be seen as a distinction in types of gaze: the 'alethetic gaze' versus the 'assertoric gaze' - an 'intertwining of gazes' that undermines an objectifying vision versus a gaze that sets up an opposition between observer and observed.[138] Further evidence for there being different constructions of what it means to be in or out of the social gaze may be seen in the structuring of domestic space. In general, houses in the East were introverted and the entrance was positioned so as to avoid the public gaze. This is in clear contrast to Italian housing. This is reflected in the use of water features for display, which is relatively common in Italy, but not part of the domestic habit outside of Antioch in the Near East.[139] The problem with using a communal latrine seems again to be a concern with animalistic behavior both of the self and others, seen through a specific cultural filter of what it means to be under the social gaze.

Overall, it seems that a Roman latrine may have provoked a variety of socio-cultural, moral, and religious concerns. The same general sets of concerns and worries appear to have been in play across the empire: fear of unknown threats of disease and a desire not to behave animalistically, particularly in the presence of others. The differences across the empire come out due to the different cultural forces that were applied to these concerns. In areas, such as Italy and North Africa, protection from these concerns manifested itself in two different, but connected ways. Firstly, hazard-precaution systems against unknown and unexplained threats of disease were set in place via protective imagery and exhortations. Secondly, specific boundaries were drawn designating where it was appropriate to defecate and urinate or what activities were deemed appropriate and what was out of place. In both cases, part or all of the protection was expressed in religious terms. In other parts of the Roman world, such as Britain and the Near East, it was not enough to call on divine protection. The potentially different constructions of where something was deemed to be a pollutant and of social rules governing the social gaze and a sense of shame seems to have meant that using communal latrines presented serious problems. Where we have the evidence, these rules and concerns seem to have resulted in clear sets of virtues that focused on cleanliness and purity, which were closely interrelated with moral and religious taboos on impurity; to break these taboos would have been to render yourself impure and potentially disgusting. This seems to have meant that using communal latrines presented serious problems. Where we have the evidence, these rules and concerns seem to have resulted in clear sets of virtues that focused on cleanliness and purity, which were closely interrelated with moral and religious taboos on impurity; to break these taboos would have been to render yourself impure and potentially disgusting. This seems to have resulted in severely restricted latrine use in these regions.

Case Study: The Red Marble Thrones of the Lateran: The Cultural Afterlife of Roman Toilet Seats

(Andrew Wilson)

Two identical elaborate red marble late Roman seats in *rosso antico* from southern Greece, each with a hole in the seat, are now to be found in the Vatican Museum and in the Louvre (*fig. 12.33*). They stood in the Lateran Palace in Rome until the 18th century, when they were moved to the Vatican Museum by Pius VI; Napoleon later removed one to Paris, which is now in the Louvre.[140]

The chairs are a matching pair, each with a semicircular curved back 44.5 cm high and stepped armrests at the sides. The seat is pierced with a circular hole 21.4 cm in diameter, with a nearly square slot (13.2 x 13.7 cm) extending to the front edge. The seat is supported by two parallel lateral supports 48 cm high decorated with volutes at the top front and back; the front of the supports are shaped like lions' legs, ending in a claw, and there is a smaller volute at the rear base. The sides of the supports are decorated with a stylized relief floral design (*fig. 12.34*).[141] To any observer familiar with the design of Roman toilets, these are clearly latrine seats, yet their function has puzzled many over the centuries and led to a series of fantastic explanations.

Bizarrely, these Roman toilet seats were used in papal investitures from at least the eleventh to sixteenth centuries as part of the ceremony of taking possession of the Lateran Palace, until the accession of Leo X in 1513. Jacopo d'Angelo's account of the coronation of Gregory XII in 1406 has the Pope sit first in one, then in the other chair, receiving a staff and the keys of St. Peter in the first, and a belt studded with twelve jewels in the second. The *sedes porphyreticae* are mentioned in accounts of ceremonial by Albinus and Cencius; they stood at the entrance to the chapel of St. Sylvester in the Lateran, under an arch supported on a pair of porphyry columns in a manner recalling an imperial throne under a porphyry baldachin.[142] Albinus and Cencius both depend here on a lost part of the *Liber Politicus* of Benedictus, written ca 1143-1444, giving a *terminus ante quem* in the 1140s for the seats' positioning and use. The thrones are probably the same as the *duae curules* mentioned in an account of the coronation of Pope Paschal II in AD 1099;[143] if they are not the same objects, they performed the same function, the new pope sitting in one and then the other as he received symbols of office. They may even be the *sedilia ... de marmoribus* placed by Leo IV (847-855) at the entrance to the Lateran palace.[144] Of their earlier history we know nothing for certain; they might have been taken from any part of Rome, but the red marble suggests an imperial connection and the simplest hypothesis would be to assume that they formed part of the furniture of Constantine's palace at the Lateran, which he gifted to the Church.

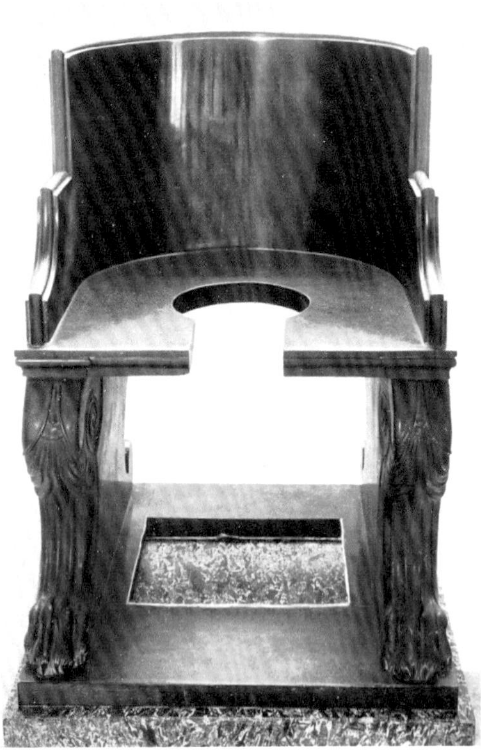

Fig. 12.33. Vatican Museum (formerly in the Lateran Palace), Roman toilet seat in rosso antico *(from Deér 1959, pl. 188).*

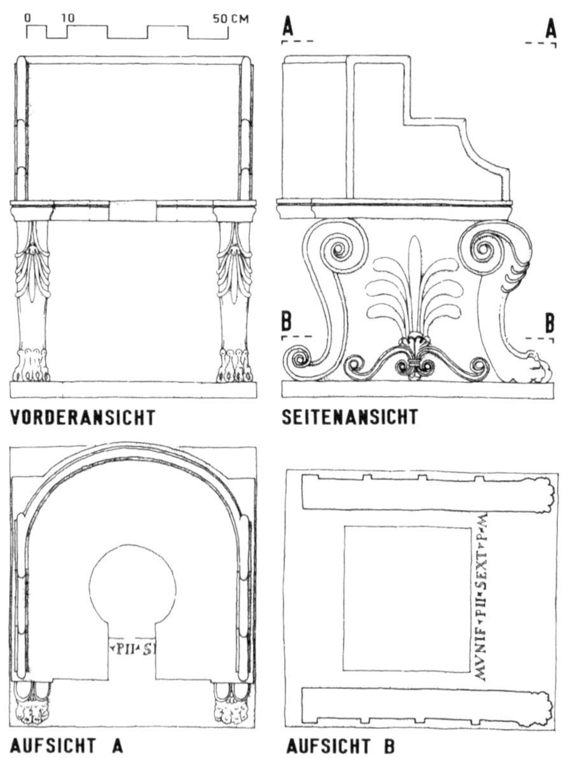

Fig. 12.34. Louvre (formerly in the Lateran Palace), Roman toilet seat in rosso antico *(from Grassnick 1992, 9).*

Why were two Roman toilet seats used in medieval papal coronations? The account in the *Liber Pontificalis* of the coronation of Paschal II in 1099 calls them *duae curulae*, 'two curule chairs', which they are not; which suggests the extent to which their original function had already become forgotten, and they had become invested instead with connotations of magisterial authority. But the red marble of *rosso antico* resembles porphyry, and indeed medieval and later sources call them *sedes porphyreticae*, 'porphyry chairs'; now the symbolism is imperial and in the coronation ceremony they seem to have functioned as a link with Roman imperial authority. Their designation as *sedes porphyreticae* thus emphasized the imperial connotations that supported part of the Church's wider claims at the time to the universal authority of the Pope.[145]

The various aetiological attempts to explain their particular morphology by those who did not recognize their true original purpose have lent these seats a curious life of their own in the imagination of popular and religious culture at different periods. Around AD 1250 emerged the myth of Pope Joan, a supposed female Pope in disguise, said to have been enthroned in 855 and discovered when she gave birth during a Papal procession. By ca 1290 this myth had become widespread and had generated its own ancillary details. Prominent among these were the rumors that the two marble pierced chairs were used during the papal investiture ceremonies to prevent a recurrence of the scandal, by checking the gender of a newly-elected Pope in a manner that allowed the rite to be performed publicly, but without compromising the Pope's dignity by revealing the object of the examination. According to these accounts, many of which erroneously set the chairs in the Church of St John Lateran rather than the palace, the new Pope sat in one of the chairs and the most junior deacon would reach up under the papal robes through the hole in the seat, to feel the Pope's genitals, and would announce: *Habet testiculos duos et bene pendentes* ('He has two testicles, and well hanging'); to which the response was *Deo gratias*, and the Pope would then process to the High Altar while the choir sang the *Te Deum*.[146] This rite never in fact happened, but importantly, from the late 13th century to the 16th century or later, lots of people believed that it did happen, from Geoffrey de Courlon to Rabelais and beyond (*fig. 12.35*).

One person correctly to identify the original function of the chairs was the humanist Bartolomeo Sacchi, called Platina, who wrote in his *Life of the Popes* (1479), in connection with the story of Pope Joan, rejecting the fable of the rite of verification of gender: 'that seat was prepared in such a manner so that the one who is invested with such great domination will know that he is not God, but a man; that as such he is subjected to the necessities of nature and must defecate. That is why that seat is rightly called the stercory (or excremental) seat.'[147] Other accounts of papal investitures mention a marble chair called *stercoraria*, in the portico of the palace, whose purpose is to remind the Pope of his humility; it is unclear whether this was also pierced and, in fact, a toilet seat, or whether it has at some stage been confused with the porphyry thrones.[148]

Even more curiously, the modern scholarly works on the myth of Pope Joan also fail to recognize the true original function of these seats. The otherwise excellent standard account by Alain Boureau has an extended treatment of the problem of the so-called 'porphyry chairs', and while he rightly rejects Cesare D'Onofrio's hypothesis that these are imperial birthing chairs, he believes them to be 'bathing chairs'.[149] This misidentification goes back to antiquarian accounts of the 18th century, based on the similarity with seats found in the Baths of Caracalla and in baths at Ostia; in reality, these parallels are actually the seats in the bath latrines, not identified as latrines at the time. Boureau's failure to identify the red marble thrones of the Lateran as Roman latrine seats thus leads him to reject Platina's opinion as humanist mischief: 'we cannot eliminate the suspicion that Platina was taking a mischievous pleasure in saving the pope from sexual impurity by plunging him into excrement.' Did the *sedia stercoraria* of other accounts of the papal coronation ceremonies, in fact, originally refer to these marble thrones, even if at an early date, the term became attached to another chair used in the investiture ceremony?

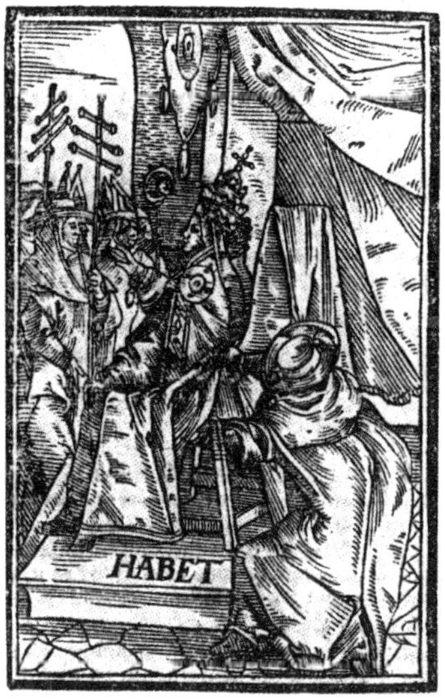

Fig. 12.35. Woodcut from Johann Wolf, Lectiones memorabiles *(Frankfurt 1600), showing the supposed rite of verification of the Pope's gender; the deacon announces* Habet *('He has [them]') (from Boureau 2000, fig. 1).*

Notes

1 For good introductions to the world of the 'Roman' pygmies, see Versluys 2002 and Clarke 2005-2006. Clarke's definition can be found on p. 293 and is used here.

2 Meyboom/Versluys 2007, 208.

3 Versluys 2002, 283-284; Meyboom/Versluys 2007.

4 Versluys 2002, 282-283, esp. n. 310.

5 Clarke 2001, 88. For a good explanation of the working of the evil eye, see Levi 1941 and Bartsch 2006, especially: the penetrating gaze on p. 139-152. For parallels in other cultures see Dundes 1981. The relation or differences between the evil eye (cast at person by a jealous other), a demon (who can also cast crazy looks), and the *malum* (evil), however, has not been explained clearly by anyone. Maybe the lines are not so clearly drawn as a scientist hopes for. The effect, however, is the same: an unexpected disaster happens ending in disease or death. Specific symbols and rituals offer protection.

6 Clarke 2001; Dunbabin 1989, 42-45, who discusses them among all other kinds of protective inscriptions and symbols in baths (like *phalli*, labyrinths, tridents, swastika's etc). She does not mention the pygmy paintings in the *frigidarium* tub and the garden room of the Pompeian Sarno Baths (VIII 2, 17-21). See for these paintings Koloski-Ostrow 1985, 337 and 1990, 64, 75 and figs 100-104; p. 75 offers also some comments on the evil eye in baths.

7 According to Clarke they were found on a toilet floor mosaic in the Baths of Neptune at Ostia (II iv, 2) (see also Versluys 2002, 43-45), on a toilet floor mosaic in the so-called southern baths of Timgad (see Versluys, 2002, 171-178) and in a wall painting above the toilet seats at Bolsena (Barbet 1982, 111-114; here p. 57, *fig. 5.15*). The one not listed by Clarke is the toilet floor mosaic in the House of the Gymnasium at Itálica, see Versluys 2002, 206-207. See also chapter 5.2 on decorations in toilets.

8 See section below on graffiti in toilets.

9 For example, at the garden toilet at the *caupona* of Euxinus (I 11, 10-11) at Pompeii.

10 Dagron 1918, 300-303. I want to thank Heidi Marx-Wolf (University of Manitoba, Winnipeg) for showing me this important text. The translation is also hers.

11 Miguel John Versluys deserves my warm thanks for helping me to compile this list. It is remarkable that all the urinating and defecating pygmies in this list are male. Was it such a taboo to see a female doing these things? As far as I know there is not one representation from Roman antiquity (also outside the pygmy context) available.
1. Colemancio, mosaic, pygmy urinates in the direction of a Nile animal (Versluys 2002, 173-174); 2. Ostia, Baths of Neptune (II iv, 2), mosaic floor, pygmy defecates in the direction of a crocodile (Versluys 2002, 43-45); 3. Ostia, tomb 22 on the Via Laurentina, wall painting, pygmy urinates in the direction of a crocodile (Versluys 2002, 51-52); 4. Pompeii, *fullonica* of Vesonius Primus (VI 14, 22), wall painting in peristyle, two defecating Aethiopians (*PPM* VI, 1991, 328-331) - I thank Miko Flohr for this reference; 5. Pompeii, Sarno Baths (VIII 2, 17-21), wall painting, pygmy defecates during a rescue action (Koloski-Ostrow 1990, 64, 75; Versluys 2002, 134-136); 6. Pompeii, House of the Sculptor (VIII 7, 24), painting in peristyle, defecating and urinating Aethiopians (Versluys 2002, 134-136; Clarke 2007, 91-96); 7. Pompeii, tomb of Vestorius Priscus, wall painting, pygmy defecates on a fish (Mols/Moormann 1993-1994, 27-29; Versluys 2002, 159-160); 8. Rome, Region IX temple of Isis on Campus Martius, relief, pygmy defecates in direction of a Nile animal (Versluys 2002, 68-69); 9. Rome, *columbarium* of the Villa Doria Pamphilj, wall paintings, on wall C XII a pygmy defecates in the direction of hippopotamus and on wall E IV a pygmy defecates in the direction of crocodile (Bendinelli 1941, 16, 22, tav. A and X; Versluys 2002, 79-81; here *fig. 12.2*) - according to Versluys (personal communication) there is also one urinating pygmy represented, which I could not trace; 10. Timgad, northwest baths, mosaic, Aethiopian bath employee urinates (Neudecker 1994, 27); 11. Zliten, Villa of Bar Duc Ammèra, mosaic floor, pygmy defecates in the direction of an attacking bird (Versluys 2002, 191-192). Possible defecating pygmies: 1. Pompeii, House of the Menander (I 10, 4), mosaic in *triclinium* (Versluys 2002, 108-109); 2. Priverno, House of the Nilotic Threshold, mosaic (Versluys 2002, 55-58).

12 Neudecker 1994, 26-27. Such an attitude is underlined by a passage in the *Meditations* of Marcus Aurelius (6.30), where he advises his readers the stoic way of life: '[...] Do all things as a disciple of Antoninus (Pius) [...] how he would remain the whole day at the same occupation, owing to his spare diet not even requiring to relieve nature except at the customary time.' (quoted from Loeb translation C.R. Haines).

13 Versluys 2002, 284.

14 This is also noted by Clarke 2007, 93: 'projectile defecation is the standard defense.' For more examples of a jet of faeces as a weapon, see Koloski-Ostrow forthcoming.

15 This bas-relief of unknown provenance (its present location is also unknown) was first published by Millingen 1821. See Bartsch (1996) for four more images of the evil eye under attack. Here no defecator is present, but all the other types of attackers (and more) show up: at fig. 3 at p. 140 on a mosaic from Antioch a hunchback with large penis, a trident, a dagger, a scorpion, a snake, a dog, a centipede, a leopard and a crow. Fig. 4 at p. 141 with a mosaic from an unknown location shows an evil eye stabbed by a spear, and as fellow aggressors, a scorpion, a snake, a leopard, a bull, a goat an owl and others. Fig. 5 on p. 142 shows an evil eye besieged by two snakes and a penis and fig. 6 also on p. 142 shows three daggers, a scorpion, a snake, two lions and a long beaked bird.

16 Ascione and Pagano (2000, 97-99) discuss this one and mention a smaller bronze statuette from Herculaneum in the same posture. The type might refer to a work of Lysippus translated to a popular garden statue in Hellenistic times.

17 Kapossy (1969, 54-55) list several statues from whose natural openings (mouth, eyes, nipples, wounds and penis) fountain water falls down. He refers on p. 26 to a Hercules *mingens* from Sousse as a fountain statue, and on p. 44 he records four children *mingentes* as fountain statues.

18 Found in the fill of a toilet in Hanghaus 1, 2 at Ephesus. It is not clear whether this fountain had actually a place in this toilet room, or elsewhere in the house. See Aurenhammer 1990, 196-197, pictures are at p. 125.

19 Langner 2001, 61 and illustrations 1257-1260. One graffito comes from a room underneath Santa Maria Maggiore, two from the *paedagogium* on the Palatine and one from a *taberna* in the Domus Tiberiana.

20 Normally on display in the picture gallery: inv. no 112285. The most important descriptions of the exca-

vation of this house and the first remarks on the painting can be found in Sogliano 1880, 394-395 and Mau 1882-1883, 196.

21 It is apparent that this defecator is depicted in a completely different context than the pygmy paintings we saw in the previous paragraph. He himself does not look funny at all (he is clearly not the Other), and he is seriously concentrating on his act. The presence of a goddess adds seriousness to the scene.

22 Above the man, the words *cacator cave malu* (*CIL* IV. 3832) are written in black. This *dipinto* is clearly of later date, see also Clarke 2005-2006, 299.

23 For House of the Greek Epigrams, see Fröhlich 1991, 40 n. 194. He cites an older description in which this figure is seen as Vesta. Fröhlich, however, regards her as Fortuna. For house V 4, 9, see Sogliano 1899, 345-346.

24 Fröhlich 1991, 301 no L114.

25 For fresh flower garlands in toilets, see Thüry chapter 4.1, p. 44 n. 12.

26 See Santa Maria Scrinari 1995, 86, 95 and fig. 79.

27 See Vaglieri 1911, 209-211.

28 *Protrepticus* 4, 51. Translated from Greek by G.W. Butterworth in Loeb translation.

29 Most Roman toilet rooms must have been very dark and were badly lit as the windows were small. In the toilets where Fortuna occurred, large windows provided a lot of light.

30 Fröhlich 1991, 40.

31 Neudecker 1994, 56; Koloski-Ostrow 2000, 292.

32 Fröhlich 1991, 56-61.

33 Clarke 2005-2006.

34 I want to express my sincere thanks to Ton Derks (Free University at Amsterdam) who discussed the subject with me several times and was of great help with the inscriptions. Translations of the inscriptions are by Eveline Vermeulen, unless stated otherwise.

35 The expression *cave* in the sense of 'watch out' or 'beware' is very widespread as, for example, in the well-known *cave canem*. A common variant of the addressed in combination with *cave malum* is the expression *fur cave malum* - 'thief, beware of the evil' also found at Pompeii: *CIL* IV. 06253 *Fur cave malu(m)*, *CIL* X. 08067, 06a (p. 1002) *(F)ur cave // malu(m)*, *CIL* X. 08067, 06b (p. 1002), *Fur cav(e) // malu(m)*. At Pompeii the same expression is used to scare off a mouse or a rat *CIL* IV. 08645 *Mus cave / malum*. That the expression *cave malum* is rather common can be deduced from two other inscriptions, one from Rome where people are warned to behave themselves near a sanctuary *CIL* VI. 22949 *Sacer / locus / sacrilege / cave malu(m) // Sacer / locus / sacrilege / cave malu(m)*, and one from Aquileia where a worker is encouraged to work faster: *CIL* V. 8110, 176 *Cave malum / si non raseris lateris DC*, 'Watch out for the evil (eye), if you have not smoothed down 600 bricks'.

36 The translation of Clarke 2005-2006, 299 'Shitter watch out' seems to me too understated. The threat, or perhaps it is even a curse, is very severe.

37 I leave out two inscriptions that do not relate to our problem. The first is *stercorari / ad murum / progredere si / pre(n)sus fueris poena(m) / patiare necesse / est cave* (CIL IV. 7038), 'You, who want to make a mess (*stercorari*), walk to the (city) wall or if you are caught (that is, dumping your load someplace inside the town), beware, (because) it is necessary to endure a punishment.' Here the *cacator* is not addressed, but the *stercorarius*, and the threat including *malum* is absent. This seems more a general announcement from the city officials not to unload rubbish here. I want to thank John Bodel for this observation. See Wilson (p. 148), who takes a different view. The other is a tiny inscription scratched in the facade of house III 5, 4, next to the house entrance on the Street of Abundance, which seems related to the *cacator dipinti*: *hospes adhuc tumuli ni meias ossa pre(cantur) / nec si vis (h)uic gratior esse caca / urticae monumenta vides discede cacator / non est hic tutum culu(m) aperire tibi* (*CIL* IV. 8899), 'Visitor, my bones beg you not to pee near my tomb, nor shit, if you want to be more agreeable. You see the tomb of "Nettle" (*urtica*). Go away shitter. It is not safe to open your anus here.' (Translation by John Bodel.) This poem in elegiac distich is rather out of place in the collection of the *cacator cave malum dipinti*, as we shall see in the following. The inscription is more of a joke, and it is a variation of the well-known poem: *Anthol. lat. carm. epigr.* n. 838. *Hospes, ad hunc tumulum meias, ossa precantur / tecta hominis <set>, si gratus homo es misce bibe da me*. 'Visitor, the buried bones of a man ask you to pee at my tomb, but if you are agracious man, mix up (the wine), drink (it), (and) give me (a drink).' Translation Ann O. Koloski-Ostrow.

38 *CIL* IV. 7714-7716. See Spinazzola 1917, 260-261 and della Corte 1929, 241. At the amphitheater, which could house several thousands of people, no sanitary provision has been found. The nearest public toilet is the twenty-seater at the large *palaestra*. It seems only logical that people went to a quiet side alley to relieve themselves.

39 See for a first analysis Wilson 2000b, 310 and Thüry 2001, 17-21.

40 Translation Eric M. Moormann and Ann O. Koloski-Ostrow.

41 *CIL* VI. 29828b. The *CIL* states that the *dipinto* was found on the facade of the Baths of Titus. I want to thank Eric Moormann for this correction. See Meyboom/Moormann forthcoming.

42 Wilson (2000b, 310) mentions a small inscription on the two piers of an honorific arch at Thigibba (Tunisia): *si qui hic urinam fecerit, habebit Martem iratum*, 'If anyonewill have urinated here, he will incur the wrath of Mars.' A marble relief slab from Aquileia (North Italy) shows a defecating man hit by Jupiter's thunderbolt, thus illustrating Jupiter's revenge. There are no words on this relief. See for a good illustration, Wilson 2000b, 311. Clarke (2007, 61-62) states that the gods are too important to interfere in such trivial matters, and considers this humor. Regarding the many gods that are mentioned in the other inscriptions and *tituli picti*, humor alone does not seems to me to be the intention.

43 *Inschriften von Ephesos* II, 567.

44 *CIL* III. 1966 *Quisq(ue) in eo vico stercus non posu/erit aut non cacaverit aut non me / iaverit habeat illas propitias / si neglexerit viderit*, 'Whoever will not have left rubbish in this alley, and will not have crapped or urinated, may he have these blessings. If he will have neglected (these things), he will see (what happens).' For a picture see Thüry 2001, 20 fig 17.

45 See Jobst 1976-1977, 61-5, and here, Wilson, p. 155 10.

46 Personal communication of Martino La Torre. For a first report on this latrine see La Torre 2006, 88.

47 See Netzer/Weiss 1994, 32 (with illustration) and Notermans 2007, 398. At p. 195 Notermans asks whether this word reflects any notion on hygiene practices.

48 As Dunbabin (1989, 19) argues, this could mean something like 'have a good bath and a safe return'. Maybe this health wish here has the same connotation.

49 Carlo Molle (personal communication) interprets these

lines of Martial differently and thinks that Martial is referring to ordinary graffiti as discussed in the next paragraph.

50 The one from Smyrna (*Anth. Pal.* 9.624) is quoted by Wilson in chapter 10.4. The one from Ephesus is quoted and translated by Moormann, p, 59.

51 For the text of the riddles, a translation and references, see Moormann, p. 60.

52 Carlo Molle deserves my sincere thanks for suggestions and adjustments to this section. I also want to thank Antonio Varone for his much appreciated help.

53 Calza (1933, 602). One wonders to what inscriptions Calza is referring to, as there are no inscriptions known from Ostian toilets.

54 For example, Tomei/Conti 1991, 63: 'incisioni e scritte erano assai frequenti nelle latrine pubbliche', and De Kind 1998, 93: 'As usual, the toilet [...] was a popular place for writing graffiti.'

55 Langner 2001, 100, 117.

56 Langner (2001, 101 Abb. 49-51) shows tables from which it is clear that most inscriptions occur in the peristyle, the *tablinum* and the *fauces*.

57 Langner 2001, 117.

58 Langner 2001, 19, 20.

59 For example the public toilet in Bolsena (Hallier/Humbert/Pomey 1982) and the private toilet in Cos (Sirano 2005).

60 For example, at the toilet of Rottenburg (Heiligmann 2003, 49), and at the toilet underneath the palace of Domitian in Rome (Tomei/Conti 1991, 63, 67 and figs 10 and 15). See for more information on those toilets the case study at chapter 5 by Hoss, p. 67 and chapter 5.2 by Moormann, pp. 57-58.

61 House of the Citharist (I 6, 5), *CIL* IV. 2375: *Ampliate, / Icarus / te pedicat. / Salvius / scripsit* ('Ampliatus, Icarus buggered you. Salvius wrote it.') together with a drawing of a man with a giant nose. House I 7, 16, *CIL* IV 8169: *Masc(u)lus vincet and vicit Iovia SH CC / n(onis?) / Apri(libus) / XXI* ('Masculus will win; Iovia won 200 sestertii on the 7th of April.'). House I 7, 18, *CIL* IV 8170: *M C I* (height of the letters 30 cm!). House of Menander (I 10, 4), *CIL* IV 8346 *IOYKOYNΔO* ('of Iucundus') with *phallus* to the left; *CIL* IV 9274: 4 initial parts of Greek alphabets varying from the first two to seven letters; *CIL* IV 8347: *Crescens Cryseroti salutem / Quid agit tibi dexter ocellus* ('Crescens greets Chryseros. What is the right eye doing to you?'). *CIL* IV 8348a: *Cre(..)*; *CIL* IV 8348b: *Verecundus* (?); *CIL* IV 8348c: *A. s(...) v(...) va(le)*; *CIL* IV 8349: *tot, tota restis, tota u[n]ita[s]* ('So much, you remain whole, an entire unity.'); *CIL* IV 8350: *Duxi / chorum* ('I led the chorus.') see Varone in press. House of Octavius Quartio (II 2, 1-3, 5, 6), *CIL* IV 8482: *(Semper) ubique fortis / hoc cum fe/m[ini]s a[gam?]... / XVVVI* ('Always and everywhere strong, I am doing this with women (fucking them?) (26 times).'); *CIL* IV 8483: *Mentula / V HS* ('Male part for sale (rent?) for five sestertii.'). *Praedia* of Iulia Felix (II 4), *CIL* IV 10126: *Crescens. Eu/antil(lus?) / Paris va(le)*; *CIL* IV 10127: *Trebenius*; *CIL* IV. 10128: *Unus amat una(m) / sa(lutem) sal(utem)* ('One boy loves one girl, hello, hello'); *CIL* IV 10129: *Li(n)ge Aspasia*, ('Lick, Aspasia') between the words a *phallus* pointing to the right; *CIL* IV 10130: *Celer[i]na Spuri f(ilia) / Se(l)inunti*; *CIL* IV 10131: *Pac[atus?] / Pom[peia]nis (salutem?)*; *CIL* IV 10132: *Iuli lingis / Pacatus* ('You are licking (the penis?) of Iulius, Pacatus') between the first two words a *phallus* pointing to the right; *CIL* IV 10133: *[A]basc[antus]*. House of Marcus Lucretius Fronto (V 4, a.11): large *phallus* (20 x 40 cm) and two adorned squares, see Peters 1993, 387. House VI 3, 5, *CIL* IV 10202: *VI k(alendas) Sep(tembres) ma(n)simus / Po(m)peis* ('We spent the night at Pompeii on the VI Kalends of September (August 27)'), together with a drawing of a *phallus* between two wraths; *CIL* IV. 10203: *lochoo eimi* ('I am a midwife'). Suburban Baths (VII 16, a): *[...] k(alendas) III Septemb[res] [...]; Habi[tus] / habitus / Issae / sal(utem); Episcrise / scrito va(le) / op[.]; Hab[i]t[u]s / [...]io [s]al(utem) / Issian[u]s / [...]s*; see Varone 2008. House of Marcus Lucretius (IX 3, 5), *CIL* IV 3146: *Secundus / hi(c) cacat / hi[---]at / Hic cacat*; *CIL* IV 3146a *Serenus*. House IX 7, 22, *CIL* IV 3832: *cacator cave malu*. House of the Centennial (IX 8, 1-7) toilet 1 *CIL* IV 3770: *Q. Lollio Paridi*. Ibidem, toilet 2 *CIL* IV 5241: *Mystice hic*; *CIL* IV 5242: *Quodam quidem testis eris, quid senserim / ubi cacaturiero. Veniam cacatum* ('Sometime indeed you will be a witness of what I have felt, when I will have shat. I shall come to shit.'); *CIL* IV 5243: *Memoria*; *CIL* IV 5244: *Marthae hoc trichlinium /est. Nam in trichlinio / cacat* ('This is the dining room of Martha, for she shits in the dining room.') See *fig 8.11* in this volume. Most of the translations in this note and in the following note are by Eric M. Moormann and Ann O. Koloski-Ostrow.

62 House of the Inn (III 19-20), *CIL* IV 10511: *Aniciae feliciter*; *CIL* IV 10512: *IIII P. Quin(tilius)* ('P. Quintilius did something four times, or has to do something four times.') The 'P' after the numeral might also refer to a weight e.g. '*IIII P(ondus)*'; *CIL* IV 10707: first twelve letters of the Greek alphabet. House of the Corinthian Atrium (V 30), *CIL* IV 10580: *Ex sept(em?)*. House of the Gem (Ins. Or. I, 1), *CIL* IV 10619: *Apollinaris medicus Titi imp(eratoris) / hic cacavit bene* ('Apollinaris, doctor of emperor Titus, had a good shit here.)' See *fig. 12.16*. Workshop Ins. Or. II, 2, *CIL* IV 10548: *Rufula P(ondo?) V s(emis?)*; *CIL* IV 10549: *eviino*; and one not in *CIL* provided by Varone: *XI*.

63 Ephesus: Hanghaus 2.2. so-called philosophers toilet SR 29: GR 146 *Salutaris / cun(n)um li(n)ge / libetr(a)e* ('Salutaris, lick the pussy of Libetra.); GR 147 ἀγαθὰ τῷ χέζο(ν)τι ('Hail the shitter!'), GR 149 *a cun(n)o Libetra(e) [py]gize / lupos / aocopos* ('After the pussy of Libetra, fuck the cheerful catamite'). See also Täuber 2005 and two drawings of birds (not published), (*fig. 12.18*). Hanghaus 2.4. toilet room 4: two concentric circles, see Thür 2005, 44. Besides, there is in the so-called Steindepot behind the Lower Agora a marble toilet seat *ex situ* with a drawing of a *phallus* (not published) (*fig. 12.17*).

64 The first is the toilet underneath the Piazza Garibaldi in Rome. Chini (1999) records eleven different inscriptions above the toilet seats of which nine are drawn in the wet stucco and, therefore, must be by one hand. Several large *phalli* occur together with Greek words *phoole* ('penis') and *leiche* (also meaning 'penis') and an ejaculating *phallus*. There is also a sketch of a man being penetrated from behind by another man with a large *phallus*, an animal, a ship, a frontal face of a man, a rough sketch of a man, and an ivy leaf. In the dry stucco, three letters of unknown meaning are inscribed (*IHP*) along with a Latin inscription: *Pos(t) tantas epulas et suava / vina / ut cunnum lingas, / quo cula, quo venter* ('After so many feasts and sweet wines, that you may lick pussy, is good (for emptying) the ass and the belly.') (Translation by Ann O. Koloski-Ostrow). The second example in Rome is the toilet of the so-called house of Domitia Lucilla, see Santa Maria Scrinari 1995, Fig. 81 and 82: many alpha-

bets and a possible caricature of Jesus as a fish.

65 This phenomenon does not occur on toilets with one row of seats, but only with more rows. The reason might be that the inscriptions on these toilets are always visible from the other row of seats. The other reason might be that the toilets were always very full so that someone standing in front of a seat and writing would clearly irritate the ones who are waiting for a seat.

66 Carettoni, 1949, 66-69, fig. 24 shows some of the inscriptions. The inscriptions are not yet published. Langner (2001) has some of them in his catalogue: a bird (no 1772) and boats (nos 2193-2195).

67 Mertens 1995, 218-219.

68 Langner 2001, 118-120.

69 This contribution is an elaboration from my PhD thesis, *Graffiti occasionali antichi con particolare riferimento ad alcuni contesti archeologici di Roma e del Lazio*, Macerata 2004, which I hope to publish. I am particularly grateful, for the access to the archaeological area, to Anna Maria Reggiani, Benedetta Adembri, and Pietro Di Croce (MiBAC, Soprintendenza Archeologica per il Lazio); for the scientific support, to Gianfranco Paci, Silvia Maria Marengo, and Stefano Tortorella; for revising my English to Claudio Malnati and Ann O. Koloski-Ostrow, the latter also making useful observations on the contents.

70 On this toilet, see also Aurigemma 1956, 68-69 and Jansen 2003, 143, fig. 15, with bibliography. The toilet is rectangular (6.65 x 2.30 m), and the door is on the eastern short side (approximate orientation); the perforated seats were along the southern and western sides. In the toilet there are also modern and contemporary graffiti that I do not consider in this article.

71 I read something like ++*V OMN*+[---?] / [---]*LL*+*V OMN*[---] // *V*. The adjective *omnis* at least seems to be repeated.

72 *SE*[---] is part of a word, perhaps '*sedebat*', or a reflexive pronoun. The most immediate interpretation 'Once upon a time, when Troy ... remained' is a possible translation but, as Virgilio Petrucci made me think, this translation is not suitable for an hexameter (the verse you would above all expect), as opposed to '*A time, when from Troy...*' (with *ā*). This makes it very suggestive to think about a scene of *nostos*, 'homecoming', and it is possible that the Trojan subject is linked with a part of the drawings (fighter and ships).

73 The animal is preceded by something on the left, but I am not able to distinguish what it is. The quadruped, as the other quadruped up ahead in the drawing, very probably had horns.

74 The text of the inscription shows [------] / [----?]*TREX* (see, for this form, *CIL* VI 33984). Like the *Thrax* gladiator, I note that the Amazons are linked to the Thracian region too. If the figure really depicts a woman, we must not exclude the possibility that this is a rare case of the representation of a female gladiator (see e.g. Gregori 2001, 24, with references: one of these women had the nickname 'Amazon'). Probably there was an adversary or a beast to the right of the fighter. The object in the hand of the figure suggests the whip of an Amazon (see e.g. Sirano 2007, 94), but the proportions are here definitely too large.

75 If it is really a person, one can think about an arbiter of gladitorial games or a vedette on a tower or on a ship.

76 Maybe there was a foresail too, and we can not exclude the possibility that remains of an illegible inscription were in the upper part of the main sail.

77 Smaller than the first; we see the mast, some ropes, part of the sails, and maybe the helm and the extremity of the stern. Because of the presence of pots, we can compare this scene with many other harbor scenes (see e.g. Casson 1995, *saltim*).

78 Maybe an amphora or a *dolium*.

79 Maybe they represent simplified shapes of dogs or horses. Their backs are not to be seen or maybe were never drawn at all. Their nice silhouettes are very unusual in ancient iconography, reminiscent rather of modern cartoons.

80 It has the form *P* (X), probably to consider a note in which (X) could be a disarticulated number 1000.

81 The interpretation of *vulvae* was suggested to me by Lidio Gasperini, who proposes to interpret the long horizontal shape as a *phallus*; the inscription could maybe read [---]*P*+*LES* or [---]*B*+*LES*. The simplified silhouettes of this wall, whose traces are partially recognizable only from a light imprint on the plaster, seem to reflect an unskilled hand and a more 'childlike' approach, compared to the drawings of the southern wall. Even on the bottom hydraulic plaster there are some charcoal traces, in two cases maybe representing a pair of legs.

82 Aurigemma 1956, 69 proposed to read, not without hesitation: *P(ublius) Vi(bius) Primus, P(ublius) V(ibius) Eros Do*(..?) and hypothesized to refer this inscription to the family of the *Vibii*. My new interpretation - I am grateful to Werner Eck and Aroldo Barbieri for their discussion with me about this - is already quoted by Gian Luca Gregori (Gregori/Massaro 2005, 134, n. 16). Gregori has suggested that I consider *do* as the beginning of an unfinished word, e.g. *do(cuit)* 'who first taught boys' rather than as a complete form of the verb *dare*. For a similar beginning, see Ovid *Am*. 2.3.3-4: *Qui primus pueris genitalia membra recidit / vulnera quae fecit debuit ipse pati*.

83 For the motifs of this graffito, whose antiquity is confirmed by the concretions, a similar iconography can be found in a graffito that I discovered in the Barracks of the Firemen at Ostia (see also Langner 2001, n. 293).

84 On the same wall, but on the upper white plaster, I read another scratched inscription too: *ACR* (?).

85 For the dating of the building see also De Franceschini 1991, 562 and Salza Prina Ricotti 2001, 263. The paintings of the contiguous rooms could be Antonine-Severan (see also Molle 2004, 387). The general palaeography of the inscriptions leads us to exclude a late-antique chronology (especially the *E* made by two vertical bars, present in the inscription *Qui primus pueros do*(---?), seems to disappear after the first decades of the 3rd century AD (see e.g. Cencetti 1954, 64; the latest dated example that I know of is *CIL* VI. 3029, AD 230).

86 The only probable exception is the graffito *P* (X). Naturally, the absence of utilitarian graffiti is normal in a toilet (if we were for example in a shop, we would expect numbers and notes of wares). As regards to the verses, I want to recall first of all the *carmina quae legunt cacantes* of Martial (12.61.7-11); for the figurative themes of our graffiti, see the rich study of Langner 2001, *saltim*, and for the general problem of graffiti in toilets see now Jansen in this chapter. See also Moormann (chapter 5.2, pp. 57-60) for figural themes and for texts as part of mural decorations in toilets.

87 The charcoal, now almost invisible (I used spurts of distilled water to see it), should originally have been undoubtedly evident, as well as the deep furrows of the graffito concerning the *pueri* (see *figs 12.24-25*); gen-

erally the graffiti 'do not command the general impression compared with painted wall decorations or painted wall inscriptions' (Langner 2001, 144).

88 It would be very interesting to know if this multi-seater toilet was used by women or men. The psychological background of the graffiti seems to suggest men, but the 'Amazon' and the 'personified *vulvae*' could provoke an interesting debate for gender archaeology. Unfortunately, the other multi-seater toilet at the northern extremity of the same building is badly preserved and a comparison of graffiti is impossible. About the problem concerning the segregation of sexes, see, however, Neudecker 1994, 64-65 and Van Vaerenbergh in chapter 8.2, pp. 117-118.

89 The translations from the walls of the Seven Sages are our own. We wish to thank Stephan Mols and Andrew Wilson for several suggestions that were extremely helpful.

90 *OCD*[3] (1996) 1397 on 'Seven Sages': The original *sophoi* belong to the early decades of the 6th century BC, and the usual list comprises four members from the eastern cities (Thales of Miletus, Bias of Priene, Cleobulus from Lindos on Rhodes, and Pittacus of Mitylene) and three from the homeland (Solon from Athens, Chilon from Sparta, and Periander the Corinthian tyrant).

91 Neudecker, 38, reviews the sad excavation history of the Baths of the Seven Sages (III.X, 2-3) under Calza.

92 Mols 1997, 72: there is no door to the street, for which there is no certainty about the function. Neudecker 1994, 35 is also cautious about assigning a function to the room. In Clarke 2007, 125-131, figs 57-59, the toilet aspect is stressed, though without explaining the function of the room.

93 Neudecker 1994, 35-38, figs. 7-8; Clarke 2006, quotation on p. 55. In the same vein Clarke 1998-1999, 2003, 170-180 and 2007, 125-131 (p. 129: 'class conflict'). Briefly mentioned in Schefold 1997, 380-381, who mentions the folkloristic and iconographic interest of the images. Clarke's hypothesis of heteroglossy is inspired by work of Bakhtin explained extensively in his book.

94 Mols 1997, 92: 'una parodia sul costume del ceto ricco di ostentare la propria *humanitas* tramite gallerie di ritratti, una parodia che trova ispirazione nel genere romano del mimo.' Clarke 2007 also arrives at this conclusion, but does not cite Mols.

95 Cf. Neudecker 37, Abb. 8. Note the word *falernum*, mentioned above, a reference to the famous wine produced in the north of Campania, visible in the uppermost register.

96 See Howes 2005.

97 Howes 2005, 7-12.

98 Taste has been excluded from this analysis as it was not felt to have played a significant part in experiencing a public latrine.

99 Barton 2002, 217; Seneca, *Naturales Quaestiones* 1.16.4.

100 Seneca, *Naturales Quaestiones* 1.16.4.

101 Bille/Sørensen 2007.

102 Tanizaki 1977.

103 Drobnick 2006, 1-12.

104 Drobnick 2006, 15; Largey/Watson 2006; Tuzin 2006.

105 See Jansen above on demons.

106 See Koloski-Ostrow and Moormann in Case Study in this chapter.

107 See Largey/Watson 2006, 31 on this subject, who also point out that even now social scientists have not discussed the taboo.

108 Curtis/Biran 2001.

109 Haidt et al. 1997, 109.

110 Frodsham 2007

111 James 2000, 77 has recognised that assumptions about the nature and boundaries of what the 'Roman military' was is not so implicit as often presented.

112 James 2000, 78 has noted that the Roman's generally wrote of the 'soldiers' or the 'legions' when we speak of 'the Roman army.' They thought in terms of a class of men rather than an institution.

113 Haynes 1999.

114 Shotter/White 1990, 32.

115 Bishop/Dore 1988

116 Hoss 2005, Beth-Guvrin Cat. no 18, 129, Beth-She'an Eastern and Western Bathhouse Cat. no 18, 129, Cat. no 21, 131, Caesarea Maritima, Cat. no 29, 134, En Hazeva Cat. No. 59, 146 . Kloner/Cohen 1999, 112-114, 78*-79*. Mazor/ Bar-Nathan, 11-14, 20-24. Porath, 1998, 42-43. Cohen/Israel 1996, 110-116.

117 Hoss 2005, 92-99.

118 Hoss 2005, Cat. No. 30. Horton 1996, 177-189.

119 Hirschfeld 1995, Beth-Yerah (3rd-2nd c. BC), 66-67, fig. 42, Umm el-Jimal (2nd-3rd c. AD) 45, fig. 22, Mampsis (2nd-3rd c. AD) 76-77, fig. 51, Sepphoris (3rd-4th c. AD) 92-94, fig. 67.

120 Shereshevski 1991, 28; Kamash 2006, 220

121 Neudecker 1994; Koloski-Ostrow 1996; Jansen 2000.

122 Neudecker 1994, 157-158.

123 Kamash 2006, 179. Levi 1947, 260; Campbell 1936, 1; Stillwell 1941, 8, 19, 25; Butcher 2003, 263; Harper/Wilkinson 1975, 328-329; Brown 1936, 71, 95; Fisher 1938, 266; Bounni/As'ad 1989, 71; Butler et al. 1907 II.B.3, 118, 121; Early/Humphrey 2003, 55-6.

124 Balty 1981, 76; Schmidt-Colinet 1984, 142.

125 Koloski-Ostrow 1996, 84 and fn. 9.

126 Hoss 2005.

127 Kamash 2006, 184-214.

128 On protective imagery in bathhouses see Dunbabin 1989; Kamash 2006, 202-206; 2008.

129 Kamash 2008.

130 Boyer/Lienard 2006.

131 Dulaney/Fiske 1994; Fiske/Haslam 1997.

132 Boyer/Lienard 2006, 8.

133 On the concept of social gaze, see e.g. Garvey 2005.

134 James 1901-2, 129; Douglas 1966, 165.

135 Kamash 2008.

136 Strang 2004, 77.

137 Barton 2002, 217.

138 Garvey 2005, 173; Reed 1999, 50; Levin 1988, 210-211.

139 Kamash 2006, 224-229.

140 Deér 1959; 142; Boureau 2000, 48.

141 Deér 1959; 142-146; Boureau 2000, 48-49.

142 Deér 1959, 144.

143 Deér 1959; 145-146; Boureau 2000, 53-57.

144 *Liber Pontificalis* II, p. 108; cited in Deér 1959, 143 (without making the equation with the 'porphyry' thrones).

145 Deér 1959; 145-146; Boureau 2000, 55-57.

146 Boureau 10-26. Early versions of this include Geoffrey de Courlon in his chronicle of the Abbey de Saint-Pierre-le-Vif at Sens ca 1290; Robert d'Uzès (ca 1291); the Anonymous continuator of the Chronicle of Johannes of Viktring ca 1379; and Adam of Usk (*Chronicon*, 1404).

147 Quoted in Boureau 2000, 22.

148 Boureau 2000, 16, citing Jacopo d'Angelo (1406).

149 Boureau 2000, 48-53; D'Onofrio 1979.

Bibliography

Ailloud, H. 1957. *Suétone. Vie des douze césars*, Paris.

Alarcão, J. de/R. Etienne 1977, *Fouilles de Conimbriga* 1. *L'architecture*, Paris.

Alba, M. 2001, Apuntes sobre la red de aguas de Mérida en época romana, *Mérida Ciudad y Patrimonio* 5, 59-78.

Álvarez Sáenz de Buruaga, J. 1983, Observaciones sobre el teatro romano de Mérida, in *Actas del Simposio "El teatro en la Hispania romana" (Badajoz, 1982)*, Badajoz, 303-311.

Amici, C.M. 1991, *Il Foro di Cesare*, Firenze.

Anderson, J.C. Jr. 1997, *Roman Architecture and Society*, Baltimore.

Annese, C./G. De Felice/M. Turchiano 2000, Ceramiche della prima e media età imperiale dai riempimenti delle latrine della *domus* A, in G. Volpe (ed.), *Ordona* X. *Ricerche archeologiche a Herdonia (1993-1998)*, Bari, 251-265.

Antoniou, G.P. 2007, Lavatories in ancient Greece, *Water Science & Technology. Water Supply* 7.1, 155-164.

Antoniou, G.P. 2010, Ancient Greek Lavatories: Operation with Reused Water, in L. Maijs (ed.), *Ancient Water Technologies*, New York. 67-86.

Aranguio-Ruiz, V. (ed.) 1943, *Fontes Iuris Romani Antejustiniani* III. *Negotia*, Florence.

Arrowsmith, W. 1994, *Petronius, The Satyricon*, Harmondsworth.

Arthur, P. 1993, Le città vesuviane: problemi e prospettive nello studio dell'ecologia umana dell'antichità, in L. Franchi dell'Orto (ed.), *Ercolano 1738-1988. 250 anni di ricerca archeologica*, Rome, 193-199.

Ascione, G./M. Pagano 2000, *The Antiquarium of Herculaneum*, Naples.

Aspöck, H./H. Auer/O. Picher 1999, Parasites and parasitic diseases in prehistoric human populations in Central Europe, *Helminthologia* 36.3, 139-145.

Aspöck, H./F.E. Barth/H. Flamm/O. Picher 1974, Parasitäre Erkrankungen des Verdauungstraktes bei prähistorischen Bergleuten von Hallstatt und Hallein (Österreich), *Mitteilungen der Anthropologischen Gesellschaft Wien* 103, 41-47.

Aspöck, H./H. Flamm/O. Picher 1973, Darmparasiten in menschlichen Exkrementen aus prähistorischen Salzbergwerken der Hallstatt-Kultur (800-350 v. Chr.), *Zentralblatt für Bakteriologie, Parasitenkunde, Infektionskrankheiten und Hygiene. 1. Abteilung. Originale A* 223, 549-558.

Ault, B.A. 1994a, Koprones and Oil Presses. Domestic installations related to agricultural productivity and processing at Classical Halieis, in N. Doukellis/L. Mendoni (eds), *Structures rurales et sociétés antiques, Congrès Korfu 1992*, Paris, 197-206.

Ault, B.A. 1994b, *Classical Houses and Households. An Architectural and Artifactual Case Study from Halieis, Greece*, Ann Arbor.

Ault, B.A. 1999, Koprones and Oil Presses at Halieis: Interactions of Town and Country and the Integration of Domestic and Regional Economies, *Hesperia* 68, 549-573.

Ault, B.A. 2005, *The Excavations at Ancient Halieis. The Houses*, Bloomington.

Aurenhammer, M. 1990, *Die Skulpturen von Ephesos. Idealplastik* 1 (FiE X/1), Vienna.

Aurigemma, S. 1956, Lavori nel Canopo di Villa Adriana – III, *BdA* 41, 57-71.

Avery-Peck, J. 1995, The Mishnah, Tosefta, and the Talmuds. The Problem of Text and Context, in J. Neusner/A.J. Avery-Peck (eds), *Judaism in Late Antiquity* I. *The Literary and Archaeological Evidence*, Leiden, 173-216.

Baccini Leotardi, P. 1978, *Pitture con decorazioni vegetali dalle terme*, Rome.

Bakker, J.-Th. (ed.) 1999, *The Mills-Bakeries of Ostia. Description and Interpretation*, Amsterdam.

Ballu, A. 1897, *Les ruines de Timgad*, Paris.

Ballu, A. 1911, *Les ruines de Timgad: Sept années de découvertes 1903-1910*, Paris.

Ballu, A. 1926, Rapport sur les travaux de fouilles et consolidations entreprises par le service des monuments historiques pendant l'exercice 1924, *BAParis*, 141-144.

Balty, J.-C. 1981, *Guide d'Apamée*, Brussels.

Barbet, A. 1982, Peintures murales trouvées dans la latrine et les boutiques près du Forum de Bolsena, in Hallier/Humbert/Pomey 1982, 103-132.

Barbet, A. 1993, Peintures murales en relation avec la fonction des pièces en Gaule, in E.M. Moormann (ed.), *Functional and Spatial Analysis of Roman Painting*, Leiden, 9-17.

Barbet, A. 2008, *La peinture murale en Gaule romaine*, Paris.

Barlow, R.S. 1992, *The Vanishing American Outhouse*, El Cajon, California.

Bartoccini, R. 1929, *Le terme di Lepcis (Leptis Magna)*, Bergamo.

Barton, C. 2002, Being in the Eyes: Shame and Sight in Ancient Rome, in D. Fredrick (ed.), *The Roman Gaze: Vision, Power and the Body*, Baltimore/London, 216-235.

Bartsch, S. 2006, *The mirror of the self: sexuality, self-knowledge and the gaze in early Roman Empire*, Chicago.

Bastianelli, S. 1942, Civitavecchia. Nuove esplorazioni eseguite nelle Terme Taurine, *NSc*, 245-252.

Becatti, G. 1961, *Mosaici e pavimenti marmorei. Scavi di Ostia* 4, Rome.

Becker, W.A./H. Göll 1881, *Gallus oder römische Scenen aus der Zeit Augusts*, 2. Teil, Berlin.

Bell, E. 1987, A Preliminary Report on Health, Hygiene, and Sanitation at the Boott Mills Boardinghouses: An Historical and Archeological Perspective, in M.C. Beaudry (ed.), *Interdisciplinary Investigations of the Boott Mills, Lowell, Massachusetts* I. *Life at the Boarding House*, Boston, Mass., 57-68.

Bellini, G.R. 2002, *Il comprensorio archeologico di Minturnae: Itinerari di visita: La città*, Marina di Minturno.

Bendinelli, G. 1941, *Le pitture del Columbario di Villa Pamphili* (MontPitt 3, Roma 5), Rome.

Bennett, C.-M. 1974, Excavations at Buseirah, Southern Jordan 1972: Preliminary Report, *Levant* 6, 1-24.

Bilicki, J. 1996, Wharves, Privies, and Pewter: Recovery at Two Colonial Period Sites on the Shawmut Peninsula, Boston, Massachusetts. Paper presented at the 1996 Conference of the Society for Historical Archaeology, Cincinnati, Ohio.

Bille, M./T.F. Sørensen 2007, An Anthropology of Luminosity: The Agency of Light, *Journal of Material Culture* 12, 263-284.

Binsfeld, W. 1994, Vasa obscena, *TrZ* 57, 129-31.

Birley, A./J. Blake, *Vindolanda Research Report: the Excavations of 2005–2006*, Bardon Mill.

Birley, R. 1970, Excavations at Chesterholm-Vindolanda 1967-69, *Archaeologia Aeliana* 48 (Series 4), 97-155.

Birley, R. 1977, *Vindolanda: A Roman Frontier post on Hadrian's Wall*, London.
Bishop, M.C./J.N. Dore 1988, *Corbridge: Excavations of the Roman Fort and Town 1947-1980*, London.
Blackman, W.S. 2000, *The Fellahin of Upper Egypt. With a new foreword by Salima Ikram* (1st ed. 1927), Cairo.
Blake, M.E. 1947, *Ancient Roman Construction in Italy from the Prehistoric Period to Augustus*, Washington, D.C.
Blanco, A. 2007, Recenti scoperte alle Piccole Terme di Villa Adriana, *BABesch* 82, 183-190.
Blümner, H. 1887, *Technologie und Terminologie der Gewerbe und Künste bei Griechen und Römern*, Leipzig.
Blümner, H. 1911, *Die römischen Privataltertümer*, Munich.
Bodel, J. 1986 [1994]. Graveyards and Groves: A Study of the Lex Lucerina, *AmJAncHist* 11, 1-133.
Boehlau, J./K. Schefold 1940, *Larisa am Hermos* I. *Die Bauten*, Berlin.
Börker, C./R. Merkelbach 1979, *Die Inschriften von Ephesos* 2, Bonn.
Boersma, J. 1985, *Amoenissima civitas. Block V, 2 at Ostia*, Assen.
Boersma, J.S. et al. 1995, *Mutatio Valentia: The late Roman bath at Valesio, Salento*, Amsterdam.
Boeswillwald, E./R. Cagnat/A. Ballu 1905, *Timgad: Une cité africaine sous l'Empire romain*, Paris.
Boethius, A./J.B. Ward Perkins 1970, *Etruscan and Roman Architecture*, Harmondsworth.
Bollmann, B. 1998, *Römische Vereinshäuser: Untersuchungen zu den Scholae der römischen Berufs-, Kult- und Augustalen-Kollegien in Italien*, Mainz.
Bollmann, B. 2001, Les collèges religieux et professionnels romains et leurs lieux de réunion à Ostie, in J.P. Descoeudres (ed.), *Ostia: Port et porte de la Rome antique. Musée Rath, Genève*, Chêne-Bourg, 172-178.
Bonini, P. 2006, *La casa nella Grecia romana. Forme e funzioni dello spazio privato fra I e VI secolo*, Rome.
Boon, G.C. 1972, *Isca. The Roman Legionary Fortress at Caerleon*, Cardiff.
Borchardt, L. 1912, Ausgrabungen in Tell el-Amarna 1911/12, *MDOG* 50, 1-40.
Borchardt, L. 1916, *Das altägyptische Wohnhaus im 14. Jahrhundert v. Chr.* (Zeitschrift für Bauwesen 66), Berlin.
Borchardt, L./H. Ricke 1980, *Die Wohnhäuser in Tell el-Amarna*, Berlin.
Bosanquet, R.C. 1904, Excavations on the line of the Roman Wall in Northumberland 1: The Roman camp at Housesteads, *Archaeologia Aeliana* 25 (Series 2), 193-300.
Bounni, A./K. As'ad 1989, *Palmyre: Histoire, Monuments et Musée*, Damascus.
Boureau, A. 2000, *The myth of Pope Joan* (translated by Lydia Cochrane), Chicago/London.
Bowen Ward, R. 1992, Women in Roman Baths, *The Harvard Theological Review* 85, 1992, 125-147.
Boyer, P./P. Lienard 2006, Why Ritualized Behaviour? Precaution Systems and Action Parsing in Developmental, Pathological and Cultural Rituals, *Behavioural and Brain Sciences* 29, 1-19.
Bradley, M. 2002. It all comes out in the wash. Looking harder at the Roman fullonica, *JRA* 15, 21-44.
Brashaer, W.M./A. Breitenbach 2006, Kot (Latrine), *RAC*, 761-810.
Breeze, D.J. 1972, Excavations at the Roman fort of Carrawburgh, 1967-1969, *Archaeologia Aeliana* 50 (Series 4), 81-144.
Breeze D.J. 1984 (ed.), *Studies in Scottish Antiquity*, Edinburgh.
Breeze D.J. 2006, *Handbook to the Roman Wall*, [14]Newcastle upon Tyne.
Brewer, D.J./D.B. Redford/S. Redford 1994, *Domestic plants and animals. The Egyptian origins*, Warminster.
Bridger, C. 1989, *Colonia Ulpia Traiana, Insula 38: Die Befunde der Grabung 1979 bis 1983* (Rheinische Ausgrabungen 31), Cologne.
Brissaud, L. 2003, Un vase de foulon sur le site de Saint-Romain-en-Gal? Hypothèses et pistes de recherche, in P. Ballet/P. Cordier/N. Dieudonné-Glad (eds), *La ville et ses déchets dans le monde romain: rebuts et recyclages. Actes du Colloque de Poitiers (19-21 septembre 2002)*, Montagnac, 61-72.
Broise, H./J. Scheid 1987, *Le balneum des Frères Arvales: recherches archéologiques à la Magliana*, Rome.
Brothwell, D.R./A.M. Pollard 2001 (eds), *Handbook of Archaeological Sciences*, Chichester.
Brown, F.E. 1936, Block F3 and The Roman Baths, in M.I. Rostovtzeff et al. (eds), *The Excavations at Dura Europos: Preliminary Report of the Sixth Season of Work October 1932 - March 1933*, New Haven, 49-105.
Brun, J.P. 1999, Laudatissimum fuit antiquitus in Delo Insula. La maison IB du Quartier du Stade et la production des parfums à Délos, *BCH* 123, 87-155.
Brun, J.P./M. Brunet 1997, Une huilerie du premier siècle avant J.-C. dans le Quartier du théâtre à Délos, *BCH* 121, 573-613.
Brunet, M. 1998, L'artisanat dans la Délos antique, *Topoi* 8, 681-691.
Bruyère, B. 1939, *Rapport sur les fouilles de Deir el-Médineh (1934-1935)* III. *Le village, les décharges publiques, la station de repos de la Vallée des rois* (FIFAO 16), Cairo.
Buckland, P.C. 1976, *The environmental evidence from the Church Street Roman sewer* (The Archaeology of York 14.1), London.
Burden, D.J. et al. 1976, The treatment of soil infested with human whipworm, *Trichuris trichiura*, *Journal of Hygiene* 77, 377-382.
Butcher, K. 2003, *Roman Syria and the Near East*, London.
Butler, H.C. et al. 1907, *Syria: Publications of the Princeton University Archaeological Expeditions to Syria in 1904-1905 and 1909*, Leiden.
Butterworth, G.W. 1919 [1999], *Clement of Alexandria, Exhortation to the Greeks. The Rich Man's Salvation. To the Newly Baptized* (Loeb Classical Library), Cambridge, Mass.
Cahill J. et al. 1991, It had to happen: Scientists Examine Remains of Ancient Bathroom, *Biblical Archaeology Review* 17.3, 64-69.
Callen E.O. 1967, Analysis of Tetuacan coprolites, in D. Dyers (ed.), *The prehistory of the Tehacan valley* 1. *Environment and substistence*, Austin, 261-289.
Calza, G. 1933, Latrina, *Enciclopedia Italiana* 20, Rome, 602.
Calza, G. 1939, Die Taverne der Sieben Weisen in Ostia, *Die Antike* 15, 99-115.
Campbell, W.A. 1936, The Third Season of Excavation at Antioch on the Orontes, *AJA* 40, 1-9.
Candilio, D. 1999, Thermae Diocletiani, in E.M. Steinby (ed.), *Lexicon topographicum urbis Romae* 5, Rome, 53-58.
Cantarella, E. 1987, *Pandora's Daughters. The Role and Status of Women in Greek and Roman Antiquity* (trans. M.B. Fant), Baltimore.
Cappel, A. 1994, *Untersuchungen zu Pygmäendarstellungen in der römischen Dekorationskunst*, PhD Würzburg.
Carandini, A. (ed.) 1973, *Ostia* III. *Le Terme del Nuotatore. Scavo degli ambienti III, VI, VII* (Studi Miscellanei 21), Rome.
Carandini, A. (ed.) 1982, *Filosofiana: la villa di Piazza Armerina*, Palermo.

Carettoni, G. 1949, Roma (Palatino) - Costruzioni sotto l'angolo sud-occidentale della Domus Flavia (triclinio e ninfeo occidentale), *NSc*, 48-79.
Carettoni, G./A.M. Colini/L. Cozza 1960, *La pianta marmorea di Roma antica: Forma Urbis Romae* 1, Rome.
Cary, E. 1927, *Cassius Dio. Roman History* 9, London.
Casson, L. 1995, *Ships and seamanship in the ancient world*, [2]Baltimore/London.
Castrén, P. 1975, *Ordo populusque Pompeianus: Polity and Society in Roman Pompeii* (Acta Instituti Romani Finlandiae 8), Rome.
Cencetti, G. 1954, *Lineamenti di storia della scrittura latina*, Bologna.
Chapman, R. 1991, A stone toilet seat found in Jerusalem in 1925, *Palestine Exploration Quarterly* 124, 4-8.
Chini, P. 1995a, Forica Romana in via Garibaldi, *Archeologia Laziale* 12.1, 207-212.
Chini, P. 1995b, Un nuovo mosaico della latrina romana di via Garibaldi, in *Atti del II Colloquio Nazionale AISCOM*, Rome, 375-382.
Chini, P. 1997, Pitture rinvenute nella forica di via Garibaldi a Roma, in D. Scagliarini Corlàita (ed.), *I temi figurativi nella pittura parietale antica (IV sec. a.C. – IV sec. d.C.)*, Bologna, 189-191.
Chini, P. 1999, Graffiti inediti nella forica di via Garibaldi a Roma, in *XI Congresso Internazionale di Epigrafia Greca e Latina, Roma 18-24 settembre 1997*, Rome, 567-578.
Christison, D./M. Buchanan/J. Anderson 1903, Excavation of Castlecary fort on the Antonine Vallum, *Proceedings of the Society of Antiquaries of Scotland* 37, 271-346.
Ciancio Rossetto, P. 1985, Circo Massimo, in *Roma: Archeologia nel centro* 1. *L'area archeologica centrale*, Rome, 214-223.
Clarke, J.R. 1998-1999, Look who's laughing: Humor in Tavern Painting as Index of Class and Acculturation, *MemAmAc* 43-44, 27-48.
Clarke, J.R. 2001, Sex, Death, and Status: Nilotic Tomb imagery, apotropaic magic, and freedman acculturation, in A. Barbet (ed.), *La peinture funéraire antique, Actes du VIIe colloque de L'AIPMA, 6-10 okt. 1998, Saint-Romain-en-Gal-Vienne*, Paris, 85-91.
Clarke, J.R. 2003, *Art in the Lives of Ordinary Romans: Visual Representation and Non-Elite Viewers in Italy, 100 B.C.-A.D. 250*, Berkeley.
Clarke, J.R. 2005-2006, Forica security: the apotropaic pygmee-other in an imperial latrine at Ostia, in S. Mucznik (ed.), *Kalathos, Studies in Honour of Asher Ovadiah* (Assaph, Studies in Art History 10-11), Tel Aviv, 293-302.
Clarke, J.R. 2006, High and Low: Mocking Philosophers in the Tavern of the Seven Sages, Ostia, in E. D'Ambra/G.P.R. Métraux (eds), *The Art of Citizens, Soldiers and Freedmen in the Roman World*, Oxford, 47-57.
Clarke, J.R. 2007, *Looking at Laughter. Humor, Power, and Transgression in Roman Visual Culture, 100 B.C – A.D. 250*, Berkeley/Los Angeles/London.
Coarelli, F. 1981, *L'area sacra di Largo Argentina* 1. *Topografia e storia*, Rome.
Coarelli, F./D. Musti/H. Solin (eds) 1982, *Delo e l'Italia* (Opuscula Instituti Romani Finlandiae 2), Rome.
Cohen, D. 1991, *Law, Sexuality, and Society: the Enforcement of Morals in Classical Athens*, Cambridge.
Cohen, R./Y. Israel 1996, 'En Hazeva – 1990-1994, *Hadaschot Arkheologiyot* 103 (= Excavations and Surveys in Israel 15), 110-116.
Collingwood, R.G. 1926, *The Archaeology of Roman Britain*, London.
Confalonieri, U.E.C. et al. 1985, The experimental approach to paleoparasitology: desiccation of Trichuris trichiura eggs, *Paleopathology Newsletter* 51, 9-11.
Coste 1902, Travaux hydrauliques romains à Dolfusville (Sufasar), sur le Chélif, in S. Gsell (ed.). *Enquête administrative sur les travaux hydrauliques anciens en Algérie*, Paris, 31-35.
Courtois, C. 1951, *Timgad, antique Thamugadi*, Alger.
Crist, T. 2000, Infanticide at Five Points: The Anthropological Analysis of Twin Neonates from a Nineteenth-Century Privy, in R. Yamin (ed.), *Tales of Five Points: Working-Class Life in Nineteenth-Century New York* II. *An Interpretive Approach to Understanding Working-Class Life*, West Chester, Pennsylvania, 405-419.
Crouch, D. 1993, *Water Management in Ancient Greek Cities*, New York/Oxford.
Crow, J. 1995, *Housesteads, a Roman fort and garrison on Hadrian's Wall*, London.
Curtis, V. 2007, Dirt, Disgust and Disease: a Natural History of Hygiene, *Journal of Epidemiology and Community Health* 61 (8), 660-664.
Curtis, V./A. Biran 2001, Dirt, Disgust and Disease: Is Hygiene in our Genes?, *Perspectives in Biology and Medicine* 44.1, 17-31.
Curtis, V./S. Cairncross/R. Yonli 2000, Domestic hygiene and diarrhoea, pinpointing the problem, *Tropical Medicine and International Health* 5.1, 22-32.
Dagron, G. 1918, *Vie et miracles de sainte Thècle: Texte grec, traduction et commentaire*, Brussels.
Dainton, M. 1992, A quick, semi-quantitative method for recording nematode gut parasite eggs from archaeological deposits, *Circaea, the Journal of the Association for Environmental Archaeology* 9, 58-63.
Dakaris, S.I. 1986, Το Όρραον. Το σπίτι στην αρχαία Ήπειρο, *AEphem*, 108-146.
Daremberg, C./E. Saglio (eds) 1912, Latrina, in *Dictionnaire des antiquités grecques et romaines* III.2, Paris, 987-991 (H. Thédenat).
Deér, J. 1959, *The Dynastic Porphyry Tombs of the Norman Period in Sicily*, Harvard.
De Franceschini, M. 1991, *Villa Adriana: mosaici, pavimenti, edifici*, Rome.
De Haan, N./G.C.M. Jansen (eds), *Cura Aquarum in Campania: Proceedings of the Ninth International Congress on the History of Water Management and Hydraulic Engineering in the Mediterranean Region, Pompeii, 1-8 October 1994*, Leiden.
De Haan, N./K. Wallat 2006, The Water Supply of the Central Baths at Pompeii, in Wiplinger 2006, 417-422.
De Kind, R.E.L.B. 1998, *Houses in Herculaneum, a new view on the town planning and the building of insulae III and IV*, Amsterdam.
De Matteis, L.M. 2004, *Mosaici di Cos, dagli scavi delle Missioni italiane e tedesche (1900-1945)* (Monografie della Scuola Archeologica di Atene e delle Missioni Italiane in Oriente, XVII), Athens.
De Romanis, A. 1822, *Le antiche camere esquiline dette comunemente delle Terme di Tito*, Rome.
De Ruyt, C. 1996, Un exemple de discontinuité des fonctions monumentales dans un quartier de la ville romaine d'Ostie (reg. III, ins. II), *RBAH* 65, 5-16.
De Vos, A. and M. 1982, *Guide archeologiche Laterza: Pompei, Ercolano, Stabia*, Rome/Bari.
Della Corte, M. 1929, Excursus II – epigrafie della via fra le isole VI e X della Reg.I, *NSc*, 455-476.
Dittenberger, W. (ed.) 1903, *Orientis graeci inscriptiones selectae: supplementum sylloges inscriptionum graecarum*, Leipzig.
Dixon, D.M. 1972, The disposal of certain personal, house-

hold and town waste in ancient Egypt, in P.J. Ucko/R. Tringham/G.W. Dimbleby (eds), *Man, settlement and urbanism*, London, 647-650.
Dörpfeld, W. (ed.) 1901, *Antike Denkmäler* II, 4, Berlin.
Donadoni Roveri, A.M. (ed.) 1997, *La civilisation des Égyptiens, La vie quotidienne*, Milan.
D'Onofrio, C. 1979, *La Papessa Giovanna: Roma e papato tra storia e leggenda*, Rome.
Douglas, M. 1966, *Purity and Danger: An Analysis of the Concepts of Pollution and Taboo*, London/New York.
Drexel, F. 1921, Das Latrinenwesen in Rom und den Provinzen, in L. Friedländer, *Darstellungen aus der Sittengeschichte Roms* 4, ²Leipzig, 310-311 (= reprint, Aalen 1979).
Drobnick, J. (ed.) 2006, *The Smell Culture Reader*, Oxford/ New York.
Dulaney, S./A.P. Fiske 1994, Cultural Rituals and Obsessive-Compulsive Disorder: Is there a Common Psychological Mechanism?, *Ethos* 22.3, 243-283.
Dunbabin, K. 1989, *Baiarum grata voluptas*: Pleasures and Dangers of the Baths, *BSR* 57, 1-46.
Dundes, A. (ed.) 1981, *The evil eye, a folklore casebook*, New York.
Dupré y Raventos, X./J. A. Remolà (eds) 2000, *Sordes Urbis. La eliminaciòn de residuos en la ciudad romana*, Rome.
EAD VIII: J. Chamonard, *Le Quartier du théâtre. Étude sur l'habitation délienne à l'époque hellénistique*, Paris 1922-1924.
EAD XIX: É. Lapalus, *L'Agora des Italiens*, Paris 1939.
EAD XXV: J. Delorme, *Les Palestres*, Paris 1961.
Early, R./J.H. Humphrey (eds) 2003, *Zeugma: Interim Reports, Rescue Excavations*, Portsmouth, R.I.
Efron, J. 1987, *Studies on the Hasmonean Period*, Leiden.
Ehrhardt, W. 1998, *Casa di Paquio Proculo* (Häuser in Pompeji 9), Munich.
Ehrhardt, W. 2004, *Casa delle Nozze d'Argento* (Häuser in Pompeji 12), Munich.
Emery, W.B. 1979, *The fortress of Buhen: The archaeological report* (EEF 49), London.
Eretria VIII: P. Ducrey/I.R. Metzger/K. Reber, *Le Quartier de la Maison aux mosaïques*, Lausanne 1993.
Eretria X: K. Reber, *Die klassischen und hellenistischen Wohnhäuser im Westquartier*, Lausanne 1998.
Eschebach, H. 1979, *Die Stabianer Thermen in Pompeji* (Denkmäler antiker Architektur 13), Berlin.
Eschebach, L. 1991, Die Forumthermen in Pompeji, Regio VII, Insula 5, *AW* 22, 4, 257-287.
Eschebach, L./J. Müller-Trollius 1993, *Gebäudeverzeichnis und Stadtplan der antiken Stadt Pompeji*, Cologne/ Weimar/ Vienna.
Evans, J./T. O'Connor 1999, *Environmental Archaeology. Principles and Methods*, Stroud.
Fagan, G.G. 1999, *Bathing in Public in the Roman World*, Ann Arbor.
Fagan, G.G. 2000, Hygienic conditions in Roman public baths, in Jansen 2000b, 281-286.
Fairlie, S. 1965, Dyestuffs in the eighteenth century, *Economic History Review* 17.3, 488-510.
Feeney, D. 1992, *Si licet et fas est*: Ovid's *Fasti* and the Problem of Free Speech Under the Principate, in A. Powell (ed.), *Roman Poetry and Propaganda in the Age of Augustus*, London, 1-25.
Fernández Uriel, P. 1995, Algunas precisiones sobre el sistema fiscal Romano, *EspacioHist*, 8, 159-181.
Fink R.O. 1971, *Roman Military Records on Papyrus*, Cleveland.
Fisher, C.L./K.J. Reinhard/M. Kirk/J. Di Virgilio 2007, Privies and Parasites: The Archaeology of Health Conditions in Albany, New York, *Historical Archaeology* 41 (4),172-197.
Fisher, C.S. 1938, The Baths of Placcus, in C.H. Kraeling (ed.), *Gerasa of the Decapolis*, New Haven, 265-269.
Fiske, A.P./N. Haslam 1997, Is Obsessive-Compulsive Disorder a Pathology of the Human Disposition to Perform Socially Meaningful Rituals? Evidence of Similar Content, *Journal of Nervous and Mental Disease* 185.4, 211-222.
Flohr, M. 2006, Organizing the Workshop. Water management in Roman Fullonicae, in Wiplinger 2006, 193-200.
Flohr, M. 2007, Nec quicquam ingenuum habere potest officina? Spatial contexts of urban production at Pompeii, AD 79, *BABesch* 82, 129-148.
Follett, W.I. 1967, Fish remains from coprolites and midden deposits at Lovelock Cave, Churchill County, Nevada, *University of California Archaeological Survey Report* 70, 94-115.
Forbes R.J. 1957, *Studies in Ancient Technology* 5, Leiden.
Forbes, R.J. 1965, *Studies in Ancient Technology* 3, ²Leiden.
Fox, A. 1940, The legionary fortress at Caerleon, Monmouthshire: Excavations in Myrtle Cottage Orchard 1939, *Archaeologia Cambrensis* 95, 101-152.
Fox, A./W. Ravenhill 1972, The Roman Fort at Nanstallon, Cornwall, *Britannia* 3, 56-111.
Frankfort H./J.D.S. Pendlebury 1933, *The City of Akhenaten* II. *The North Suburb and the desert altars* (MEES 40), London.
Freed, R./Y.J. Markowitz/S.H. D'Auria (eds) 1999, *Pharaohs of the sun, Akhenaten, Nefertiti, Tutankhamen*, Boston.
Frodsham, P. (ed.) 2007, *Archaeology in Northumberland National Park*, York.
Fröhlich, Th. 1991, *Lararien- und Fassadenbilder in den Vesuvstädten*, Mainz am Rhein.
Fry, G.F. 1980, Prehistoric diet and parasites in the desert west of North America, in D.L. Bowman (ed.), *Early Native Americans*, The Hague, 325-339.
Garbrecht, G./H. Manderscheid, Die Wasserbewirtschaftung römischer Thermen. Archäologische und hydrotechnische Untersuchungen, *Mitteilungen Leichtweiss-Institut der Universität Braunschweig* 118 A-C.
Garvey, P. 2005, Domestic Boundaries: Privacy, Visibility and the Norwegian Window, *Journal of Material Culture* 10, 157-176.
Gaubatz-Sattler, A. 2005, Rottenburg am Neckar. Römische Stadt Sumelocenna, in D. Planck (ed.), *Die Römer in Baden-Württemberg*, Stuttgart, 281-289.
Geel, J. 1828, *Dav. Ruhnkenii scholia in Suetonii vitas Caesarum*, Leiden.
Gethke, K. et al. 2006, Phosphorus recovery from human urine, *Water Practice & Technology* 10.2166, WPT.2006070.
Ginouvès, R. 1962, *Balaneutike techne*, Paris.
Gonçalves, M.L.C./A. Araújo/L. F. Ferreira 2003, Human Intestinal Parasites in the Past: New Findings and a Review, *Memórias do Instituto Oswaldo Cruz* 98 (Suppl. I), 103-118.
Goppelsröder, A./C.S. Sommer 1996, Die organischen Reste einer römerzeitlichen Latrinenverfüllung und anderer Befunde in Ladenburg, Merkurplatz 5, *FuBerBadWürt* 21, 401-412.
Goulet, C.C. 2001-2002, The "Zebra Stripe" Design: An Investigation of Roman Wall Paintings in the Periphery, *RStPomp* 12-13, 53-94.
Gräzer, A. 2009, Hygiène et sécurité dans l'habitat égyptien d'époque pharaonique, in M.F. Boussac/T. Fournet/ B. Redon (eds), *Le bain collectif en Égypte* (IFAO - Études Urbaines 7), Cairo, 33-63.

Grahame, M. 1997, Public and Private in the Roman House: the Spatial Order of the *Casa del Fauno*, in R. Laurence/ A. Wallace-Hadrill (eds), *Domestic Space in the Roman World: Pompeii and Beyond* (JRA Supplement 22), Portsmouth, R.I., 137-164.

Grandjean, Y. 1988, *Recherches sur l'habitat thasien à l'époque grecque* (Études thasiennes XII), Paris.

Greene, K. 1979, *The Preflavian Wares (Report on the excavations at Usk 1965-1976)*, Cardiff.

Gregori, G.L. 2001, Aspetti sociali della gladiatura romana, in A. La Regina (ed.), *Sangue e Arena* (cat. of the exhibition), Rome, 15-27.

Gregori, G.L./M. Massaro 2005, Brescia, domus delle fontane: i graffiti del «passaggio del kantharos», *Epigraphica* 67, 129-157.

Gülbay, O. 2006, Western Anatolian Public Latrines, in Wiplinger 2006, 461-466.

Guéraud, O. 1931, *Enteuxeis. Requêtes et plaints adressées au roi d'Égypte au IIIe siècle avant J.-C.*, Kairo.

Guidobaldi, M.P. et al. 2006, Indagini archeologiche nella Casa dell'Atrio a Mosaico di Ercolano (IV, 2;1), *Fasti Online* 61-2006, 1-13.

Guidoboni, E. (ed) 1989, *I terremoti del Mille in Italia e nell'area mediterranea*, Bologna.

Guillaume, E. 1887, Cloaca, in Daremberg/Saglio I.2, 1260-1264.

Hänggi, R. 1989, Zur Baustruktur der Strassen von Augusta Rauricorum, *JberAugst* 10, 73-96.

Hänggi, R./C. Doswald/K. Roth-Robi 1994, *Die frühen römischen Kastelle und der Kastell-Vicus von Tenedo-Zurzach* (Veröffentlichungen der Gesellschaft Pro Vindonissa 11), Brugg.

Haidt, J. et al. 1997, Body, Psyche and Culture: The Relationship between Disgust and Morality, *Psychology and Developing Societies* 9, 107-131.

Hall, A.R. (ed.) 2002. *Environmental Archaeology: A guide to the theory and practice of methods, from sampling and recovery to post-excavation*, London.

Hall, A.R./H.K. Kenward 1990, *Environmental evidence from the Colonia* 14/6. *The Archaeology of York*, London.

Hall, R. 1986, *Egyptian textiles*, Oxford.

Hallier, G./M. Humbert/P. Pomey 1982, *Fouilles de l'École Française de Rome à Bolsena (Poggio Moscini)* VI. *Les abords du Forum*, Rome.

Harper, R.P./T. Wilkinson 1975, Excavations at Dibsi Faraj, Northern Syria 1972 1974: A Preliminary Note on the Site and its Monuments, *DOP* 29, 319-338.

Harris, E.C. 1979, 1989, *Principles of Archaeological Stratigraphy*, [1-2]New York.

Hauschteck, E. 2004, Goats in houses on Elephantine during the Middle Kingdom and the Second Intermediate Period, *Göttingische Miszellen* 202, 59-70.

Haynes, D.E.L. 1981, *The antiquities of Tripolitania*, [4]Tripoli.

Haynes, I. 1999. Introduction: the Roman army as a community, in A.K. Goldsworthy/I. Haynes (eds), *The Roman Army as a Community* (JRA Supplementary series 34), Portsmouth, Rhode Island, 7–14.

Heck, D./J. Bilicki 1996, Katherine Naylor's 'House of Office:' Data Recovery of a Seventeenth-Century Privy. Paper presented at the 1996 Conference of the Society for Historical Archaeology, Cincinnati, Ohio.

Heiligmann, K. 2003, *Sumelocenna: Römisches Stadtmuseum Rottenburg am Neckar*, Esslingen.

Heinonen-Tanski, H./C. Van Wijk-Sijbesma 2005, Human excreta for plant production, *Bioresource Technology* 96, 403-411.

Henderson, J. 1975, *The maculate muse*, London.

Herrmann, J.J. 1976, Observations on the baths of Maxentius in the Palace, *RM* 83, 403-424.

Hezser, C. 1998, „Privat" und „Öffentlich" im Talmud Yerushalmi und in der griechisch-römischen Antike, in P. Schäfer (ed.), *The Talmud Yerushalmi and Graeco-Roman Culture* I (TSAJ 71), Tübingen, 423-579.

Hilgers, W. 1969, *Lateinische Gefäßnamen. Bezeichnungen, Funktion und Form römischer Gefäße nach den antiken Schriftquellen*, Düsseldorf.

Hischfeld, Y. 1995, *The Palestinian Dwelling in the Roman-Byzantine Period* (Studium Biblicum Franciscanum. Collectio Maior 34), Jerusalem.

Hobson, B. 2009, *Latrinae et Foricae: Toilets in the Roman World*, London.

Hodder, P.A. 1982, *The Roman Army in Britain*, London.

Hodge, A.T. 1992, *Roman aqueducts and water supply*, London.

Hoepfner, W. (ed.) 1999, *Geschichte des Wohnens* I. *5000 v. Chr.-500 n. Chr.*, Stuttgart.

Hoepfner, W./E.-L. Schwandner 1994, *Haus und Stadt im klassischen Griechenland*, [2]Munich.

Hoeppli, R. 1959, *Parasites and Parasitic Infection in Early Medicine and Science*, Singapore.

Honigsberg, P. 1940, Sanitary installations in ancient Egypt, *The Journal of the Egyptian Medical Association* 23.4, 1-48.

Hornung, E. 1968, *Altägyptische Höllenvorstellungen*, Berlin.

Hoss, S. 2005, *Baths and Bathing: The culture of bathing and the baths and thermae in Palestine from the Hasmoneans to the Moslem Conquest. With an Appendix on Jewish Ritual baths* (miqva'ot) (BAR Int. Ser. 1346), Oxford.

Howell, P. 1989, *A commentary on Book One of the Epigrams of Martial*, London.

Howes, D. (ed.) 2005, *Empire of the Senses: The Sensual Culture Reader*, Oxford/New York.

Hufschmid, Th./H. Sütterlin 1992, Zu einem Lehmfachwerkbau und zwei Latrinengruben des 1. Jahrhunderts in August, *JberAugst* 13, 129-176.

Jacobelli, L. 1987, Lo scavo delle Terme Suburbane. Notizie Preliminari, *RStPomp* 1, 151-154.

Jacobelli, L. 1988, Terme Suburbane: Stato attuale delle conoscenze, *RStPomp* 2, 202-208.

Jacomet, S./A. Kreuz 1999, *Archäobotanik*, Stuttgart.

James, S. 2001, Soldiers and civilians: identity and interaction in Roman Britain, in S. James/M. Millett (eds), *Britons and Romans: advancing an archaeological agenda*, York, 187-209.

James, W. 1901-1902, *The Varieties of Religious Experience*, London.

Jansen, G. 1991, Water Systems and Sanitation in the Houses of Herculaneum, *MededRom* 50, 149-166.

Jansen, G. 1993, Paintings in Roman Toilets, in E.M. Moormann (ed.), *Functional and Spatial Analysis of Roman Painting*, Leiden, 29-33.

Jansen, G. 1997, Private toilets at Pompeii: appearance and operation, in S.E. Bon/R. Jones (eds), *Sequence and Space in Pompeii*, Oxford, 121-134.

Jansen, G.C.M. 2000a, Studying Roman Hygiene: The Battle between the Optimists and the Pessimists, in Jansen 2000b, 275-280.

Jansen, G. (ed.) 2000b, *Cura Aquarum in Sicilia: Proceedings of the Tenth International Congress on the History of Water Management and Hydraulic Engineering in the Mediterranean Region*, Leiden.

Jansen, G. 2000c, Systems for the disposal of waste and excreta in Roman cities. The situation in Pompeii, Herculaneum and Ostia, in Dupré/Remolà 2000, 37-49.

Jansen, G. 2000d, Urban water transport and distribution,

in Ö. Wikander (ed.), *Ancient water technology* (Technology and change in history 2), Leiden, 103-125.

Jansen, G. 2002a, *Water in de Romeinse stad. Pompeji – Herculaneum – Ostia*, Louvain.

Jansen, G. 2002b, Toilets of the Villa Adriana and Roman Privacy. A Research in Progress, in A.M. Reggiani (ed.), *Villa Adriana. Paesaggio antico e ambiente moderno: elementi di novità e ricerche in corso*, Milan, 76-83

Jansen, G. 2002c, Toilets of Hadrian's Villa at Tivoli (Italy) and Roman Privacy, *AJA* 106, 257.

Jansen, G. 2003, Social distinctions and issues of privacy in the toilets of Hadrian's Villa, *JRA* 16, 137-152.

Jansen, G. 2005, Stiller Ort mit Aussicht, *AW* 36, 3, 55-60.

Jansen, G. 2006a, The Unknown Urban Water System at Roman Ostia (Italy), in Wiplinger 2006, 189-196.

Jansen, G. 2006b, The Toilets of Ephesus. A Preliminary Report, in Wiplinger 2006, 109-112.

Jansen, G. 2007, Toilets with a View. The Luxurious Toilets of the Emperor Hadrian at his Villa near Tivoli, *BABesch* 82, 165-181.

Jobst, W. 1976-1977, Das „öffentliche Freudenhaus" in Ephesos, *OeJh* 51, 61-84.

Johnson, A. 1983, *Roman Forts of the 1st and 2nd Centuries AD in Britain and the German Provinces*, London.

Johnson, W. 1998, The myth of Jewish male menses, *Journal of Medieval History* 24.3, 273-295.

Jones, A.K.G. 1982. Human parasite remains: prospects for a quantative approach, in A.R. Hall/H.K. Kenward (eds), *Environmental archaeology in the urban context*, London.

Jones. A.K.G. 1983. Report on a coprolite from 6-8 Pavement, York, in A.R. Hall et al., *Environmental and living conditions at two Anglo-Scandinavian sites. The Archaeology of York* 14/4, London, 157-240.

Jones, A.K.G. 1986, Parasitological investigations on Lindow Man, in I.M. Stead et al., *Lindow Man: The body in the bog*, London, 136-139.

Jones, A.K.G. 1990, Coprolites andiaecal concretions, in M. Bell (ed.), *Brean Down excavations 1983-87*, London, 242-245.

Jones, A.K.G. 1991, *Fish remains from Freswick Links*, PhD York.

Jones, A.K.G./A.R. Hutchinson/C. Nicolson 1988, The worms of Roman horses and other finds of intestinal parasite eggs from unpromising deposits, *Antiquity* 62, 275-276.

Jones, B./D. Mattingly 1990, *An Atlas of Roman Britain*, Oxford.

Joshi, D./S. Ferron 2007, Manual scavenging - a life of dignity?, *Waterlines* 26.2, 24-27.

Juan-Tresseras, J. 2000, El uso de plantas para el lavado y teñido de tejidos en época romana. Análisis de residuos de la fullonica y tinctoria de Barcino, *Complutum* 11, 245-252.

Kadish, G.E. 1978-1979, The scatophagous Egyptian, *Journal of the Society for the Study of Egyptian Antiquities* 9, 203-217.

Kalopissi-Verti, S. 1991, Kos tardoantica e bizantina nelle scoperte archeologiche dal IV secolo al 1314, in *XXXVIII Corso di Cultura sull'arte Ravennate e Bizantina*, Ravenna, 233–251.

Kamash, Z. 2006, *Water supply and management in the Near East 63 BC – AD 636*, PhD, University of Oxford.

Kamash, Z. 2008, What Lies Beneath? Perceptions of the Ontological Paradox of Water, *WorldA* 40, 224-237.

Kandler, M. et al. 2004, Carnuntum, in M. Šašel Kos/P. Scherrer (eds), *The Autonomous Towns in Noricum and Pannonia – Die autonomen Städte in Noricum und Pannonien: Pannonia* II, Ljubjana, 11-66.

Kapossy, B. 1969, *Brunnenfiguren der hellenistischen und römischen Zeit*, Zürich.

Keil, J. 1929, 13. vorläufiger Bericht über die Ausgrabungen in Ephesos, *ÖJh* 24, Beiblatt, 6-67.

Kenward, H.K./A.R. Hall/A.K.G. Jones 1980, A tested set of techniques for the extraction of animal and plant macrofossils from waterlogged archaeological deposits, *Science and Archaeology* 22, 3-15.

Kienast, H. 1978, Zur Wasserversorgung griechischer Städte, *DiskAB* 3, 1978, 114-125.

Kilmer, M.F. 1993, *Greek erotica on Attic Red-Figure vases*, London.

Kliks, M.M. 1982, Parasites in archaeological material from Brazil, *Transactions of the Royal Society of Tropical Medicine and Hygiene* 76, 701.

Köhler, J. 2000, Zur Wasserbewirtschaftung der Terme Taurine bei Civitavecchia, in Jansen 2000b, 185-194.

Köhler, J./A. Rapone 2002, Die Terme Taurine bei Civitavecchia: Untersuchungen zur Chronologie und Funktion der zentralen Thermalbadesäle, *Boreas* 25, 125-132.

Kloner, A./M. Cohen 1999, Bet Guvrin, Area 750, *Hadaschot Arkheologiyot* 104 (= Excavations and Surveys in Israel) 19, 112-114, 78*-79*.

Kolb, F. 1984, *Die Stadt im Altertum*, Düsseldorf.

Kolling A. 2000, Latinum in latrina (Latein in der Latrine). Erstmals ausgewiesen: Ein Nachtgeschirr für den Mann (matella) im römischen Schwarzenacker, in *2000 Jahre Römerstadt Homburg* (http://www.hom.shuttle.de/hom/spg/roep-092.htm).

Koloski-Ostrow, A.O. 1985, Pygmies in the Cold Plunge: The Sarno Bath Paintings at Pompeii, abstract of paper given at 1984 meeting of AIA-APA, *AJA* 89, 337.

Koloski-Ostrow, A.O. 1990, *The Sarno Bath Complex*, Rome.

Koloski-Ostrow, A.O. 1996, Finding Social Meaning in the Public Latrines of Pompeii, in De Haan/Jansen 1996, 79-86.

Koloski-Ostrow, A.O. 1997, Violent Stages in Two Pompeian Houses: Imperial Taste, Aristocratic Response, and Messages of Male Control, in A.O. Koloski-Ostrow/C.L. Lyons (eds), *Naked Truths: Women, Sexuality, and Gender in Classical Art and Archaeology*, London/New York, 243-266.

Koloski-Ostrow, A.O. 2000, Cacator cave malum: the subject and object of Roman public latrines in Italy during the first centuries BC and AD, in Jansen 2000b, 289-295.

Koloski-Ostrow, A.O. (ed.) 2001, *Water Use and Hydraulics in the Roman City* (Colloquia and Conference papers, No. 3), Dubuque, Iowa.

Koloski-Ostrow, A.O. forthcoming, *The Archaeology of Sanitation in Roman Italy: Water, Sewers and Toilets*, Chapel Hill (University of North Carolina Press).

Krause, C. 1994, *Domus Tiberiana* I. *Gli scavi* (*BA* 25-27), Rome.

Krause, C. 2004, Die Domus Tiberiana – Vom Wohnquartier im Kaiserpalast, in A. Hoffmann/U. Wulf (eds), *Die Kaiserpaläste auf dem Palatin in Rom: das Zentrum der römischen Welt und seine Bauten*, Mainz am Rhein, 33-58.

Kwintner, M. 1992, Plautus Pseudolus 782: A fullonious assault, *ClPhil* 87, 232-233.

La Torre, M. 2006, Das Vediusgymnasium in Ephesos, in Wiplinger 2006, 87-93.

Labisch, A./U. Koppitz 2005, Hygiene, in K.-H. Leven (ed.), *Antike Medizin, Ein Lexikon*, Munich, 443-447.

Laken, L. 2003, Zebrapatterns in Campanian wall painting: a matter of function, *BABesch* 78, 167-189.

Lang, M. 1968, *Waterworks in the Athenian Agora* (Excavations of the Athenian Agora, Picture Books 11), Princeton NJ.

Lang-Auinger, C. 2003, *Hanghaus 1 in Ephesos. Funde und Ausstattung* (FiE VIII, 4), Vienna.

Langner, M. 2001, *Antike Graffitizeichnungen, Motive, Gestaltung und Bedeutung*, Wiesbaden.

Largey, G./R. Watston 2006, The Sociology of Odors, in Drobnick 2006, 29-40.

Lassus, J. 1969, *Visite à Timgad*, Alger.

Laur-Bélart, R. 1948, *Führer durch Augusta Raurica*, Basel.

Lauter, H. 1986, *Die Architektur des Hellenismus*, Darmstadt.

Lawrence, A.W. 1957, *Greek Architecture*, Harmondsworth/ Baltimore/Mitcham.

Le Clère, M. 1985 (ed.), *Paris de la préhistoire à nos jours*, Paris.

Leblanc, O. 1995, Le décor des latrines des „Thermes des lutteurs" à Sain-Romain-en-Gal (Rhône), *Revue archéologique de Picardie* numéro spécial 10, 239-263.

Lendon, J.E. 1997, Social Control at Rome, *CJ* 93, 83-92.

Levi, D. 1941, The Evil Eye and the Lucky Hunchback, in Stillwell 1941, 220-232.

Levi, D. 1947, *Antioch Mosaic Pavements*, Princeton/London.

Levin, D.M. 1988, *The Opening of Vision: Nihilism and the Postmodern Situation*, London.

Levitan, B. 1982, *Excavations at West Uley: the sieving and sampling programme*, Gloucester.

Lewis, C./C. Short, 1969. *A Latin Dictionary*, Oxford.

Lézine, A. 1968, *Carthage, Utique. Etudes d'architecture et d'urbanisme*, Paris.

Lézine, A. 1969, *Les Thermes d'Antonin à Carthage*, Tunis.

Lichtheim, M. 1975, *Ancient Egyptian Literature* I. *The Old and Middle Kingdoms*, Berkeley/Los Angeles/London.

Liedtke, C. 2003, *Nebenraumdekorationen des 2. und 3. Jahrhunderts in Italien*, Berlin/New York.

Lintott, A. 1993, *Imperium Romanum: Politics and Administration*, London.

Livadiotti, M./G. Rocco (eds) 1996, *La presenza italiana nel Dodecaneso tra il 1912 ed il 1948. La ricerca archeologica. La conservazione. Le scelte progettuali*, Catania.

Lloyd, J.A. (ed.) 1977, *Excavations at Sidi Khrebish, Benghazi (Berenice)* 1. *Buildings, coins, inscriptions, architectural decoration* (Supplements to Libya Antiqua 5), Tripoli.

Löfstedt, E. 1933, *Syntactica. Studien und Beiträge zur historischen Syntax des Lateins* II. *Syntaktisch-stilistische Gesichtspunkte und Probleme*, Lund.

Loewental, A.I./D.B. Harden/ C.E.N. Bromehead 1949, Vasa Murrina, *JRS* 39, 31-37.

Love, M. 2007, *Analysis of calcareous deposits from the down pipes of first century Pompeii*, Unpublished Undergraduate Dissertation, University of Bradford.

Luis, M.R. 1943, Les fouilles des Fontaines salées (1942), *Gallia* 2, 26-28.

Lynch, K.M./J.K. Papadopoulos 2006, Sella cacatoria. A study of the potty in archaic and classical Athens, *Hesperia* 75, 1-32.

MacDonald, W.L. 1982, *The Architecture of the Roman Empire: An Introductory Study*, New Haven.

MacDonald, W.L./J.A. Pinto 1995, *Hadrian's Villa and its Legacy*, New Haven/London.

MacMullen, R. 1980, Women in public in the Roman empire, *Historia* 19, 208-218.

Magness, J. 1998, Two Notes on the Archaeology of Qumran, *BASOR* 312, 37-44.

Mahjoubi, A. 1978, *Recherches d'histoire et archéologie à Henrichir el Faouar*, Tunis.

Maiuri, A. 1939, Pompei, Regione I, *NSc* 1935-1939, 188-193.

Maiuri, A. 1958, *Ercolano. I nuovi scavi (1927-1958)*, Rome.

Manacorda, D. 1993, Crypta Balbi, in E.M. Steinby (ed.), *Lexicon topographicum urbis Romae* 1, Rome, 326-329.

Manacorda, D. 2001, *Crypta Balbi. Archeologia e storia di un paesaggio urbano*, Milan.

Manderscheid, H. 1988, Römische Thermen. Aspekte von Architektur, Technik und Ausstattung, in *Die Wasserversorgung antiker Städte, Geschichte der Wasserversorgung* 3, Mainz am Rhein, 99-125.

Manderscheid, H. 1993, Bemerkungen zur Wasserbewirtschaftung der Suburbanen Thermen. *AKorrBl* 23, 3, 337-346.

Manderscheid, H. 2000, The Watermanagment of Greek and Roman Baths, in *Handbook of Ancient Water Technology* (Technology and Change in History 2), Leiden/ Boston/Cologne, 467-538.

Manderscheid, H. 2009, *Dulcissima aequora. Wasserbewirtschaftung und Hydrotechnik der Terme Suburbane in Pompeii* (BABesch Suppl. 13), Leuven.

Manning, W.H. 1981, *The Fortress Excavations 1968-1971* (Report on the Excavations at Usk 1965-1976), Cardiff.

Marangou, L. 1986a, *Gymnasium of Minoa*, Athens.

Marangou, L. 1986b, Anaskafe Minoas Amorgou, *Prakt*, 226-228.

Marangou, L. 1987, Anaskafe Minoas Amorgou, *Prakt*, 255-266.

Mansel, A.M. 1963, *Die Ruinen von Side*, Berlin.

Martin, R. 1957, Sur deux expressions techniques de l'architecture grecque, *RPhil* 31, 66-81.

Martins, M. 2006, Bracara Augusta: A Roman Town in the Atlantic Area, in L. Abdad Casal (ed.), *Early Roman Towns in Hispania Tarraconensis* (JRA Suppl. 62), Portsmouth, 213-222.

Mattelaer, J.J. 1999, Some historical aspects of urinals and urine receptacles, *World Journal of Urology* 17.3 June, 145-150.

Mau A. 1882-1883, Scavi di Pompei 1880-1881, *BdI*, 196.

Mazor, G./R. Bar-Nathan 1998, The Bet-She'an Excavation Project – 1992-1994 Antiquities Authority Expedition, *Hadaschot Arkheologiyot* 105 (= Excavations and Surveys in Israel 17), 11-14.

McGuire, R./M.B. Schiffer 1983, A Theory of Architectural Design, *Journal of Anthropological Archaeology* 2, 227-303.

McPeake, J.C./M. Bulmer/J.A. Rutter 1980, Excavations in the garden of No 1 Abbey Green, Chester 1975-77: interim report 1975-77, *Journal of the Chester Archaeological Society* 63, 22-31.

Meeks, D. 1976, Pureté et purification en Égypte, in *Dictionnaire de la Bible, Supplément* 9, Paris, col. 430-452.

Meeuwssen, J.C.L./ G. Boer/ R.P. Exaltus/ H. Kars 1997, Effects of Soil Acidification and Declining Groundwater Tables on the Decay of Buried Archaeological Features, *BerRijksdOudhBod* 42, 475-491.

Mélida, J.R. 1921, El anfiteatro y el circo romanos de Mérida: memoria de las excavaciones practicadas en 1919 y 1920, *Junta Superior de Excavaciones y Antigüedades* 39, 1-17.

Menéndez-Pidal, J. 1976, Algunas notas sobre la restauración y atención prestadas a los monumentos emeritenses, in *Augusta Emerita. Actas del Simposio Internacional Conmemorativo del Bimilenario de Mérida (Mérida, 1975)*, Madrid, 199-216.

Merletto, A. 2000, Public toilets in the Roman world: peculiarities and diffusion, in Jansen 2000b, 297-305.

Merletto, A. 2001, The Latrine near the Western Baths, in *Ιστορία, Τέχνη, Αρχαιολογία της Κω*, Athens, 165-170.

Merletto, A. 2004, The latrine near the Western Bath of Kos: excavation and reconstruction, in *ΧΑΡΙΣ ΧΑΙΡΕ. Μελέτες στη Χάρης Κάντζα*, Athens, I, 251-262.

Mertens, D. et al. 2005, *Selinous* I. *Die Stadt und ihre Mauern*, Mainz.
Mertens, D. 2006, *Städte und Bauten der Westgriechen. Von der Kolonisation bis zur Krise am Ende des 5. Jahrhunderts v. Chr.*, Munich.
Mertens. J. (ed.) 1995, *Herdonia: scoperta di una città*, Bari.
Meyboom, P.G.P./ E.M. Moormann, *Le decorazioni dipinte e marmoree della Domus Aurea di Nerone a Roma*, BABESCH supplement, in print.
Meyboom, P.G.P./M.J. Versluys, 2007, The meaning of dwarfs in nilotic scenes, in L. Bricault/M.J. Versluys/ P.G.P. Meyboom (eds), *Nile into Tiber, Egypt in the Roman World, Proceedings of the IIIrd International Conference on Isis studies, Leiden, May 11-14, 2005*, Leiden, 170-208.
Michel, D., *Casa dei Cei* (Häuser in Pompeji 3), Munich.
Miket, R. 1983, *The Roman Fort at South Shields: Excavation of the Defences, 1977-81*, Newcastle upon Tyne.
Miller, S.N. 1928, *The Roman Fort at Old Kilpatrick*, Glasgow.
Millingen, J. 1821, Some observations on an Antique Bas-relief on which the evil eye, or fascinum, is presented, *Archaeologia* 19, 70-74.
Moeller, W.O. 1976. *The Wool Trade of Ancient Pompeii*, Leiden.
Molle, C. 2004, La decorazione pittorica delle volte delle sostruzioni occidentali del Canopo di Villa Adriana, in L. Borhy (ed.), *Plafonds et voûtes à l'époque antique. Actes du VIIIe Colloque international de l'Association internationale pour la peinture murale antique* (AIPMA), Budapest, 385-388.
Mols, S.T.A.M. 1997, I "Sette Sapienti" ad Ostia, in D. Scagliarini Corlàita (ed.), *I temi figurativi nella pittura parietale antica (IV sec. A.C. – IV sec. D.C.)*, Bologna, 89-96.
Mols. S.T.A.M./E.M. Moormann 1993-1994, 'Ex parvo crevit' Proposta per una lettura iconografica della tomba di Vestorius Priscus fuori Porta Vesuvio a Pompei, *RSt Pomp* 6, 15-52.
Mols. S.T.A.M./E.M. Moormann 2010, L'edificio romano sotto S. Maria Maggiore a Roma e le sue pitture: proposta per una nuova lettura, *RM* 116, 469-506.
Mooney, C. 1930, *Suetoni Tranquilli De vita Caesarum libri VII-VIII, with introduction, translation and commentary*, New York.
Morricone, L. 1955, Scavi e ricerche a Coo (1935-1943), Relazione Preliminare, *BdA* 1, 54-75, 219-246, 316-331.
Morris, S.P. 1985. Λάσανα. A contribution to the ancient Greek kitchen, *Hesperia* 54, 393-409.
Mygind, H. 1921 Hygienische Verhältnisse im alten Pompeji, *Janus* 22, 251-281.
Nash-Williams, V.E. 1969, *The Roman Frontier in Wales*, Cardiff.
Netzer, E./Z. Weiss 1994, *Zippori*, Jerusalem.
Neudecker, R. 1994, *Die Pracht der Latrine: zum Wandel der öffentlichen Bedürfnisanstalten in der kaiserzeitlichen Stadt*, Munich.
Neueburg, N. 1965, *L'architettura delle fontane e dei ninfei dell'Italia antica*, Naples.
Neusner, J. 1973, *The Idea of Purity in Ancient Judaism* (Studies in Judaism in Late Antiquity 1), Leiden.
Neusner, J. 1991, *The Talmud of the Land of Israel: A preliminary Translation and Explanation: Shabbat*, London/Chicaco.
Nielsen, I. 1990, *Thermae et Balnea: The Architecture and Cultural History of Roman Public Baths*, Aarhus.
Nieto-Galan, A. 2001, *Colouring Textiles. A History of Natural Dyestuffs in Industrial Europe*, Dordrecht.
Notermans, A. 2007, *Sprekende mozaïeken. Functie en betekenis op Romeinse vloermozaïeken*, PhD Nijmegen.
Nutton, V. 2000, Did the Greeks have a Word for It? Contagion and Contagion Theory in classical Antiquity, in L.I. Conrad/D. Wujastyk (eds), *Contagion: Perspectives from Pre-Modern Societies*, Aldershot, 137-162.
O'Connor, T. 2003, *The analysis of urban animal bone assemblage* (Archaeology of York 19.2), York.
Oder, E. (ed.) 1901, *Claudii Hermeri Mulomedicina Chironis*, Leipzig.
Oder, E./C. Hoppe 1924, *Corpus hippiatricorum Graecorum* 2. *Hippiatrica Parisina Cantabrigiensia Londiniensia Lugdunensia; Appendix*, Leipzig.
Oleson, J.P. 1996, Water-Lifting Devices at Herculaneum and Pompeii in the Context of Roman Technology, in De Haan/Jansen 1996, 67-77.
Outschar U./H. Thür, 1997, Latrinegerüch(t)e aus Ephesos. Ein stiller Ort?, *Forum Archaeologiae - Zeitschrift für klassische Archäologie* 4.8, http.farch.net.
Owens E.J. 1983, The Koprologoi at Athens in the Fifth and Fourth Century B.C., *CQ* 33, 44-50.
Packer, J.E. 1998, Mire exaedificavit: Three Recent Books on Hadrian's Tiburtine Villa, *JRA* 11, 583-596.
Pandermalis, D. 1997, *Dion. Archäologische Stätte und Museum*, Athens.
Pagano, M. 1993, Ricerche sull'impianto urbano di Ercolano, in L. Franchi dell'Orto (ed.), *Ercolano 1738-1988 250 anni di ricerca archeologica*, Atti Convegno Internazionale Ravello-Ercolano-Napoli-Pompei 1988, Rome, 595-608.
Pantalacci, L. 1983, Wnm-Hw33t: Genèse et carrière d'un génie funéraire, *BIFAO* 83, 297-311.
Papadopoulous, J.K. 2002, Παίζων ἢ χέζω? A contextual approach to *pessoi* (gaming pieces, counters or convenient wipes?), *Hesperia* 71, 423-427.
Parslow, Ch. 1998, Preliminary report of the 1997 fieldwork project in the Praedia Iuliae Felicis (regio II, 4), Pompeii, *RStPomp* 9, 199-207.
Parslow, Ch. 2000, The hydraulic system in the 'balneum venerium et nongentum' of the Praedia Iuliae Felicis in Pompeii, in Jansen 2000b, 201-209.
Payne, S. 1972, Partial recovery and sample bias: the results of some sieving experiments, in E.S. Higgs (ed.), *Papers in economic prehistory*, Cambridge, 49-64.
Peet, T.E./C.L. Wooley 1923, *The City of Akhenaten* I. *Excavations of 1921 and 1922 at El-'Amarnah*, London.
Pellicioni, G. 1973, Le nuove scoperte sulle origini del Battistero Lateranense, *MemPontAc* 12, 1.
Peňa, E.S./J. Demnon 2000, The Social Organization of a Boardinghouse: Archaeological Evidence from the Buffalo Waterfront, *Historical Archaeology* 34.1, 79-96.
Pendlebury, J.D.S. 1951, *The city of Akhenaten* III. *The central city and the official quarters* (MEES 44), London.
Peters, W.J.Th. 1993, *La casa di Marcus Lucretius Fronto a Pompei e le sue pitture*, Amsterdam.
Petrie, W.F. 1891, *Illahun, Kahun and Gurob. 1889-1890*, London.
Petrie, W.F. 1907, *Gizeh and Rifeh*, London.
Petznek, B./S. Radbauer 2008, Römische Nachttöpfe aus der Zivilstadt von Carnuntum, *CJb*, 51-92.
Philp, B. 1981. *The Excavation of the Roman Forts of the Classis Britannica at Dover, 1970-1977*, Dover.
Pietrogrande, A. 1976, *Scavi di Ostia* VII: *Le fulloniche*, Rome.
Pillet, M. 1952, Les scènes de naissance et de circoncision dans le temple nord-est de Mout, à Karnak, *Annales du Service des Antiquités de l'Égypte* 52, 77-104.
Piranomonte, M. 1999, Thermae Antoninianae, in E.M. Steinby (ed.), *Lexicon topographicum urbis Romae* 5, Rome, 42-48.
Pirson, F. 1999, *Mietwonungen in Pompeji und Herculaneum*, Munich.

Poinssot, C. 1983, *Les ruines de Dougga*, ²Tunis.
Porath, Y. 1997, Expedition of the Antiquities Authority, *Hadaschot Arkheologiyot* 105 (= Excavations and Surveys in Israel 17), 42-43.
Quibell, J.E. 1923, *Excavations at Saqqara (1912-1914). Archaic Mastabas*, Cairo.
Radbauer, S./F. Humer 2004, Die Ausgrabungen an der Weststraße in der Zivilstadt von Carnuntum, *AÖ* 15.2, 40–44.
Radbauer, S./F. Humer 2005, Ausgrabungen an der Weststraße 2002–2003, *FÖ* 43, 903–906.
Rallo, A. 1977, Scavi e ricerche nella città antica di Selinunte (Relazione preliminare), *Kokalos* 22-23, 720-733.
Rebuffat, R. 1970, *Thamusida. Fouilles du service des antiquités du Maroc* II, Rome/Paris.
Reed, A. 1999, Anticipating Individuals: Modes of Vision and their Social Consequences in a Papua New Guinea Prison, *Man* 5, 43-56.
Reid, D. 1991, *Paris Sewers and Sewermen, Realities and Representations*, Cambridge.
Ricciardi, M.A./V. Santa Maria Scrinari 1996, *La civiltà dell'acqua in Ostia Antica* 1-2, Rome.
Richardson, G.H. 1936, Excavations at the Roman fort of Piercebridge, 1933-4, *Transactions of the Architectural and Archaeological Society of Durham and Northumberland* 7, 235-266.
Richardson, J./G. Thompson/A. Genovese 1997, New directions in economic and environmental research at Pompeii, in S.E. Bon/R. Jones (eds.), *Sequence and space in Pompeii*, Oxford, 88-101.
Ricke, H. 1932, *Der Grundriss des Amarna Wohnhauses*, Leipzig.
Riggsby, A.M. 1997, 'Private' and 'Public' in Roman Culture: The Case of the cubiculum, *JRA* 10, 36-56.
Rizqallah F./K. Rizqallah 1978, *La préparation du pain dans un village du Delta égyptien*, Cairo.
Roberts, D./D. Barrett 1984, Nightsoil Disposal Practices of the Nineteenth Century and the Origin of Artifacts in Plowzone Provenience, *Historical Archaeology* 18.1, 108-115.
Robinson, D.M. 1946, *Excavations at Olynthus* XII. *Domestic and Public Architecture*, Baltimore/London/Oxford.
Robinson, D.M./J.W. Graham 1938, *Excavations at Olynthus* VIII. *The Hellenic House*, Baltimore/London/Oxford.
Robinson, O.F. 1992, *Ancient Rome: City Planning and Administration*, London/New York.
Rolfe, J.C. 1914, *Suetonius* I, London.
Salza Prina Ricotti, E. 1995, Lavacra pro sexibus separavit, *RendPontAc* 66, 77-110.
Salsa Prina Ricotti, E. 2001, *Villa Adriana. Il sogno di un imperatore*, Rome.
Santa Maria Scrinari, V. 1995, *Il Laterano Imperiale* II. *Dagli 'horti Domitiae' alla Cappella cristiana*, Rome
Satlow, M.L. 1997, Jewish Constructions of Nakedness in Late Antiquity, *Journal of Biblical Literature* 116.3, 429-454.
Schatzmann, P. 1923, *Das Gymnasion* (Altertümer von Pergamon VI.2), Berlin.
Schefold, K. 1997, *Die Bildnisse der antiken Dichter, Redner und Denker*, ²Basle.
Scheibelreiter, V. 2005, Ein schwarzfiguriges Mosaik aus dem Vediusgymnasium von Ephesos, *Römische Historische Mitteilungen* 47, 55-79.
Scherrer, P./E. Trinkl 2006, *Die Tetragonos Agora in Ephesos: Grabungsergebnisse von archaischer bis in byzantinische Zeit: Ein Überblick: Befunde und Funde klassischer Zeit* (FiE 13, 2), Vienna.
Schiaparelli, E. 1927, *Relazione sui lavori della missione archeologica italiana in Egitto (Anni 1903-1920)* II. *La tomba intatta dell'architetto "Cha" nella necropoli di Tebe*, Turin.
Schiffer, M.B. 1987, *Formation Processes of the Archaeological Record*, Albuquerque.
Schmidt-Colinet, A. 1984, Die sogennante Maison à Atrium, in J.-C. Balty (ed.), *Apamée de Syrie: Bilan des Recherches Archéologiques, 1973-1979: Aspects de l'Architecture Domestique d'Apamée*, Brussels, 141-149.
Schnalke, T., 2005, Hygieia, in: K.-H. Leven (ed.), *Antike Medizin, Ein Lexikon*, Munich, 443.
Schneider, J. 1987, The anthropology of cloth, *Annual Review of Anthropology* 16, 409-448.
Schönbeck, G. 1962, *Der locus amoenus von Homer bis Horaz*, PhD Heidelberg.
Schwartz, J./H. Wild 1950, *Fouilles Franco-Suisses. Rapports* I, *Qasr-Qarun/Dionysias 1948*, Cairo.
Scobie, A. 1986, Slums, Sanitation and Mortality in the Roman World, *Klio* 68, 399-433.
Sear, F. 1982, *Roman Architecture*, Ithaca.
Seiler, F. 1992, *Casa degli Amorini Dorati* (Häuser in Pompeji 5), Munich.
Shaw, I. 1984, Report on the 1983 excavations, The animal pens (building 400), *AR* 1, 40-59.
Shereshvski, J. 1991, *Byzantine Urban Settlements in the Negev Desert*, Beer-Sheva.
Shotter, D.C.A./A.J. White 2001, *The Roman Fort and Town of Lancaster*, Lancaster.
Sirano, F. 2005, The 'House of the Rape of Europa' at Cos, *BABesch* 80, 145-162.
Sirano, F. 2007, Amazzone seduta, in M.L. Nava/R. Paris/R. Friggeri (eds), *Rosso Pompeiano. La decorazione pittorica nelle collezioni del Museo di Napoli e a Pompei* (catalogue of the exhibition), Rome, 94-95.
Smith, M.S. (ed.) 1990, *Petronius, Cena Trimalchionis*, Oxford.
Smith, W. 1875, *A dictionary of Greek and Roman Antiquities*, London.
Sogliano, A. 1880, Pompei, *NSc*, 394-395.
Sogliano, A. 1899, Pompei – Relazione degli scavi durante il mese di settembre 1899, *NSc*, 339-358.
Sokolowski, F. 1962, *Lois sacrées des cités grecques: supplément*, Paris.
Solin, H. 1982, *Die griechischen Personennamen in Rom. Ein Namenbuch* 1, Berlin/New York.
Sparkes, B.A./L. Talcott 1958, *Pots and pans of Athens*, Princeton.
Spinazzola, V. 1917, Scavi in Via dell'Abbondanza a Pompei, *NSc*, 217-264.
Stambaugh, J.E. 1988, *The ancient Roman City*, Baltimore.
Steuernagel, D. 2005, Öffentliche und private Aspekte von Vereinskulten am Beispiel von Ostia, in R. Neudecker/P. Zanker (eds), *Lebenswelten: Bilder und Räume in der römischen Stadt der Kaiserzeit*, Wiesbaden, 73-80.
Stillwell, R., 1941 *Antioch-on-the-Orontes* III, Princeton.
Strang, V. 2004, *The Meaning of Water*, Oxford/New York.
Strickland, T.J. 1982, Defences of Roman Chester: Note on Discoveries made on North Wall, 1982, *Journal of the Chester Archaeological Society* 65, 25-36.
Strocka, V.M. 1977, *Die Wandmalereien der Hanghäuser in Ephesos* (FiE VIII, 1), Vienna.
Szaivert, W./R. Wolters 2005, *Löhne, Preise, Werte. Quellen zur römischen Geldwirtschaft*, Darmstadt.
Täuber, H. 2005, C. Vibius Salutaris - Wohnungsbesitzer im Hanghaus 2?, in B. Brandt/V. Gassner/S. Ladstätter (eds), *Synergia, Festschrift für Friedrich Krinzinger* 1, 349-353.
Tagliamonte, G. 1988, *The Baths of Diocletian*, Milan.
Talcott, L. 1935, Pottery from a Fifth Century Well, *Hesperia* 4, 476-523.

Tanizaki, J. 1977, *In Praise of Shadows*, New Haven.

Taylor, E.L. 1955, Parasitic helminths in medieval remains, *Veterinary Record* 67, 216-8.

Thédenat, H. 1904, latrina, in Daremberg/Saglio III.2, 987-991.

Thera I: F. Hiller von Gaertringen (ed.), *Die Insel Thera in Altertum und Gegenwart, mit Ausschluß der Nekropolen*, Berlin 1899.

Thera III: F. Hiller von Gaertringen/P. Wilski, *Die Stadtgeschichte von Thera*, Berlin 1904.

Thera V: W. Hoepfner (ed.), *Das dorische Thera*, Berlin 1997.

Thienpont, D./F. Rochette/O.F.J. Van Parijs 1986, *Diagnosing helminthiasis by coprological examination*, Becrse.

Thompson, D.B. 1971, *The Athenian Agora: an ancient shopping center* (Excavations of the Athenian Agora, Picture Book 12), Princeton, N.J.

Thompson, H.A. 1959, Activities in the Athenian Agora 1958, *Hesperia* 28, 91-108.

Thür H. 2005, *Hanghaus 2 in Ephesos, die Wohneinheit* 4 (FiE 8.6), Vienna.

Thüry, G.E. 2001, *Müll und Marmorsäulen. Siedlungshygiene in der römischen Antike*, Mainz.

Tietze, C. 1985, Amarna, Analyse der Wohnhäuser und soziale Struktur der Stadtbewohner, *ZÄS* 112, 48-84.

Tölle-Kastenbein, R. 1990, *Antike Wasserkultur*, Munich.

Tomei, M.A./C. Conti 1991, Domus Tiberiana. Pitture con scene gladiatorie, *BA* 10, 57-67.

Torrence, R./H. Barton (eds) 2006, *Ancient Starch Research*, Left Coast.

Traunecker, C. 1988, Les maisons du domaine d'Aton à Karnak, *Cahiers de Recherches de l'Institut de Papyrologie et d'Égyptologie de Lille* 10, 73-93.

Travlos, J. 1971, *Bildlexikon zur Topographie des antiken Athen*, Tübingen.

Trümper, M. 1998, *Wohnen in Delos. Eine baugeschichtliche Untersuchung zum Wandel der Wohnkultur in hellenistischer Zeit*, Rahden/Westfalen.

Trümper, M. 2002, review of *Eretria* X, *Gnomon* 74, 627-638.

Trümper, M. 2006a, Negotiating Religious and Ethnic Identity: the Case of Clubhouses in Late Hellenistic Delos, *Hephaistos* 24, 113-150.

Trümper, M. 2006b, Baden im späthellenistischen Delos I: Die öffentliche Badeanlage im Quartier du Théâtre, *BCH* 130, 143-229.

Trümper, M. 2008, *Die ‚Agora des Italiens' in Delos. Baugeschichte, Architektur, Ausstattung und Funktion einer späthellenistischen Porticus-Anlage*, Rahden/Westfalen.

Trümper, M. 2010, Where the Non-Delians met in Delos: The meeting-places of foreign associations and ethnic communities in Late Hellenistic Delos, in O.M. van Nijf/R. Alston/ (eds), *Political Culture in the Greek City after the Classical Age*, Leuven, 49-100.

Tsakirgis, B. 1984, *The domestic architecture of Morgantina in the Hellenistic and Roman periods*, PhD University of Princeton.

Tuzin, D. 2006, Base Notes: Odor, Breath and Moral Contagion in Ilahita, in Drobnick 2006, 59-67.

Vaglieri, D. 1911, Osta, *NSc*, 207-213.

Valbelle, D. 2007, *Tell el-Herr: Les niveaux hellénistiques et du Haut-Empire*, Paris.

Van Vaerenbergh, J. 2001, *De latrines in of nabij de Romeinse badcomplexen van Italië. Het discrete secreet* 1-3, unpublished master thesis of the Catholic University Leuven.

Van Vaerenbergh, J. 2006, The Latrines in and near the Roman Baths of Italy. A Nice Compromise with a Bad Smell, in Wiplinger 2006, 453-459.

Van Vaerenbergh, J. forthcoming, The Stunning Latrine of the Smaller Baths. Smelly or not?, in *Atti del Convegno "Rileggere l'antico", Roma 13-15 dicembre 2004*, Rome.

Varone, A. 2008, Inseguendo un'utopia. L'apporto delle nuove tecnologie informatiche alla lettura 'obiettiva' delle iscrizioni parientali, in O. Brandt (ed.), *Unexpected voices. The graffiti in the cryptoporticus of the horti Sallustiani, and papers from a conference on graffiti at the Swedish Institute in Rome March 7, 2003 (Acta Instituti Romani Regni Sueciae)*, Stockholm, 125-135.

Varone, A. in press, *Insula of the Menander at Pompeii* V. *The Inscriptions.*

Vatin, C. 1976, Jardins et services d'évoirie, *BCH* 100, 555-564.

Versluys, M.J. 2002, *Aegyptiaca romana. Nilotic Scenes and the Roman Views of Egypt*, Leiden.

Vogel, M. 2000, Warum „nicht nackt"? Sozioanthropologische Erwägungen zu 2 Kor 5,3, in A. von Dobbeler/K. Erlemann/R. Heiligenthal (eds), *Religionsgeschichte des Neuen Testaments. Festschrift Klaus Berger*, Tübingen, 445-463.

Volpe G. (ed.) 2000, *Ordona* X. *Ricerche archeologiche a Herdonia (1993-1998)*, Bari.

Von Pilgrim, C. 1996, *Elephantine* VIII. *Untersuchungen in der Stadt des Mittleren Reiches und der Zweiten Zwischenzeit* (AV 91), Mainz.

Wacher, J.S. 1969, *Excavations at Brough-On-Humber 1958-1961* (Reports of the Research Committee of the Society of Antiquaries of London 25), London.

Walker, S.F.C. 1979, *The Architectural Development of Roman Nymphaea in Greece* I-II, PhD London.

Wallace-Hadrill, A. 1988, The Social Structure of the Roman House, *BSR* 56, 43-97.

Wallace-Hadrill, A. 1994, *Houses and Society in Pompeii and Herculaneum*, Princeton.

Ward, J.1903, *The Roman Fort at Gellygaer in the County of Glamorgan*, London.

Ward, P. 1970, *Sabratha: a guide for visitors*, London.

Ward, S./T.J. Strickland 1978, *Excavations on the site of the Northgate Brewery, Chester 1974-5; A Roman centurion's quarters and barrac'* (Chester Excavations 1), Chester.

Waslander, C.T. 1994, Romeinse openbare latrines: Openbare latrines, gemeenschappelijk gemak of noodzakelijk kwaad?, in S. Piras (ed.), *Latrines. Antieke toiletten - modern onderzoek*, Amsterdam, 14-23.

Wb = A. Erman /H. Grapow, *Wörterbuch der aegyptischen Sprache* 1-5, Leipzig, 1926-1963.

Weisshäuptl, R. 1902, Ephesische Latrinen-Inschriften, *OeJh* 5, Beiblatt, 33-34.

Wheeler, A./A.K.G. Jones 1989, *Cambridge Manuals in archaeology: Fishes*, Cambridge.

Wheeler, K. 2000, Theoretical and Methodological Consideration for Considering Privies, *Historical Archaeology* 34.1, 3-19.

Wiblé, F. 1977, Fouilles gallo-romaines de Martigny. Recherches archéologiques aux Morasses en 1975 et 1976, *AnnVall*, 199-214.

Wiegand, Th./H. Schrader 1904, *Priene. Ergebnisse der Ausgrabungen und Untersuchungen in den Jahren 1885-1898*, Berlin.

Wilfand, Y. 2009, Did the Rabbis Reject the Roman Public Latrine?, *BABESCH* 84, 183-196.

Wilkes, J. 1961, Excavations in Housesteads Fort, 1960, *Archaeologia Aeliana* 39 (Series 4), 279–301.

Williams, H. 1996, Excavations at Stymphalos 1995, *Echos du Monde Classique/Classical News and Views* 15, 75-98.

Williams, H. et al. 1997, Excavations at Stymphalos 1996, *Echos du Monde Classique/Classical News and Views* 16, 23-73.

Willis, S./R. Hingley 2007, Roman Finds: Context and Theory, in R. Hingley/S. Willis (eds), *Roman Finds. Context and Theory*, Oxford, 2-17.
Wilson, A.I. 1995, Running water and social status in North Africa, in M. Horton/T. Wiedemann (eds), *North Africa from Antiquity to Islam*, Bristol, 52-56.
Wilson, A.I. 2000a, Drainage and Sanitation, in O. Wikander (ed.), *Handbook of Ancient Water Technology*, Leiden, 151-179.
Wilson, A.I. 2000b, Incurring the wrath of Mars: sanitation and hygiene in Roman North Africa, in Jansen 2000b, 307-12.
Wilson, A.I. 2009, Villas, horticulture and irrigation infrastructure in the Tiber Valley, in F. Coarelli/H. Patterson (eds), *Mercator Placidissimus: The Tiber Valley in Antiquity. New research in the upper and middle river valley (Proceedings of the Conference held at the British School at Rome, 27-28 Feb. 2004)*, Rome, 731-768.
Wilson, R.J.A. 1980, *Roman Forts: an illustrated introduction to the garrison posts of Roman Britain*, London.
Wilson, R.J.A. 2002, *A Guide to the Roman Remains in Britain*, [4]London.
Winkelmann, O. 1988, Hygienische Aspekte der Wasserversorgung antiker Städte, in *Die Wasserversorgung antiker Städte, Geschichte der Wasserversorgung* 3, Mainz am Rhein, 157-170.
Wiplinger, G. (ed.) 2006, *Cura Aquarum in Ephesos. Proceedings of the 12th International Conference on the History of Water Management and Hydraulic Engineering* (BABESCH Supplement 12), Louvain.
Wiplinger, G. forthcoming, Der Gebrauch des xylospongium - eine neue Theorie zu den hygienischen Verhältnissen in römischen Latrinen, in *Proceedings of SPA - SANITAS PER AQUAM. Internationales Frontinus-Symposium zur Technik- und Kulturgeschichte der antiken Thermen", Aachen*, 2009, BABESCH supplement in preparation.
Wöhrle, G. 1990, *Studien zur Theorie der antiken Gesundheidslehre* (Hermes Einzelschriften 56), Stuttgart.
Wörrle, M./P. Zanker (eds) 1995, *Stadtbild und Bürgerbild im Hellenismus*, Munich.
Wolf, M. 2003, *Die Häuser von Solunt und die hellenistische Wohnarchitektur* (DAI Rom Sonderschriften 14), Mainz.
Wright, D. P. 1992, Unclean and Clean, in D.N. Freedman (ed.), *The Anchor Bible Dictionary*, New York, VI, 729-741.
Young, R.S. 1951 An Industrial District in Athens, *Hesperia* 20, 135-288.
Youtie, H.C./J.G. Winter 1951, *Papyri and Ostraca from Karanis. Second Series* (Michigan Papyri, VIII), Ann Arbor.
Yoyotte, J./P. Vernus 2005, *Bestiaire des Pharaons*, Paris.
Zanier, W. 1992, *Das Römische Kastell Ellingen* (Limesforschungen 23), Berlin.
Zanker, P. 1998, *Pompeii: Public and Private Life* (translated by Deborah Lucas Schneider), Harvard.
Ziller, E. 1877, Untersuchungen über die Wasserleitungen Athens, *AM* 2, 107-131.
Zimmermann, N. 2002, Ausstattung von Haupt- und Nebenräumen. Zur Datierung der Wandmalereien des Hanghauses 2 in Ephesos, in F. Krinzinger (ed.), *Das Hanghaus 2 in Ephesos. Studien zur Baugeschichte und Chronologie*, Vienna, 101-117.

List of Authors and Addresses

JESÚS ACERO is a research student at the Instituto de Arqueología-Mérida (CSIC-Junta de Extremadura-Consorcio de Mérida). His PhD study is on waste management in Lusitanian Roman cities, with a particular focus on Augusta Emerita. Here he is conducting research on latrines there as a part of the overall systems of waste disposal (i.e. solid and liquid refuse) in the Roman city.

Instituto de Arqueología de Mérida
Plaza de España, 15
ES-06800 Mérida, Spain
alconetar@hotmail.com

HORST ASPÖCK is a retired Full Professor of Medical Parasitology and former head of the Department of Medical Parasitology, Clinical Institute of Hygiene, Medical University of Vienna, and still active there in research and teaching. One of his research fields is paleoparasitology. He has investigated intestinal parasites of the prehistoric saltminers of Hallstatt (Iron Age) and has examined the famous glacier mummy 'Ötzi' for parasites.

Department of Medical Parasitology
Clinical Institute of Hygiene and Medical Microbiology
Medical University of Vienna
Kinderspitalgasse 15
A-1095 Vienna, Austria
horst.aspoeck@meduniwien.ac.at

DOMENICO CAMARDO gained postgraduate qualifications in archaeology from the Università degli Studi di Roma La Sapienza. He is the scientific director of Sosandra Heritage Services, a company specializing in archaeological and geological investigations. Since 2001 he has been the lead archaeologist of the Herculaneum Conservation Project, where he coordinates archaeological investigations and examines specific research questions, such as those related to the water supply and drainage of ancient Herculaneum.

Via Vittorio Veneto, 90
I-80054 Gragnano (NA), Italy
d.camardo@herculaneum.org

INGRID FEUEREIS is a trained specialist in laboratory medicine. She is working in the laboratories of the Department of Medical Parasitology, Clinical Institute of Hygiene, Medical University Vienna, mainly doing laboratory diagnosis of human parasites.

Department of Medical Parasitology
Clinical Institute of Hygiene and Medical Microbiology
Medical University of Vienna
Kinderspitalgasse 15
A-1095 Vienna, Austria
ingrid.feuereis@utanet.at

MIKO FLOHR is a classical archaeologist who holds a PhD from Radboud University Nijmegen, with a dissertation about *fullones* and *fullonicae* in Roman Italy. For this project, he also investigated the role of urine in the fulling process and the way fullers assembled and stored it. He is currently working as assistant director of the 'Oxford Roman Economy Project' at Oxford.

Faculty of Classics
66 St Giles', Oxford
OX1 3LU, UK
miko.flohr@classics.ox.ac.uk

ADAM GOLDWATER is a Learning Officer at Tyne & Wear Museums. He has an MA in Roman Archaeology from the University of Nottingham, where

Tyne & Wear Museums
Blandford Square
Newcastle upon Tyne

he studied latrines in the Roman military context. His independent research in this area extends to the social interaction between civilians and the army in the frontier zone, particularly Hadrian's Wall.

NE1 4JA, UK
adam.goldwater@twmuseums.org.uk

AUDE GRÄZER is about to finish her PhD in Egyptology under the supervision of Professor Emeritus Claude Traunecker (University of Strasbourg and UMR 7044 Laboratory, CNRS). Her work focuses on Egyptian concept of domestic comfort in all its facets (criteria, concrete implementation and socio-ideological implications) by studying archaeological remains of Pharaonic houses and palaces as well as iconographic and textual evidence. Latrines are a part of her investigations.

2, Rue Saint Arbogast
F-67000 Strasbourg, France
aude.grazer@gmail.com

ELLY N.A. HEIRBAUT works as an archaeologist for the city of Nijmegen. Among other projects, she is studying the Roman occupation of the city. Recent excavations have revealed several private cesspits and drainage systems. She holds an MA in Art History and Archaeology, and an MA in Eastern Mediterranean Archaeology, both from the Catholic University Leuven, Belgium. She is currently working on a PhD on Roman cesspits from Nijmegen (Leiden University).

Bureau Archeologie en Monumenten
Postbus 9105
NL-6500 HG Nijmegen, The Netherlands
eheirbaut@ruudvanbeekstichting.nl

J. BARRY HOBSON was a medical practitioner who took up archaeology after he retired in 1996. Inspired by Gemma Jansen and by his work with the Anglo American Project in Pompeii, he produced an MPhil from The University of Bradford on the latrines of Pompeii. His book, *Latrinae et Foricae: Toilets in the Roman World*, has been published by Duckworth and Co., London (2009).

235 Huddersfield Rd, Thongsbridge
Holmfirth, HD9 3TT, UK
barry_hobson@talk21.com

STEFANIE HOSS is an independent scholar who has researched baths and the social meaning behind Roman bathing in Palestine. This research developed into an interest in understanding the Roman way of defecating. She holds an MA in Provincial Roman Archaeology and Jewish studies and a PhD in Provincial Roman Archaeology from the University of Cologne.

Small finds archaeology
Weurtseweg 133
NL-6541 AR Nijmegen, The Netherlands
Stefanie.Hoss@tele2.nl

GEMMA C.M. JANSEN is an independent scholar who researches water and drainage systems in Roman Italy and Turkey. During this research she discovered that toilets have not got much scientific attention and from that moment on she has devoted a lot of time and energy to promoting toi let research. Her PhD is in Classical Archaeology from Radboud University Nijmegen.

Weustenraadstraat 3
NL-6217 HZ Maastricht, The Netherlands
gemma.jansen@rubico.nu

ANDREW K.G. JONES has recently retired as a Lecturer in Bioarchaeology at the University at Bradford. He has a PhD from the University of York for work on biological remains, including coprolites, from a Viking Age site in Caithness. He is currently studying fish remains and calcareous deposits from recent excavations in Pompeii to learn more about diet, disease and the relationship between humans and ecosystems. He now works part-time for the York Archaeological Trust.

York Archaeological Trust
47 Aldwark
York, YO1 7BX
bone@yorkat.co.uk

ANNE-MARIE JOUQUAND, engeneer, working as a researcher in the Institut national de recherches archéologiques préventives, leads rescue excavations in towns in the Centre Ouest of France. In one of her digs, at Poitiers, the unique system of drainage of latrines in the Ilot de Cordeliers de Poitiers, has been unearthed.

INRAP
148 avenue André Maginot
F-371000 Tours, France
anne-marie.jouquand-thomas@inrap.fr

ZENA KAMASH is the Research Assistant to the Professor of European Archaeology at the University of Oxford. She has a PhD from Oxford on Water Supply and Management in the Near East 63 BC-AD 636. Her interest in latrines forms part of her research into the social and cultural roles of water supply and management facilities in the Roman East.

Institute of Archaeology
36 Beaumont St
Oxford, OX 1 2PG, UK
zena.kamash@arch.ox.ac.uk

JENS KOEHLER is Adjunct Professor at the American University of Rome and at John Cabot University in Rome. His PhD is in Classical Archaeology from Munich University, Germany. The research on Roman spa-baths lead to an increasing interest in questions related to ancient water management.

Largo Somalia 13
I-00199 Roma, Italia
j.koehler@aur.edu
jkoehler@johncabot.edu

ANN OLGA KOLOSKI-OSTROW is Associate Professor and chair of Classical Studies at Brandeis University in Waltham, Massachusetts. She holds an MA in Latin and Greek and a PhD in Classical Art and Archaeology from the University of Michigan. Her interest in Roman toilets derives from earlier work on baths and sanitation on the Bay of Naples.

Chair, Department of Classical Studies
M.S. 016, Brandeis University
415 South Street
Waltham, MA 02454-9110, USA
aoko@brandeis.edu

GUENTHER KARL KUNST is researcher for archaeozoology at the Vienna Institute of Archaeological Science at the University of Vienna. He has a Dr.rer.nat. from the University of Vienna on animal bones studies from various Austrian sites. His involvement in the study of the *Carnuntum* sewers is part of an interest in comparing faunal samples from different Roman contexts.

VIAS University of Vienna
c/o Institut für Palaeontologie
Althanstr. 14
A-1090 Wien, Austria
guenther.karl.kunst@univie.ac.at

ANTONELLA MERLETTO is Adjunct Professor at the Richmond University in Rome. She holds a MA in Architecture from the Politecnico di Torino, and her interests in Roman latrines developed when she studied the latrine in the Western Baths of Kos as her thesis for her specialization in ancient Greek and Roman architecture at the Italian Archaeological School in Athens.

via Pompei 21
I-00183 Rome, Italy
antonella.merletto@tiscali.it

CARLO MOLLE is an independent researcher, whose main interests are the history of Roman Latium and Latin epigraphy. He studied classical archaeology in Rome and completed a PhD in Ancient History and Classical Archaeology at the University of Macerata. His special focus was on ancient graffiti. Toilets are a special place to find and study these particular inscriptions and drawings.

via Tagliamento 14
I-03038 Roccasecca (FR), Italy
carlo.molle@libero.it

ERIC M. MOORMANN studied Classics and Classical Archaeology at Nijmegen, where he received his PhD. After working in Amsterdam and Rome he is now Professor of Classical Archaeology at Nijmegen. His research circles around living in ancient towns (Rome, Pompeii, Herculaneum) and Roman figural arts. He also works on the reception of classical antiquity in western culture. The study of ancient toilets is a new area of his research.

Institute for Historical, Literary and Cultural Studies
Radboud University Nijmegen
Postbus 9103
NL-6500 HD Nijmegen, The Netherlands
e.moormann@let.ru.nl

RICHARD NEUDECKER is researcher at the Deutsches Archäologisches Institut in Rome and teaches Classical Archaeology at Munich University. His PhD and Habilitation are from Munich University. The theme of his postdoctoral thesis on Roman public latrines falls within a wider research interest in the cultural history of Roman imperial times.

Deutsches Archäologisches Institut
via Curtatone, 4D
I-00185, Rome, Italy
neudecker@rom.dainst.org

EDDIE OWENS is senior lecturer in Ancient History at Swansea University (Wales, UK). He holds an MA in Roman history and a PhD from Sheffield University in urban development. His research on water supply and technology and sanitation stems from his interest in the development of ancient cities and their associated problems.

The Department of Classics, Ancient History and Egyptology
Swansea University
Singleton Park
GB Swansea SA2 8PP, UK
e.j.owens@swansea.ac.uk

BEATRIX PETZNEK is a freelance archaeologist, who works on finds from Pannonia and Noricum. She holds a D.Ph. from the Alma Mater Rudolphina Universität at Vienna on ceramics from the Roman era found at *Carnuntum*. Her specific interest regards the study of Roman ceramic. In the civil town of *Carnuntum* she elaborates the finds of the excavations in the *Weststraße*. Here several chamberpots have found in a drain.

Mühlgasse 6A
A-2460 Bruck/Leitha, Austria
Beatrix.Petznek@gmx.at

SILVIA RADBAUER is an independent researcher mainly on Roman projects about streets, water systems, ceramics, and interdisciplinary field and laboratory analysis in Austria, Germany, and Italy. She holds a MA in Classical Archaeology and Ancient History from the University of Vienna. Her interest in Roman streets, their sanitary infrastructures, and ceramics derives from her continuous work in the excavations at *Carnuntum*.

Institut für Klassische Archäologie
Universität Wien
Franz Klein-Gasse 1
A-1190 Wien, Austria
Silvia.Radbauer@univie.ac.at

ROMAN SAUER studied geology at the University of Vienna (PhD). He is currently team leader of the Geological Laboratory, OMV AG in Vienna. Besides his main profession, he has general interests in archaeometry and archaeology. He has made contributions to numerous archaeological projects, mainly concerning the study of ceramics, sedimentology, and material analysis. He also gives lectures at the University of Applied Arts at Vienna.

Institut für Kunst und
Technologie/Archäometrie
Universität für angewandte Kunst Wien
Salzgrieß 14
A-1013 Wien, Austria
roman.sauer@uni-ak.ac.at

JACQUES SEIGNE is Director of Studies in the CNRS. He holds a title of architect DPLG (Bordeaux) and a PhD in history and archaeology (Université de Versailles St Quentin en Yvelines). He teaches Gallo-Roman archaeology in the Université François Rabelais at Tours. Director of the French archaeological expedition at Jerash (Jordanie), he works on urbanism, sanctuaries and water monuments of the Hellenistic and Roman era.

LAT, UMR 6173 CITERES – B.P. 60449
CNRS-Université de Tours
F-37201 Tours (cedex 03), France
Jacques.seigne@wanadoo.fr

GUENTHER E. THÜRY is Roman-Provincial archaeologist and classical philologist. The history of ancient environment and hygiene belongs to his main fields of interest. He holds a Lizentiat and an honorary doctorate of the Universität Basel.

Weilerbergstrasse 38
D-71111 Waldenbuch, Germany
www.gethuery.at; guenther.e.thuery@web.de

MONIKA TRÜMPER is Associate Professor of Classical Archaeology at the University of North Carolina at Chapel Hill. She has a PhD from the University of Munich on the Hellenistic houses of Delos, and a Habilitation from the University of Heidelberg on the 'Agora of the Italians' in Delos. Her research on Greek latrines is part of her current research on bathing culture and sanitation in the Mediterranean world.

Department of Classics
University of North Carolina at Chapel Hill
CB # 3145, 212 Murphey Hall
Chapel Hill NC 27599-3145, USA
truemper@email.unc.edu

JEROEN VAN VAERENBERGH is a field archaeologist and researcher at a Belgian regional archaeological service (Archeologische Dienst Waasland). During his MA studies at the Catholic University of Leuven he specialized in the research of latrines in and near the Roman baths of Italy. As a field archaeologist, he strongly believes in a methodological, multidisciplinary approach to the data.

Nederstraat 5
B-9150 Kruibeke-Rupelmonde, Belgium
jeroen.van.vaerenbergh@telenet.be
jeroenvanvaerenbergh@hotmail.com

KATHLEEN WHEELER is Director and Principal Archaeologist for her company, Independent Archaeological Consulting in Portsmouth, New Hampshire. She holds both an MA and PhD in Anthropology/Archaeology from the University of Arizona in Tucson, Arizona. As a student of Michael Schiffer, she applies behavioral principles to the study of the end process of human consumption in New England privies.

Independent Archaeological Consulting, LLC
97 Morning St
Portsmouth, NH 03801, USA
kwheeler@iac-llc.net

ANDREW WILSON is Professor of the Archaeology of the Roman Empire at the University of Oxford. He has a PhD from Oxford on water management in Roman North Africa. His research on ancient hydraulic technology and sanitation is part of a wider interest in the interactions between technology and society in the ancient world.

Institute of Archaeology
36 Beaumont St, Oxford
OX1 2PG, UK
andrew.wilson@arch.ox.ac.uk

GABRIEL ZUCHTRIEGEL is a Fellow of the Studienstiftung des deutschen Volkes. He holds an MA in Classical Archaeology from Humboldt-University at Berlin and has written his MAthesis on latrines and sewers in Greek houses. His interest in this field derives from his participation in the excavations at Selinunte (Sicily) carried out by the German Archaeological Institute. In 2010 he has received his PhD with his study *Das Ostheiligtum von Gabii. Die eisenzeitlichen und archaischen Funde der Ausgrabungen 1976-1977. Studien zu Kultpraxis und Urbanisierung in Latium.*

Institut für Klassische Archäologie
Universität Bonn
Am Hofgarten 21
53113 Bonn, Germany
gabrielzuchtriegel@yahoo.de

Index

Compiled by Nancy Zibman